TUMORS
OF THE
KIDNEY, RENAL PELVIS, AND URETER

by

JAMES L. BENNINGTON, M.D.
and
J. BRUCE BECKWITH, M.D.

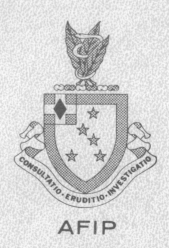

AFIP

TUMORS
OF THE
KIDNEY, RENAL PELVIS, AND URETER

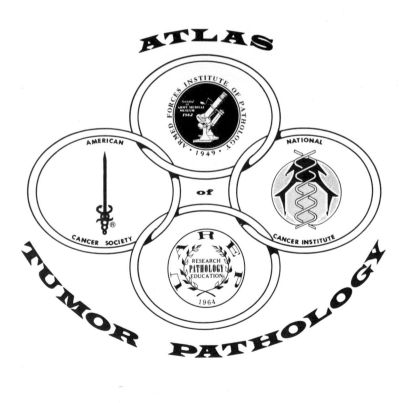

ATLAS

of

TUMOR PATHOLOGY

AMERICAN CANCER SOCIETY

ARMED FORCES INSTITUTE OF PATHOLOGY · 1949 ·
founded ARMY MEDICAL MUSEUM 1862

NATIONAL CANCER INSTITUTE

RESEARCH PATHOLOGY EDUCATION 1964

ATLAS OF TUMOR PATHOLOGY

Second Series
Fascicle 12

TUMORS OF THE KIDNEY, RENAL PELVIS, AND URETER

by

JAMES L. BENNINGTON, M. D.

Chairman
Department of Anatomic and Clinical Pathology
Children's Hospital of San Francisco
San Francisco, California 94119
and
Associate Clinical Professor of Pathology
University of California
San Francisco Medical Center

and

J. BRUCE BECKWITH, M. D.

Professor of Pathology and Pediatrics
University of Washington School of Medicine
and
Director of Laboratories
The Children's Orthopedic Hospital and Medical Center
Seattle, Washington 98105

Published by the
ARMED FORCES INSTITUTE OF PATHOLOGY
Washington, D. C.

Under the Auspices of
UNIVERSITIES ASSOCIATED FOR RESEARCH AND EDUCATION IN PATHOLOGY,INC.
Bethesda, Maryland
1975

Accepted for Publication
1975
....
For sale by the American Registry of Pathology
Armed Forces Institute of Pathology
Washington, D. C. 20306

ATLAS OF TUMOR PATHOLOGY

Sponsored and Supported by

AMERICAN CANCER SOCIETY*
NATIONAL CANCER INSTITUTE, NATIONAL INSTITUTES OF HEALTH*

and

ARMED FORCES INSTITUTE OF PATHOLOGY

EDITOR
HARLAN I. FIRMINGER, M. D.

Professor, Department of Pathology
University of Maryland School of Medicine
Baltimore, Maryland 21201
and
Scientist Associate, Universities Associated for
Research and Education in Pathology, Inc.
9650 Rockville Pike
Bethesda, Maryland 20014

EDITORIAL ADVISORY COMMITTEE

Lauren V. Ackerman, M.D.

State University of New York
Stony Brook, Long Island, New York

David G. Freiman, M.D.

Harvard Medical School
Boston, Massachusetts

John K. Frost, M.D.

The Johns Hopkins School of Medicine
Baltimore, Maryland

James C. Harkin, M.D.

Tulane University School of Medicine
New Orleans, Louisiana

Dante G. Scarpelli, M.D.

University of Kansas Medical Center
Kansas City, Kansas

Robert E. Scully, M.D.

The Massachusetts General Hospital
Boston, Massachusetts

Philippe Shubik, M.D.

University of Nebraska College of Medicine
Omaha, Nebraska

Harlan J. Spjut, M.D.

Baylor University College of Medicine
Houston, Texas

*(Supported by Public Health Service grant no. CA08575 from the
National Cancer Institute and American Cancer Society grant no. MG-122)

EDITOR'S NOTE

The Atlas of Tumor Pathology was originated by the Committee on Pathology of the National Academy of Sciences—National Research Council in 1947. The form of the Atlas became the brainchild of the Subcommittee on Oncology and was shepherded by a succession of editors. It was supported by a long list of agencies; many of the illustrations were made by the Medical Illustration Service of the Armed Forces Institute of Pathology; the type was set by the Government Printing Office; and the final printing was made by the press at the Armed Forces Institute of Pathology. The American Registry of Pathology purchased the fascicles from the Government Printing Office and sold them at cost, plus a small handling and shipping charge. Over a period of 20 years, 15,000 copies each of 40 fascicles were produced. They provided a system of nomenclature and set standards for histologic diagnosis which received worldwide acclaim. Private contributions by almost 600 pathologists helped to finance the compilation of an index by The Williams & Wilkins Company to complete the original Atlas.

Following the preparation of the final fascicle of the first Atlas, the National Academy of Sciences—National Research Council handed over the task of further pursuit of the project to Universities Associated for Research and Education in Pathology, Inc. Grant support for a second series was generously made available by both the National Cancer Institute and the American Cancer Society. The Armed Forces Institute of Pathology has expanded and improved its press facilities to provide for a more rapid and efficient production of the new series. A new Editor and Editorial Advisory Committee were appointed, and the solicitation and preparation of manuscripts continues.

This second series of the Atlas of Tumor Pathology is not intended as a second edition of the first Atlas and, in general, there will be variation in authorship. The basic purpose remains unchanged in providing an Atlas setting standards of diagnosis and terminology. Throughout the rest of this new series, the term chosen for the World Health Organization's series "International Histological Classification of Tumours" (when available) is shown by an asterisk if it corresponds to the authors' choice, or as the first synonym in bold print if it differs from the authors' heading. Hematoxylin and eosin stained sections still represent the keystone of histologic diagnosis; therefore, most of the photomicrographs will be of sections stained by this technic, and only sections prepared by other technics will be specifically designated in the legends. It is hoped that in many of the new series a broader perspective of tumors may be offered by the inclusion of special stains, histochemical illustrations, electron micrographs, data on biologic behavior, and other pertinent information for better understanding of the disease.

The format of the new series is changed in order to allow better correlation of the illustrations with the text, and a more substantial cover is provided. An index will be included in each fascicle.

It is the hope of the Editor, the Editorial Advisory Committee, and the Sponsors that these changes will be welcomed by the readers. Constructive criticisms and suggestions will be appreciated.

Harlan I. Firminger, M. D.

PREFACE AND ACKNOWLEDGMENTS

In the nearly two decades since the publication of the First Series of the Fascicle on Tumors of the Kidney, Renal Pelvis, and Ureter, there has been a virtual explosion of new information on tumors of the upper urinary tract. Many significant contributions concerning nearly all of the tumors covered in the First Series Fascicle, as well as the recognition of important new entities, have been made during this time. The authors have attempted to incorporate into this text the new well established findings in the areas of epidemiology, histogenesis, histochemistry, morphology, classification, diagnosis, treatment, and prognosis, as well as our own views on unproved and controversial theories relating to this field. While this has been largely a joint effort, Dr. Beckwith was responsible primarily for those sections relating to embryonal tumors of the kidney and Dr. Bennington for the remainder.

We wish to acknowledge the excellent First Series Fascicle by Dr. Balduin Lucké and Dr. Hans G. Schlumberger, which was such a tremendous help in the development of our manuscript and the illustrations that we have been permitted to use. They are our current figure numbers 40, 57, 58, 67, 175, 176, 201, 206, 216–218, 247, 257, and 259.

The classification and nomenclature used in this fascicle are based on our understanding of the histogenetic origin of the various tumors of the kidney, renal pelvis, and ureter. This terminology, with minor exceptions, is in general use in English speaking countries and conforms to that proposed (but not yet adopted) by the World Health Organization (WHO).

The authors wish to express their gratitude for the support in part by the U. S. Public Health Service, Grant No. R10-CA 11722, of the National Wilms' Tumor Study.

The majority of the material used in the preparation of this text was gathered at the University of Washington Medical School, Seattle, Washington; Children's Orthopedic Hospital, Seattle, Washington; King County Hospital, Seattle, Washington; Kaiser Foundation Hospital, Oakland, California; Children's Hospital, San Francisco, California; and from the National Wilms' Tumor Registry. We are particularly grateful to Dr. Seth L. Haber, Santa Clara, California; Dr. George Farrow, Rochester, Minnesota; Dr. Roger Pugh and Dr. Noel Gowing, London, England for their kindness and generosity in providing much unusual and important material. We are also indebted to the following other contributors of materials and illustrations:

Figures 9, 10, 11 - Dr. Craig Tisher, Durham, N. C.
Figure 19 - Dr. Ruth E. Bulger, Baltimore, Md.
Figure 24 - Dr. Benjamin H. Landing, Los Angeles, Calif.
Figure 25 - Dr. Nathan B. Friedman, Los Angeles, Calif.

Figures 26, 27, 75—77, 185, 186, and Plates IV-A, B, and VII-B - Dr. Seth L. Haber, Santa Clara, Calif.

Figure 29 - Dr. Warren W. Johnson, Memphis, Tenn.

Figures 32, 33 - Dr. Howard Ricketts, St. Louis, Mo.

Figures 39, 220, 222, and Plates X-D, and XI-A, B - Armed Forces Institute of Pathology

Figure 67 - Dr. Sidney Farber, Boston, Mass.

Figures 68, 145 - Dr. Joseph B. Crawford, San Francisco, Calif.

Figure 83 - Dr. H. L. Ratcliffe, Philadelphia, Pa.

Figure 89 - Dr. Louis Komarmy, San Francisco, Calif.

Figures 90, 91, 92 - Dr. J. S. Ansell, Seattle, Wash.

Figures 94, 96, 188, 200 - Dr. Joachim Burhenne, San Francisco, Calif.

Figure 97 - Dr. George Annes, San Francisco, Calif.

Figure 98 - Dr. R. M. Shishido, San Diego, Calif.

Figure 101 - Dr. James L. McRea, Sydney, Australia

Figure 126 - Dr. M. D. Lagios, San Francisco, Calif.

Figure 133 - Dr. R. Seljelid, Tromso, Norway

Plate VI-A - Dr. Vivian Gildenhorn, Los Angeles, Calif.

Figure 138 - Dr. Bruce Mackay, Houston, Tex.

Figures 140, 157 - Dr. Noel Gowing, London, England

Figures 142, 203, 248 - Dr. Roger Pugh, London, England

Figure 143 - Dr. A. Lazar, Leonia, N. J.

Figure 144 - Dr. N. L. Morgenstern, Oakland, Calif.

Figure 152 - Dr. Averill A. Liebow, San Diego, Calif.

Figures 196, 221 - Dr. P. N. Cowen, Leeds, England

Figures 197, 215 - Dr. Bradford Young, San Francisco, Calif.

Figure 231 - Dr. Carlos Perez-Mesa, Columbia, Mo.

Figure 249 (lower) - Dr. P. W. Graff, Chicago, Ill.

Figures 251—253 - Dr. R. Kempson, Stanford, Calif.

Figures 257, 259 - Dr. Beecher-Smith, Columbus, Ohio

Figure 267 - Dr. B. L. Pear, Denver, Colo.

Plate XI-D - Dr. D. C. Schneiderman, Montreal, Canada

The following illustrations have also been used. They appeared in Renal Carcinoma by Drs. J. L. Bennington and R. Kradjian, published by W. B. Saunders Co. in 1967, and cover the following subjects:

Embryology and Anatomy of the Kidney: Our figures 1 and 4 (modified), 5, 9—11.

Histogenesis of Renal Carcinoma: Our figure 80.

Epidemiology and Etiology: Our figures 85, 86.

Morphology: Our figures 83, 87, 104—107, 109, 113, 116—118, 125, 129, 143, 144, 147, plates III-B and V, and tables V and VI (modified).

Distribution of Metastases from Renal Carcinoma: Our figures 139, 141, 155, and tables VII and VIII (modified).

Diagnostic Techniques: Our figures 90—92.

We gratefully acknowledge the secretarial assistance of Judy Fletcher and Nondis Barrett who have patiently and cheerfully carried the burden of preparing the manuscript. We also wish to thank Sheila Concannon for preparation of photographic illustrations, Dr. Michael Lagios for the original electron micrographs, Dr. John Azzopardi who kindly reviewed the manuscript and made many helpful suggestions, and the Armed Forces Institute of Pathology for the use of their facilities. Our special thanks go to Dr. Harlan I. Firminger, his editorial staff, and the reviewers chosen by the Editorial Advisory Committee for all their encouragement, kindness, and much needed patience.

Permission to use copyrighted illustrations has been granted by:

Copyright 1973 by: American Association for the Advancement of Science:
    Science 179:393-395, 1973. For our figure 195.
American Cancer Society, Inc.:
    Cancer 21:727-742, 1968. For our figure 81.
    Cancer 22:545-550, 1968. For our figures 169, 171, 173, 177.
    Cancer 22:556-563, 1968. For our figure 121.
    Cancer 22:564-570, 1968. For our figure 161.
    Cancer 24:535-542, 1969. For our figure 249.
    Cancer 29:1597-1605, 1972. For our figure 34.
    Cancer 32:1030-1042, 1973. For our figure 158.
    Cancer 32:1078-1083, 1973. For our figures 202, 204.
American Medical Association:
    Arch. Pathol. 76:277-289, 1963. For our figures 2, 3.
    J.A.M.A. 204:753-757, 1968. For our figure 93.
British Medical Association: London
    J. Clin. Pathol. 23:472-474, 1970. For our figure 78.
    J. Clin. Pathol. 23:681-689, 1970. For our figures 260–263.
Churchill Livingstone (Longman Group, Ltd.): Edinburgh
    Br. J. Urol. 44:517-527, 1972. For our figure 102.
    Monograph on Neoplastic Diseases at Various Sites, Vol. V.
    Tumors of the Kidney and Ureter, 1964. For our figure 35 and graph VII (modified).
H. K. Lewis & Co., Ltd.: London
    Br. J Cancer 12:507-516, 1958. For our table I (modified).
Harper & Row, Publishers, Inc.-Hoeber Medical Division:
    Lab. Invest. 14:435-447, 1965. For our figure 132 A, B.
    Lab. Invest. 15:1357-1394, 1966. For our figures 6, 7.
Lea & Febiger:
    Renal Diseases, 2d Ed., 1950. For our graph V (data).
Mayo Clinic:
    Mayo Clin. Proc. 45:161-169, 1970. For our figure 88.
The National Foundation—March of Dimes: (Ed.) Bergsma, D. Part II
Malformation Syndromes. Vol. V(2): White Plains, N. Y.
    Birth Defects: Orig. Art. Ser. 191, 193, 1969. For our figures 28, 31.
New York Academy of Sciences:
    Ann. N. Y. Acad. Sci. 126:188-203, 1965. For our figure 84.

Oliver & Boyd, Ltd.: Edinburgh
   J. Pathol. 87:424-425, 1964. For our figure 250.
Penrose Cancer Hospital:
   Penrose Cancer Seminar, Vol. IV, No. 5, 1971. For our figure 266.
Prentice-Hall, Inc.: Sheldon C. Sommers, Englewood Cliffs, N. J.:
   Pathol. Annu. 3:213-224, (c) 1968. For our figure 18.
The Reuben H. Donnelley Corp.:
   Am. J. Med. 43:963-976, 1967. For our figures 179, 180.
   Am. J. Med. 55:86-92, 1973. For our plate IX-A, B, C.
The Royal Veterinary College: London
   J. Comp. Pathol. 78:335-339, 1968. For our figure 82.
Springer-Verlag: Berlin-Heidelberg-New York
   Virchows Arch. (Pathol. Anat.) 341:204-223, 1966. For our figure 134.
W. B. Saunders Co.:
   Renal Carcinoma, 1967. For our figures 1, 5, 9—11, 80, 83, 85—87, 90—92,
   104—107, 109, 113, 116—118, 125, 129, 139, 141, 143, 144, 147, 155,
   plates III-B and V, and tables V, VI, VII, VIII (modified).
   A Textbook of Histology, 8th Ed., 1962. For our figure 4 (modified).
The Williams & Wilkins Co.:
   J. Urol. 93:139-143, 1965. For our figure 17.
   J. Urol. 94:356-361, 1965. For our figure 254.
   J. Urol. 101:297-301, 1969. For our graph VI.
   J. Urol. 102:291-293, 1969. For our figure 16.
   J. Urol. 102:678-682, 1969. For our figure 258.
   J. Urol. 104:528-531, 1970. For our figures 183, 184.
   J. Urol. 106:515-517, 1971. For our figure 99.
   J. Urol. 109:101-103, 1973. For our figure 74.
   J. Urol. 109:567-568, 1973. For our figure 209.
The Wistar Institute of Anatomy and Biology:
   Am. J. Anat. 116:237-255, 1965. For our figure 8.

James L. Bennington, M. D.
J. Bruce Beckwith, M. D.

TUMORS OF THE KIDNEY, RENAL PELVIS, AND URETER

Contents

TUMORS OF THE KIDNEY, RENAL PELVIS, AND URETER

EMBRYOLOGY AND ANATOMY OF THE UPPER URINARY TRACT

EMBRYOGENESIS

The definitive or metanephric kidney in man has its beginnings in the second month of gestation. It is formed jointly from two different mesodermal structures; the ureteric bud, and the metanephric blastema (Hamilton et al.). The ureter, renal pelvis, renal calices, and the collecting tubules are derived from the ureteric bud, an outgrowth of the mesonephric (wolffian) duct. The nephron is composed of Bowman's capsule and glomerulus, the proximal and distal convoluted tubules and loop of Henle, all of which develop from a mesenchyme-like tissue, the metanephric blastema, located at the caudal end of the nephrogenic ridge (fig. 1).

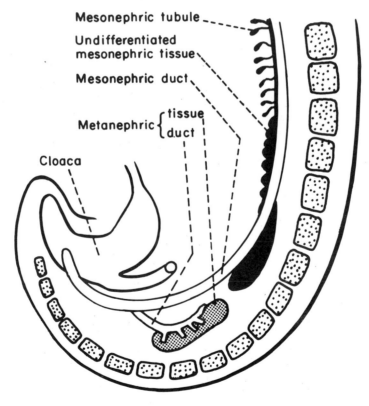

Figure 1
DEVELOPMENT OF METANEPHRIC KIDNEY
The metanephric tissue (stipple) which originates from the caudal end of the nephrogenic ridge gives rise to the nephron. The ureter, renal pelvis, and calices develop from the metanephric duct which is an outgrowth of the mesonephric duct.

The ureteric bud stretches to reach the metanephric blastema and in the process forms the ureter. The cranial end of the bud penetrates the metanephric blastema and undergoes a succession of branching. At the origin of the first several branches, a coalescence forms the renal pelvis (fig. 2) while subsequent orders of branches form the calices and collecting tubules (fig. 3; Osathanondh and Potter). Simultaneously, the metanephric blastema differentiates into two types of cells. The nephrogenic cells, characterized by scanty cytoplasm and prominent oval nuclei, orient themselves in compact masses around the growing ends of the collecting tubules, eventually differentiating into nephrons (fig. 4). Between the masses of nephrogenic cells

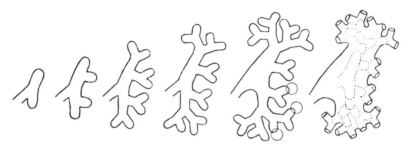

Figure 2
DEVELOPMENT OF RENAL PELVIS
Expansion of early generations of branches of the ureteral bud form the renal pelvis. The diagram represents coalescence of the third to fifth generations of branches (circled). (Fig. 9 from Osathanondh, V., and Potter, E. L. Development of human kidney as shown by microdissection. Arch. Pathol. 76:277-289, 1963.)

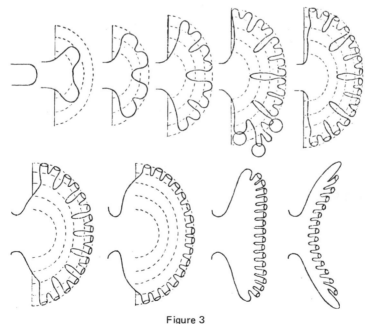

Figure 3
DEVELOPMENT OF RENAL CALICES AND PAPILLAE
Coalescence of the third to fifth generations of branches of the ureteral bud (circled) forms the primordial calix. (Fig. 10 from Osathanondh, V., and Potter, E. L. Development of human kidney as shown by microdissection. Arch. Pathol. 76:277-289, 1963.)

are widely spaced stromagenic cells with small naked-appearing nuclei, which will eventually give rise to the renal interstitial tissue. By the 36th week of gestation, nephrogenesis is usually completed and the embryonic nephrogenic and stromagenic cells are no longer recognizable.

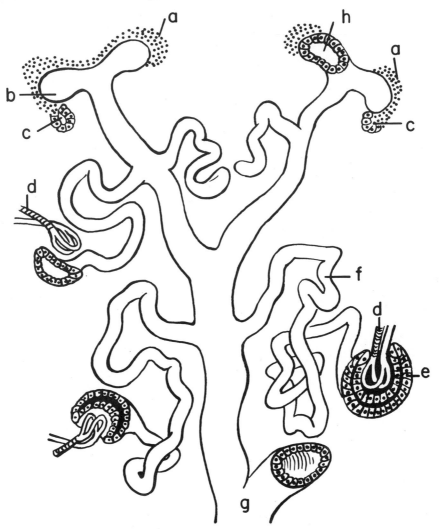

Figure 4
DIAGRAM OF DEVELOPMENT OF A METANEPHRIC KIDNEY
a. Metanephrogenic tissue capping ampulla of collecting tubule.
b. Enlarged blind end of ampulla.
c. Primordium of uriniferous tubule just formed from metanephrogenic tissue.
d. Vessel which forms the glomerulus.
e. Bowman's capsule cut open.
f. Uriniferous tubule in later stage of development.
g. Collecting tubule formed from ureteric bud of the mesonephric duct.
h. Ampulla of collecting tubule cut open. (Fig. 28-22 from Bloom, W., and Fawcett, D. W. A Textbook of Histology, 8th ed. Philadelphia: W. B. Saunders Co., 1962. [Modified from Corning])

HISTOLOGIC STRUCTURE
OF THE NEPHRON

LIGHT MICROSCOPIC FEATURES. The glomerulus consists of a number of groups of capillary loops or lobules each arranged about a mesangial axis which merges with the media of the afferent arteriole at the hilum or vascular pole. Three cell types comprise the capillary loops: (1) A reflection of the visceral epithelium covers the urinary surface of the capillary loop and is arranged as short processes or podocytes which abut on the glomerular basement membrane; (2) a fenestrated endothelium which lines the vascular space; and (3) mesangial cells which are seen in the axial area where several capillaries are conjoined. The glomerular basement membrane consists of two immunochemically distinct basement membranes which are derived from the visceral epithelium and from the endothelium.

The juxtaglomerular apparatus (complex) consists of two elements: vascular and tubular (Barajas, 1970; 1971). The vascular component comprises a specialized secretory (endocrine) smooth muscle (the granular epithelioid cells) intercalated in the media of the afferent and occasionally efferent arterioles (Takeshita), and an extraglomerular mesangium, representing the polkissen of Zimmerman or lacis cells. The granular epithelioid cells have been shown by appropriate immunohistochemical technics to be the source of the protein, renin (Edelman and Hartroft; Hartroft et al.). The extraglomerular mesangium exhibits phagocytic activity similar to that of the glomerulus and in some species may contain granular epithelioid cells as well. It occupies the triangular space between the afferent and efferent arterioles and the macula densa, a specialized segment of the distal convoluted tubule. The latter represents the tubular component of the juxtaglomerular apparatus (complex).

The granular epithelioid cells of the juxtaglomerular apparatus which synthesize the protein, renin, are thought to give rise to a distinctive renin-producing tumor of the kidney resembling hemangiopericytoma (Schambelan et al.; see mesenchymal tumors of the kidney on page 201). The visceral cells of Bowman's capsule have been shown recently by in vitro and immunohistochemical studies to be the source of erythropoietin (Busuttil et al., 1971, 1972; Burlington et al.) This new evidence suggesting synthesis of erythropoietin by the glomerular epithelial cells, developmentally a tubular portion of the nephron, may account for the production of erythropoietin by renal adenocarcinomas.

Where the proximal convoluted tubule emerges from the glomerulus, the tubular cells are similar to the parietal cells lining Bowman's capsule. In the remainder of its random tortuous course through the renal cortex, the proximal convoluted tubule is lined by a single layer of long, truncated pyramidal cells containing numerous mitochondria and abundant amounts of cytoplasm. The free surfaces of the proximal convoluted tubular cells are covered by elaborate microvilli which form the brush border seen in a light microscopic section. No such brush border is evident in the distal or collecting tubules.

The proximal convoluted tubules extend deep into the medulla and terminate as the narrowed loop of Henle. The epithelial cells of Henle's loop are squamoid in the descending portion and somewhat cuboidal in the ascending limb. After Henle's loop returns to the cortex, the nephron continues as the distal convoluted tubule which in turn subsequently empties into one of the branches of the collecting tubules. A short specialized segment of the distal convoluted tubule comprises the macula densa, which is closely applied to the afferent arteriole and the extraglomerular mesangium. Its previously described close association with the **afferent** arteriole and granular epithelioid cells has recently been shown to be a less constant feature (Barajas, 1970;1971). Relative to the adjacent segments of the distal convoluted tubule, the cells of the macula densa exhibit poorly developed basal cisternae

and apical microvilli, contain fewer mitochondria, and show a more haphazard nuclear polarity. These features suggest that this specialized segment is not engaged in resorptive processes to the same degree as seen elsewhere in the distal tubule. There is a suggestion that the segment merely serves as an electrolyte leak facilitating monitoring of distal tubular sodium.

The coalescing peripheral tributaries of the collecting tubules join to form common straight collecting ducts which descend into the medulla and empty through the apex of a renal papilla into a renal calix. The microscopic appearance of the collecting tubular cells varies with the size of the tubule. In

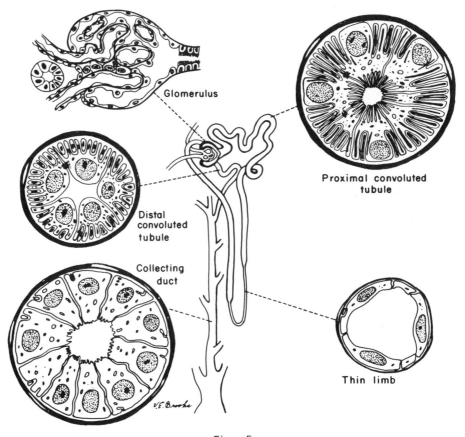

Figure 5
GENERAL HISTOLOGIC FEATURES OF THE NEPHRON
Cross sections of the various segments of the tubule roughly indicate the cellular morphologic features and the relative size of cells and tubules at these sites. (Fig. I-5 from Bennington, J. L., and Kradjian, R. Renal Carcinoma. Philadelphia: W. B. Saunders Co., 1967.)

general, the cells of the collecting tubules have sharp outlines with distinct hyperchromatic nuclei and clear pale cytoplasm. Cells of the smaller branching ducts are cuboidal, while those of the straight collecting tubules are more elongated. Surfaces of both are convex and bulge into the duct lumens (fig. 5).

ELECTRON MICROSCOPIC FEATURES. Cells of the proximal convoluted tubules have characteristic ultrastructural morphologic features which are distinctly different from those of the loop of Henle, distal convoluted tubule, and collecting ducts (Trump et al.). They are identified by their characteristic fine structure including: (1) The tall columnar shape; (2) elaborate tightly packed microvilli coated with glycocalix; (3) pinocytotic apical vesicles, vacuoles, and tubules of characteristic structure in the apical cytoplasm; and (4) abundant elongated tortuous mitochondria intimately associated with basal and lateral cisternae (elaborate invaginations of the cell membrane) (figs. 6, 7). These features are demonstrated in the three dimensional diagrammatic reconstruction of a portion of the proximal convoluted tubule (fig. 8).

In contrast, the distal convoluted tubular cells are tall and cuboidal with scattered short microvilli (fig. 9). Extensive lateral and basal cisternae are present, but they enclose several mitochondrial profiles rather than the individual mitochondria seen in the proximal convoluted tubule cells. Apical pinocytotic vesicles and vacuoles are rare.

Cells of the loop of Henle tend to be squamoid with ovoid nuclei which have folded nuclear margins (fig. 10). Basal and lateral cell interdigitations are absent and cytoplasmic organelles are scanty.

Cells of the collecting ducts (fig. 11) are cuboidal, but become more elongated in the renal medulla. Sparse microvilli are seen on cell surfaces, but no brush border is present. The elaborate system of apical pinocytotic vesicles, tubules, and vacuoles, prominent features of proximal convoluted tubules, are absent. Mitochondria are shorter and have a more rounded configuration than those of the proximal convoluted tubular cells. They are rarely associated with the infrequent basal cisternae. Droplets of membrane-bound lipid (lipofuscin) are abundant in the basal cytoplasm.

Figure 6
PROXIMAL CONVOLUTED TUBULAR CELL

The apical part of the proximal convoluted tubular cell is covered by tightly packed microvilli forming the brush border (BB). In the apical cytoplasm, apical tubules (AT), vacuoles (V), and cytosomes (C) are evident. Mitochondria (M). Tubular Lumen (TL). Nucleus (N). X9300. (Fig. 5 from Tisher, C. C. Human renal ultrastructure. I. Proximal tubule of healthy individuals. Lab. Invest. 15:1357-1394, 1966.)

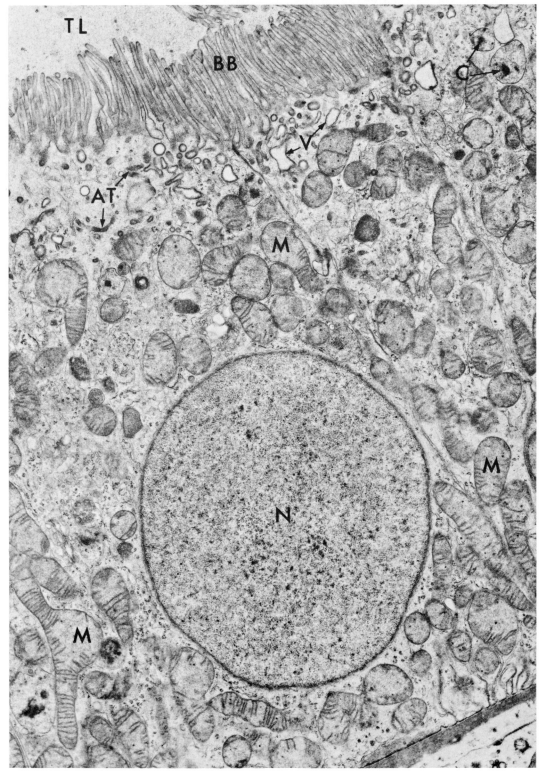

Figure 6

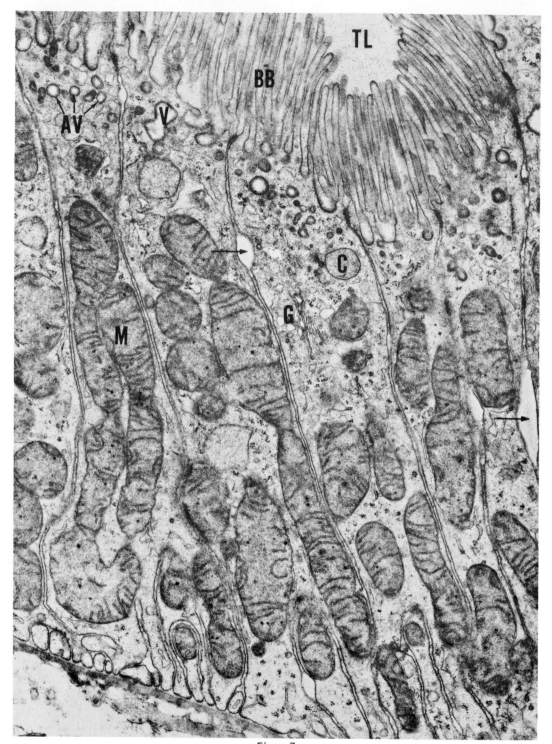

Figure 7
PROXIMAL CONVOLUTED TUBULAR CELL

In the proximal convoluted tubular cells, the mitochondria (M) are often elongated and tortuous. Deep invaginations of the apical cell membrane form apical tubules, vesicles, and vacuoles (V). Note the presence of dense homogenous material in some apical vacuoles and the presence of similar dense bodies in the apical cytosomes (C). Golgi (G). Brush Border (BB). Tubular Lumen (TL). X18,800. (Fig. 7 from Tisher, C. C. Human renal ultrastructure. I. Proximal tubule of healthy individuals. Lab. Invest. 15:1357-1394, 1966.)

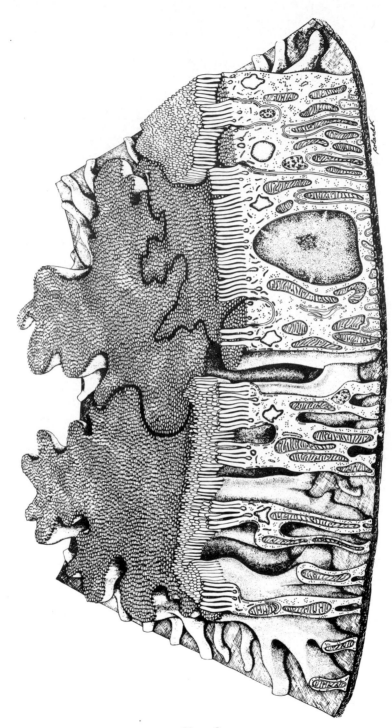

Figure 8
PROXIMAL CONVOLUTED TUBULE
This three dimensional diagram shows reconstruction of the proximal convoluted tubule. (Pl. 5 from Bulger, R. E. The shape of rat kidney tubular cells. Am. J. Anat. 116:237-255, 1965.)

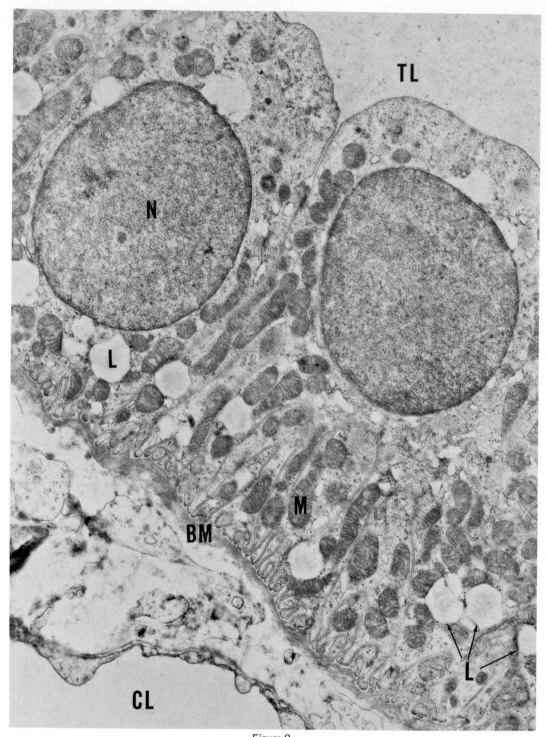

Figure 9
DISTAL CONVOLUTED TUBULAR CELLS

The distal convoluted tubular cells are tall and cuboidal. Note the lack of tubules, vacuoles, and vesicles in the apical cytoplasm. Droplets of lipid (L) are present in the basal cytoplasm. Mitochondria (M). Basement Membrane (BM). Nucleus (N). Tubular Lumen (TL). Capillary Lumen (CL). X10,600. (Courtesy of Dr. C. Craig Tisher, Durham, N. C.)

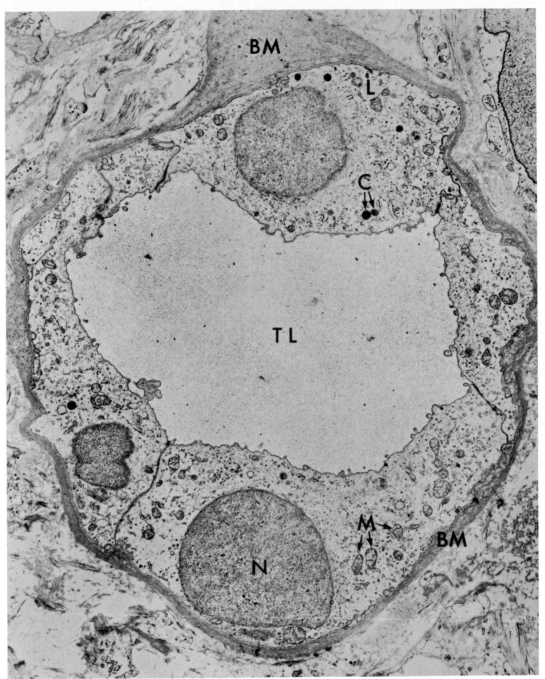

Figure 10
LOOP OF HENLE

In the thin limb of the loop of Henle, the cells assume a more squamoid configuration with nuclei (N) which often display infolding. Basal and lateral cell interdigitations are infrequent. The basement membrane (BM) is often quite variable in thickness. Occasional small mitochondria (M), cytosomes (C), and droplets of lipid (L) are present. Tubular Lumen (TL). X6700. (Courtesy of Dr. C. Craig Tisher, Durham, N. C.)

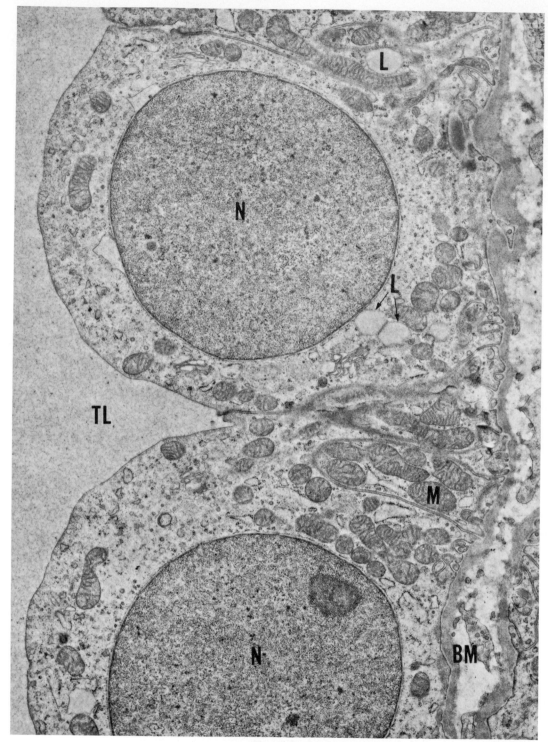

Figure 11
CORTICAL COLLECTING TUBULAR CELLS

Note the absence of microvilli, apical tubules, vesicles, and vacuoles. Mitochondria (M) are round to ovoid and are less concentrated than in the proximal convoluted tubular cells. Few basal interdigitations are present. Membrane-bound lipid (L) is present in the basal cytoplasm. Tubular Lumen (TL). Nucleus (N). Basement Membrane (BM). X12,700. (Courtesy of Dr. C. Craig Tisher, Durham, N. C.)

HISTOLOGIC STRUCTURE OF THE RENAL CALIX, PELVIS, AND URETER

LIGHT MICROSCOPIC FEATURES. The renal calices, pelvis, and ureter are structurally similar with a wall containing smooth muscle and a lining of transitional epithelium attached to the muscularis by a lamina propria composed of both elastic and collagenous fibers (fig. 12). In the calices and pelvis, the transitional epithelium is 2 to 3 cells thick and the ureter is 4 to 5 cells in thickness.

ELECTRON MICROSCOPIC FEATURES. There have been very few studies on the electron microscopic appearance of the transitional epithelium of the human renal pelvis and ureter (Bloom and Fawcett; Flaks et al.). However, there appear to be certain basic similarities between the fine structural features of the transitional epithelium of the human renal pelvis (figs. 13, 14) and that of the rat as well as other types of epithelia (Fulker et al.; Hicks; Zelickson).

1. Basal cells are attached by regularly spaced hemidesmosomes to an underlying dense basement membrane.

2. Lateral cell surfaces are connected at varying intervals by discrete attachments called desmosomes (maculae adherentes), which are specialized thickenings of the plasma membrane. Fine cytoplasmic tonofilaments converge on, and appear to terminate at these attachment sites.

3. The tonofilaments (keratin filaments) are aggregated in dense ramifying bundles throughout the cytoplasm. In addition, characteristic complex interdigitations of the lateral cell surfaces of adjacent cells are noted, particularly in the calix. Luminal cells are bound together by circumferential watertight junctional complexes of the zonula occludens type.

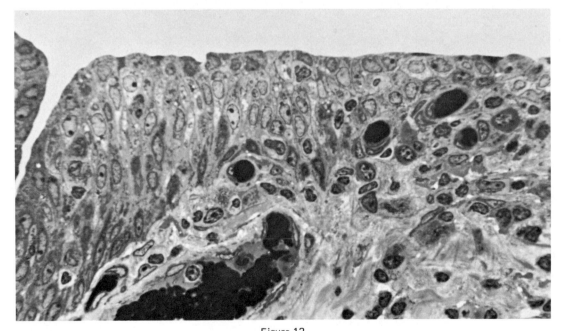

Figure 12
NORMAL TRANSITIONAL EPITHELIUM OF HUMAN URETER
A stratified pavement-like epithelium is composed of regular basal cells and larger superficial cells. Numerous small capillaries are present in the lamina propria. Epon 0.5 micron section. Toluidine blue. X700.

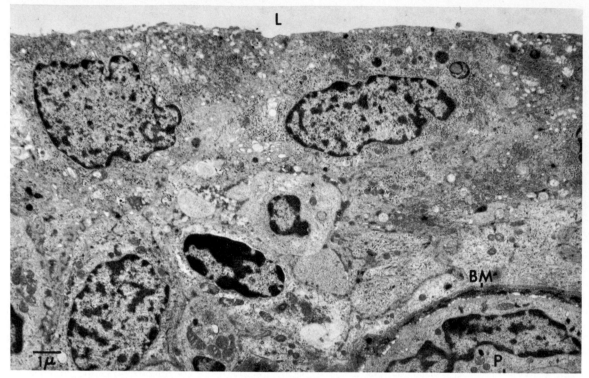

Figure 13
URETERAL EPITHELIUM

This electron micrograph was taken of an area comparable to that in figure 12. Transitional epithelial cells exhibit relatively few desmosomes in comparison to squamous epithelium. Lumen of Ureter (L). Basement Membrane (BM). Portion of Pericyte (P). Scale 1 micron.

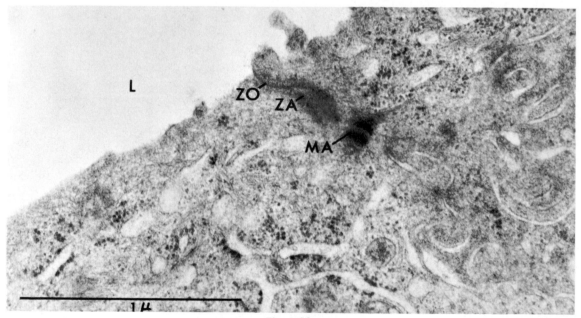

Figure 14
TRANSITIONAL EPITHELIUM

This electron micrograph demonstrates a typical tripartite junctional complex between the apical borders of adjoining transitional cells. Lumen (L). Zonula Occludens (ZO). Zonula Adherens (ZA). Macula Adherens (MA). Arrows indicate the elaborately interdigitating borders of adjoining cells. Scale 1 micron.

While the transitional epithelia of the renal pelvis and ureter cannot be differentiated from that of the bladder at the light microscopic level, certain distinguishing ultrastructural features are evident (Flaks et al.; Fulker et al.). Transitional epithelial cells of the bladder contain numerous small, dense bodies regarded as lysosomes, and the superficial transitional cells contain many flattened fusiform vesicles in their cytoplasm. These features are less evident in the epithelium of the renal pelvis or ureter.

The presence of keratin filaments within the transitional epithelial cells of the ureter and bladder is consistent with the known capacity of these cells to undergo squamous metaplasia and keratin formation under the influence of such stimuli as inflammation and irritation.

HETEROTOPIC TISSUE IN THE KIDNEY

Heterotopic adrenal tissue is encountered in the kidney more frequently through routine inspection at autopsy than is generally appreciated. Apitz found accessory adrenal tissue in the kidney of 261 of 4309 individuals examined at autopsy. In 20 of the 261 instances, two nodules were present and in six instances, there were three. Ectopic adrenal tissue in the kidney is found with the same frequency in both sexes (Risdon).

The adrenal tissue is usually located at the superior pole of the kidney along the lateral margin as a subcapsular, yellow-orange, rounded nodule or plaque, which may range up to 2 cm. in size. Ectopic adrenal tissue is not found in the renal medulla.

The heterotopic adrenal cortical tissue may superficially resemble a small renal adenocarcinoma or so-called adenoma because of the subcapsular location, and because, in both cases, intracellular lipid gives the tissue a yellow to orange coloration.

In small masses of adrenal tissue, the cells and architecture are reminiscent of the normal outer adrenal cortex. At the periphery, the organization may mimic that of the normal zona glomerulosa, while deeper in the mass the pattern is usually more like that of the zona fasciculata, with long cords of cells separated by thin-walled sinusoidal blood vessels arranged perpendicular to the capsule. In large masses of adrenal tissue, all three cortical zones and even medullary tissue may be present (Risdon). Rarely, no adrenal tissue can be located in the usual sites and the entire adrenal gland may be located beneath the renal capsule (O'Crowley and Martland).

The adrenal tissue may be separated from the renal parenchyma by a thin fibrous capsule, but usually it merges gradually with the underlying renal tubules. Dilated renal tubules, some dilated to cystic proportions, foci of fibrosis, and scattered infiltrates of lymphocytes are often present at the junction of the accessory adrenal tissue and renal parenchyma (fig. 15).

The incorporation of accessory adrenal tissue and, less frequently, the entire adrenal gland into the subcapsular area of the renal cortex is generally ascribed to displacement early in embryonic life when the adrenal and renal primordia develop in close proximity.

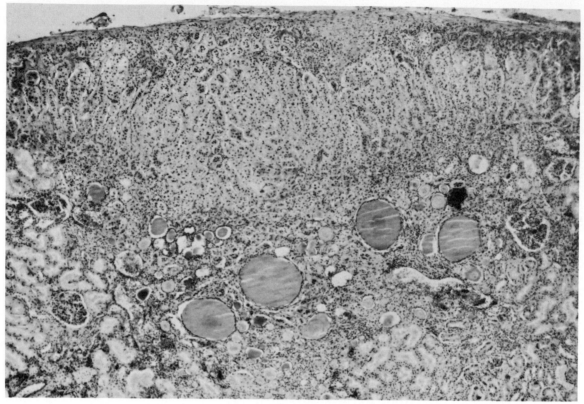

Figure 15
ECTOPIC ADRENAL CORTICAL TISSUE
Ectopic adrenal tissue is located subcapsularly in the superior pole of an adult human kidney. The histologic pattern mimics that of zona fasciculatum with the long cords of cells separated by thin, long sinusoidal blood vessels arranged perpendicular to the capsule. Cystic tubules with a fair amount of fibrosis and lymphocytic infiltration are seen at the interface with the renal cortex. X55.

ENDOMETRIAL TISSUE IN THE KIDNEY, RENAL PELVIS, AND URETER

Symptomatic involvement of the urinary tract by endometriosis is relatively infrequent. Only 151 instances were reported up to 1960, and the majority were found in the bladder (Abeshouse and Abeshouse). The bladder, ureter, and kidney are involved with relative frequencies of approximately 25 to 3 to 1.

Presenting symptoms in patients with endometriosis of the ureter include flank pain, abdominal pain, urinary frequency, dysuria, and gross hematuria (Ochsner and Markland). Excretory urograms generally disclose hydroureter and hydronephrosis proximal to the region of the affected side. Too few cases of endometriosis of the kidney have been recorded to allow a generalization on the symptomatic conditions, although gross hematuria has been reported (Miles and Falconer).

Endometriosis of the urinary tract may be extrinsic, representing extension from endometriosis in adjacent pelvic organs, or may be intrinsic with no continuity to other areas of involvement. Rarely, the focus in the ureter (fig. 16) or kidney (fig. 17) is the only demonstrable area of endometriosis.

The histologic diagnosis depends upon the presence of typical endometrial glands with accompanying endometrial stroma. While the entity is not common, it is important to keep the possibility of endometriosis in mind to avoid misdiagnosing the condition as a primary or metastatic adenocarcinoma.

Old and recent bleeding, or inflammation and fibrosis may partially or completely obliterate the usual histologic features of endometriosis, making it difficult or impossible to render a definitive diagnosis. In the absence of typical glands, such a diagnosis may be suspected if foci of decidual change are present.

A number of theories have been proposed to explain the origin of endometriosis and include: (1) Embryonic rests; (2) implantation following retrograde tubal menstruation; (3) benign metastases from endometrium by lymphatic or vascular dissemination; and (4) metaplasia of celomic epithelium. The reasons for rejecting the first three theories concerning the origin of extra-uterine endometriosis have been nicely summarized by Willis and by Hertig and Gore. It seems most likely that endometriosis arises by metaplasia of the celomic epithelium in an attempt to recapitulate development of the müllerian duct (Ferguson et al.). Search of the literature has not revealed reports of the malignant counterpart of endometriosis (endometrioid carcinoma) of the kidney or ureter.

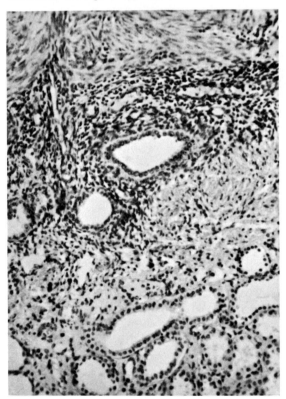

Figure 16

Figure 16
ENDOMETRIOSIS OF RENAL PARENCHYMA
Endometrial glands are illustrated having characteristic accompanying endometrial stroma with surrounding fibrosis. Endometriosis was also present in the renal pelvis. X80. (Fig. 2 from Miles, H. B., and Falconer, K. W. Renal endometriosis associated with hematuria. J. Urol. 102:291-293, 1969.)

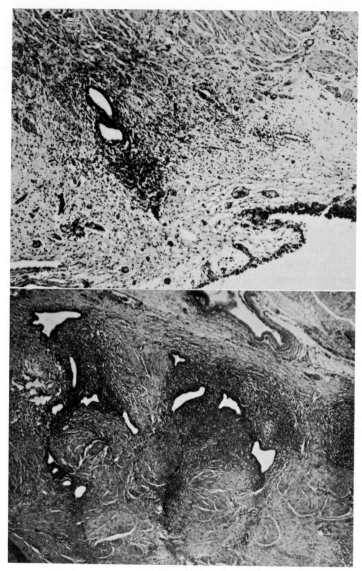

Figure 17
ENDOMETRIOSIS OF URETER
Endometrial glands are shown with accompanying endometrial stroma
present in the submucosa and muscular wall of the ureter. X15. (Fig.3 A, B
from Bulkley, G. J., Carrow, L. A., and Estensen, R. D. Endometriosis of
the ureter. J. Urol. 93:139-143, 1965.)

CARTILAGE IN RENAL STROMA

Islands of benign cartilage are found occasionally in the renal parenchyma (fig. 18). The involved kidney is usually small and cystic, and its lower urinary tract is frequently the site of partial or complete obstruction. Bigler and Killingsworth first noted this association. Subsequently, a constellation of gross and histologic abnormalities was recognized which makes up the entity of renal dysplasia. Now it is recog-

nized that instead of hypoplasia, at times the kidneys may be normal in size or grossly enlarged, externally normal or grossly malformed, and dysplasia may be total or segmental, involving only a portion of one or several contiguous developmental lobules. The cortex and/or the medulla may be involved (Bernstein; Reese and Winstanley). The cardinal histologic features of renal dysplasia are:

1. Islands of metaplastic cartilage, and occasionally bone

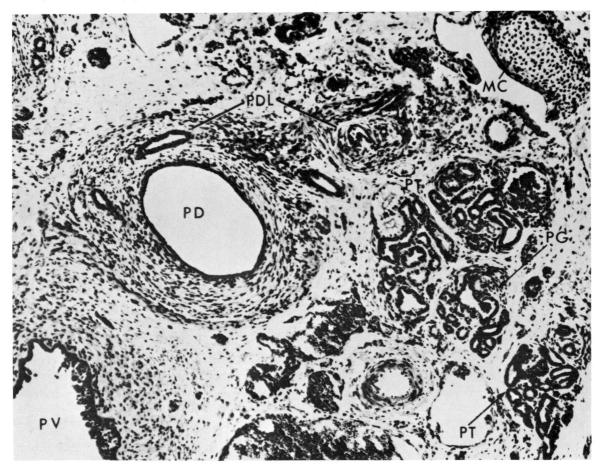

Figure 18
RENAL DYSPLASIA

This photomicrograph demonstrates the characteristic histologic features of renal dysplasia, including primitive ducts (PD) surrounded by a fibromuscular collar; a rudimentary pelvis (RP); primitive ductules (PDL); metaplastic cartilage (MC); primitive glomeruli (PG); and clusters of adjacent primitive tubules (PT). X105. (Fig. 10 from Bernstein, J. Developmental abnormalities of the renal parenchyma: renal hypoplasia and dysplasia. Pathol. Annu. 3: 213-247, 1968.)

2. Primitive ducts lined by columnar epithelium which are frequently ciliated and surrounded by collarettes of fibromuscular tissue (ciliated primitive ducts are frequently misinterpreted and reported as epididymal vestiges in the kidney)

3. Primitive glomeruli, convoluted tubules, and collecting ducts

4. Cysts arising in the nephron or collecting tubules.

While nearly 90 percent of dysplastic kidneys are associated with lower urinary tract obstruction, familial forms of renal dysplasia have been reported, and apparently an increased frequency occurs in patients with multiple congenital anomalies, primarily those involving the gastrointestinal tract and cardiovascular system. In those cases in which associated lower urinary tract obstruction occurs, the dysplasia is thought to be mediated through injury to the developing kidney in the form of altered inductive effects between the collecting tubules and nephrons during early nephrogenesis (Bernstein). Cartilaginous metaplasia usually appears to be initiated by some form of injury occurring early in nephrogenesis.

The multipotentiality of the metanephric blastema and its derivatives, the stomogenic and nephrogenic blastema, is manifested in a wide variety of benign and malignant tissue types which may arise in the kidney during nephrogenesis and in the mature kidney.

Possible genetic and histogenetic relationships among renal dysplasia, nodular renal blastema, mesoblastic nephroma, and nephroblastoma are discussed on pages 32—52.

ADIPOSE TISSUE AND SMOOTH MUSCLE

At autopsy, small islands of adipose tissue and/or smooth muscle are not infrequently found in the renal cortex. These incidentally discovered nodules are usually unilateral, solitary lesions ranging from 0.1 to 1 cm. in greatest diameter. They lack a capsule, but are fairly well circumscribed and do not appear to compress the adjacent cortex or invade blood vessels of the renal capsule or adjacent parenchyma.

While some of the nodules are composed completely of adipose tissue (lipomas) and others of smooth muscle (myomas), many contain both adipose tissue and smooth muscle (myolipomas) (Reese and Winstanley). Within the same kidney containing multiple nodules, one may find nodules of pure adipose tissue and others formed only of smooth muscle (Reese and Winstanley). Multiple mixed lesions are also occasionally found. In any of these forms, a vascular component consisting of tortuous thick-walled vessels suggesting an angiomatous pattern may be present. Within the small vessels, there is a thickened muscular layer and a collarette of smooth muscle which is continuous with the smooth muscle found in the lesion. In the presence of this vascular component, the lesion is referred to as an angiomyolipoma. The histologic continuum observed in these lesions suggests that there is basically one entity—the mixed lesion which in the extreme form may contain only one element, smooth muscle or adipose tissue.

Irrespective of the predominant histologic component, these lesions are rarely found in patients before middle age and are much more frequent in women than men (Table I; Reese and Winstanley). Histologically, they are indistinguishable from the angiomyolipoma associated with tuberous sclerosis. In the presence of tuberous sclerosis, lesions may be discovered at a much earlier age and found in as high as 80 percent of patients with this disease complex (Critchley and Earl). While the majority of patients with renal angiomyolipoma show no stigmata of tuberous sclerosis, as high as 38 percent will show some degree of expression of this disease (Hajdu and Foote; Farrow et al.). The possibility must be considered that the presence of such a lesion indicates a carrier state or a *forme fruste* of this disease.

The adipose tissue found in an angiomyolipoma is usually composed of adult fat cells with large cytoplasmic vacuoles and small peripheral nuclei. Occasionally, the lesions can be quite bizarre with active nuclei appearing in the adipose tissue and hyperchromatic, pleomorphic nuclei, with occasional mitotic figures, appearing in the smooth muscle cells. Because documented malignant behavior of angiomyolipomas is rare to the point of being nonexistent, one must guard against misdiagnosing such lesions as liposarcoma, malignant mesenchymoma, myosarcoma, or a variant of nephroblastoma (Farrow et al.).

Table I

AGE AND SEX DISTRIBUTION OF RENAL CORTICAL NODULES CONTAINING SMOOTH MUSCLE, ADIPOSE TISSUE, OR BOTH*

Age	Males		Females	
	Number	Number with Nodules	Number	Number with Nodules
0-10	0	—	1	0
11-20	9	0	1	0
21-30	9	0	1	0
31-40	7	0	1	1
41-50	12	0	3	0
51-60	22	0	9	4
61-70	36	3	16	6
71-80	29	2	32	8
81-90	9	0	14	1
91-100	0	—	1	0
Total	133	5 (4%)	79	20 (25%)

*Modified from Reese, A. J. M., and Winstanley, D. P. The small tumour-like lesions of the kidney. Br. J. Cancer 12:507-516, 1958.

How smooth muscle and fat make their appearance in the renal cortex has not been satisfactorily explained. Fatty infiltration of the renal cortex from the peripelvic or perirenal fat is a possibility, although many lesions show no continuity with the renal capsule, and such an explanation does not account for the frequent association with muscle elements. The suggestion that such lesions arise in smooth muscle and fat in the renal capsule (Colvin) is untenable, since neither smooth muscle nor adipose tissue are found in the adult renal capsule. An origin in the smooth muscle of arteriole walls does not account for lesions containing adipose tissue. There is no convincing evidence that such lesions are dysplastic— the lack of any associated renal abnormalities argues against this possibility. While these lesions are frequently referred to as lipomas, leiomyomas, and angiomyolipomas depending upon their histologic features, thus implying a neoplastic origin, such designations do not help to explain why fat or smooth muscle should be present in the renal cortex unless by metaplasia of stromal cells within the renal parenchyma.

Most authors have invoked Albrecht's concept of a hamartomatous origin and have drawn heavily on the known association between the tuberous sclerosis complex and renal angiomyolipomas for support for this theory (Hajdu and Foote). Because of the lack of smooth muscle and fat in the stroma of the normal kidney, the use of the term hamartoma would seem to be a poor one and the term choristoma, also coined by Albrecht, denoting a tumor-like formation composed of tissues displaced to an abnormal position is more appropriate. The possibility that angiomyolipomas may occasionally behave as neoplasms and rarely become malignant is discussed under mesenchymal tumors of the kidney on page 204.

INTERSTITIUM OF THE KIDNEY

The interstitium of the kidney is best developed in the medulla and is composed of cells resembling fibroblasts, with long processes which are situated mainly between the vasa recta and limbs of Henle.

Morphologic differences from fibroblasts found elsewhere in the body are largely qualitative. Interstitial cells are characterized by a cytoplasm rich in: (1) rough-surfaced endoplasmic reticulum, mitochondria, and Golgi; (2) perinuclear cisternae, and (3) lipid droplets (fig. 19). Interstitial spaces contain basement membrane material, debris, myelin figures, and collagenous fibrils (Lerman et al.; Bulger and Nagle).

The role of the interstitial cell in the production of the renomedullary interstitial cell tumor (medullary fibroma) is discussed under mesenchymal tumors on page 231.

References

Abeshouse, B. S., and Abeshouse, G. Endometriosis of the urinary tract: A review of the literature and a report of four cases of vesical endometriosis. J. Int. Coll. Surg. 34:43-63, 1960.

Albrecht, E. Ueber hamartome. Verh. Dtsch. Ges. Pathol. 7:153-157, 1904.

Apitz, K. Die Geschwülste und Gewebsmissbildungen der Nierenrinde. I. Die intrarenalen Nebenniereninseln. Virchows Arch. (Pathol. Anat.) 311:285-305, 1944.

Barajas, L. Renin secretion: an anatomical basis for tubular control. Science 172:485-487, 1971.

.... The ultrastructure of the juxtaglomerular apparatus as disclosed by three-dimensional reconstructions from serial sections. The anatomical relationship between the tubular and vascular components. J. Ultrastruct. Res. 33:116-147, 1970.

Bernstein, J. Developmental abnormalities of the renal parenchyma: renal hypoplasia and dysplasia. Pathol. Annu. 3:213-247, 1968.

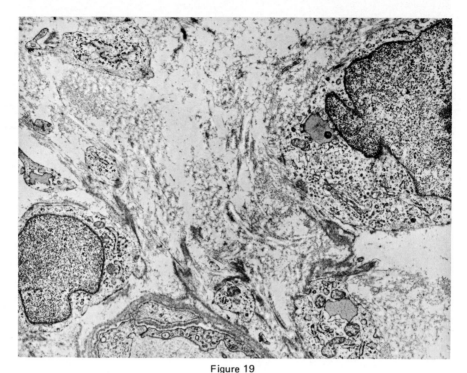

Figure 19
HUMAN KIDNEY—NORMAL VESSEL AND INTERSTITIAL CELLS
The electron microscopic appearance of the renal medullary interstitium shows portions
of interstitial cells with fibroblast-like cytoplasm and intercellular collagenous fibrils.
Approx. X4700. (Courtesy of Dr. Ruth E. Bulger, Baltimore, Md.)

Bigler, J. A., and Killingsworth, W. P. Cartilage in the kidney. Arch. Pathol. 47:487-493, 1949.

Bloom, W., and Fawcett, D. W. A Textbook of Histology, 9th ed., p. 674. Philadelphia: W. B. Saunders Co., 1968.

Bulger, R. E., and Nagle, R. B. Ultrastructure of the interstitium in the rabbit kidney. Am. J. Anat. 136:183-204, 1973.

Burlington, H., Cronkite, E. P., Reincke, U., and Zanjani, E. D. Erythropoietin production in cultures of goat renal glomeruli. Proc. Natl. Acad. Sci. 69:3547-3550, 1972.

Busuttil, R. W., Roh, B. L., and Fisher, J. W. Localization of erythropoietin in the glomerulus of the hypoxic dog kidney using a fluorescent antibody technique. Acta Haematol. (Basel) 47:238-242, 1972.

............, Roh, B. L., and Fisher, J. W. The cytological localization of erythropoietin in the human kidney using the fluorescent antibody technique. Proc. Soc. Exp. Biol. Med. 137:327-330, 1971.

Colvin, S. H., Jr. Certain capsular and subcapsular mixed tumors of the kidney herein called "capsuloma." J. Urol. 48:585-600, 1942.

Critchley, M., and Earl, C. J. C. Tuberose sclerosis and allied conditions. Brain 55:311-346, 1932.

Edelman, R., and Hartroft, P. M. Localization of renin in juxtaglomerular cells of rabbit and dog through the use of the fluorescent-antibody technique. Circ. Res. 9:1069-1077, 1961.

Faarup, P. Morphological aspects of the renin-angiotensin system. Acta Pol. Microbiol. Scand. (A) (Suppl.) 222:1-96, 1971.

Farrow, G. M., Harrison, E. G., Jr., Utz, D. C., and Jones, D. R. Renal angiomyolipoma. A clinicopathologic study of 32 cases. Cancer 22:564-570, 1968.

Ferguson, B. R., Bennington, J. L., and Haber, S. L. Histochemistry of mucosubstances and histology of mixed müllerian pelvic lymph node glandular inclusions. Obstet. Gynecol. 33:617-625, 1969.

Flaks, B., Cooper, E. H., and Knowles, J. C. Observations on the fine structure of human ureteric tumours. Eur. J. Cancer 6:145-149, 1970.

Fulker, M. J., Cooper, E. H., and Tanaka, T. Proliferation and ultrastructure of papillary transitional cell carcinoma of the human bladder. Cancer 27:71-82, 1971.

Hajdu, S. I., and Foote, F. W., Jr. Angiomyolipoma of the kidney: Report of 27 cases and review of the literature. J. Urol. 102:396-401, 1969.

Hamilton, W. J., Boyd, J. D., and Mossman, H. W. Human Embryology (Prenatal Development of Form and Function), 3rd ed., p. 271. Baltimore: Williams & Wilkins Co., 1962.

Hartroft, P. M., Sutherland, L. E., and Hartroft, W. S. Juxtaglomerular cells as the source of renin: further studies with the fluorescent antibody technique and the effect of passive transfer of antirenin. Canad. Med. Assoc. J. 90:163-166, 1964.

Hertig, A. T., and Gore, H. Tumors of the Female Sex Organs, Part 3, Tumors of the Ovary and Fallopian Tube, pp. 83 and 94. Fascicle 33, Atlas of Tumor Pathology. Washington: Armed Forces Institute of Pathology, 1961.

Hicks, R. M. The fine structure of the transitional epithelium of rat ureter. J. Cell Biol. 26:25-48, 1965.

Lerman, R. I., Pitcock, J. A., Stephenson, P., and Muirhead, E. E. Renomedullary interstitial cell tumor (formerly fibroma of renal medulla). Hum. Pathol. 3:559-568, 1972.

Miles, H. B., and Falconer, K. W. Renal endometriosis associated with hematuria. J. Urol. 102:291-293, 1969.

Ochsner, T., and Markland, C. Endometriosis obstructing the ureter. J. Urol. 98:462-465, 1967.

O'Crowley, C. R., and Martland, H. S. Adrenal heterotopia, rests, and the so-called Grawitz tumor. J. Urol. 50:756-768, 1943.

Osathanondh, V., and Potter, E. L. Development of human kidney as shown by microdissection. II. Renal pelvis, calyces, and papillae. Arch. Pathol. 76:277-289, 1963.

Reese, A. J. M., and Winstanley, D. P. The small tumour-like lesions of the kidney. Br. J. Cancer 12:507-516, 1958.

Risdon, R. A. Renal dysplasia. Part I. A clinico-pathological study of 76 cases. J. Clin. Pathol. 24:57-71, 1971.

Schambelan, M., Howes, E. L., Jr., Noakes, C. A., Stockigt, J. R., and Biglieri, E. G. Role of renin and aldosterone in hypertension due to a renin-secreting tumor. Am. J. Med. 55:86-92, 1973.

Takeshita, K. The fine structure of the juxtaglomerular apparatus from the human and bat kidney. Arch. Histol. Jap. 29:237-270, 1968.

Trump, B. F., and Bulger, R. E. Morphology of the Kidney, pp. 1-43. In: Structural Basis of Renal Disease. (Ed.) Becker, E. L. New York: Harper and Row, 1968.

............, Tisher, C. C., and Saladino, A. J. The Nephron in Health and Disease, pp. 387-494. In: The Biological Basis of Medicine. (Eds.) Bittar, E. E., and Bittar, N. New York and London: Academic Press, 1969.

Willis, R. A. The Borderland of Embryology and Pathology, 2d ed., p. 336. London: Butterworth & Co., Ltd., 1962.

Zelickson, A. S. Ultrastructure of Normal and Abnormal Skin. Philadelphia: Lea & Febiger, 1967.

TUMORS OF THE UPPER URINARY TRACT

INTRODUCTION

Primary malignant neoplasms of the renal parenchyma include **renal adenocarcinoma, nephroblastoma,** and various **sarcomas** of different histologic types. Since malignant tumors of the upper urinary tract are relatively infrequent, many epidemiologic and pathologic studies of such tumors are based on data obtained by grouping the various malignant tumors of the kidney together with those of the renal pelvis. An immediate objection to this is that such data are of no use to one interested in studying a particular tumor of the kidney parenchyma or renal pelvis; i.e., such a grouping masks important differences in the epidemiology of these various tumors. For example, nephroblastoma and renal adenocarcinoma both arise in the kidney, but occur in different age groups and are etiologically unrelated, while carcinoma of the renal pelvis arises in a structure which is embryologically and morphologically dissimilar to the renal parenchyma, but may share with renal adenocarcinoma certain etiologic factors.

Because of the way in which epidemiologic data have been gathered in the past, there is very little information available on the effect of race or geography on the tumors of the upper urinary tract. It has been reported that countries may be divided into three groups: Those countries showing low rates—Ireland, Italy, Japan, Venezuela; intermediate rates—Australia, Belgium, France, Netherlands, England, Northern Ireland, and white and nonwhite populations in the United States; and high

rates—Denmark, New Zealand, Norway, and Scotland. On the other hand, within the same country, racial background may show no influence on the incidence of malignant tumors of the upper urinary tract. The relative frequency of malignant tumors of the kidney and renal pelvis for Whites, Blacks, American Indians, Chinese, and Japanese living in California is directly proportional to the numbers of persons in each group in the population (Graph I; Case).

GRAPH I

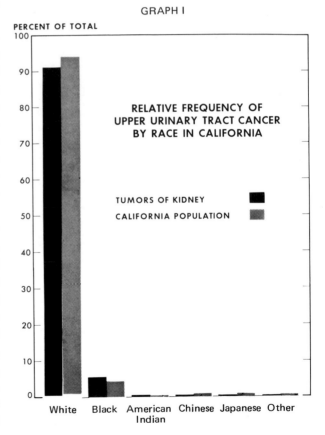

Currently, most major tumor registries throughout the world are beginning to record tumors of the renal parenchyma separately from those of the renal pelvis and are classifying these tumors by their histologic types. Hopefully, data gathered in this way will provide greater insight into the epidemiology of the various malignant tumors of the upper urinary tract.

Malignant tumors of the kidney constitute approximately 2.5 percent of all necropsies on patients with malignant neoplasms, 0.3 to 0.35 percent of all necropsies, and rank about thirteenth in order of frequency among all carcinomas (Abrams et al.; Lucké and Schlumberger; Steiner; Willis). However, none of these figures indicate either the relation of age to incidence of nephroblastoma and renal adenocarcinoma nor reflects the relative importance of these two tumors in the age groups in which they occur.

While nephroblastoma is relatively frequent among malignant tumors in children (constituting 13 to 20 percent of malignant tumors other than leukemia and lymphoma found in patients under the age of 15 years) and is almost exclusively limited to this age group, the overall incidence of nephroblastoma in children is low (Graph II; Cresson and Pilling; Ledlie et al.).

In contrast, renal adenocarcinoma is relatively infrequent among malignant tumors in adults, comprising no more than 3 percent of malignant tumors in this age group (Bennington and Kradjian); it is

GRAPH II

RATES PER 100,000 POPULATION

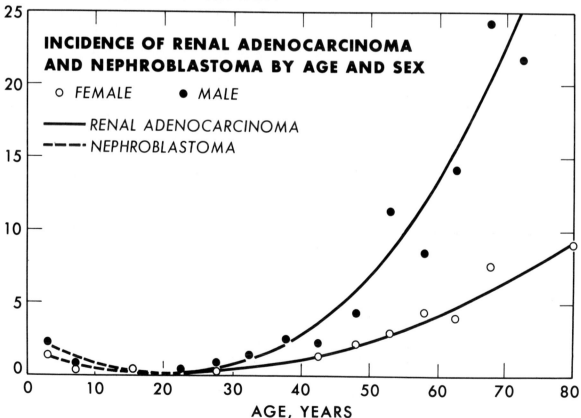

rarely found in children, and its incidence increases with advancing age (Graph II). Since the overall incidence of malignant tumors in adults is substantially greater than in children, renal adenocarcinoma makes up the great majority of all malignant renal tumors. Approximately 86 percent of clinically manifest primary malignant renal tumors are renal adenocarcinomas, and 12 percent are nephroblastomas (Table II). If one were to include the renal cortical glandular tumors histologically indistinguishable from renal adenocarcinoma, but less than 3 cm. in greatest diameter, usually discovered incidentally at the time of autopsy, the frequency of adenocarcinoma would be considerably higher.

Sarcomas of the renal parenchyma which make up the remainder of malignant tumors of the kidney are distinctly uncommon. The incidence is usually reported

Table II

RELATIVE FREQUENCY OF MALIGNANT TUMORS OF THE KIDNEY BY RACE AND SEX*
(NOT INCLUDING TUMORS OF UNDETERMINED HISTOLOGIC TYPE)

Race	Renal Adenocarcinoma		Nephroblastoma		Sarcoma		Total
	Males	Females	Males	Females	Males	Females	
White	1378	768	147	131	33	33	2490 (91.2%)
Black	82	58	14	19	3	3	179 (6.6%)
American Indian	3	2	0	0	0	0	5 (0.2%)
Chinese	4	0	2	1	0	0	7 (0.2%)
Japanese	3	3	0	2	0	0	8 (0.3%)
Other	8	0	0	0	0	1	9 (0.3%)
Unspecified	22	9	0	1	0	0	32 (1.2%)
Subtotal	1500	840	163	154	37	36	2730
Total	2340(85.7%)		317(11.6%)		73(2.7%)		(100%)

*Courtesy of Mr. George Linden, Chief, State of California Department of Public Health, California Tumor Registry, 1942–1969.

as 2 to 3 percent of all primary malignant tumors (Lucké and Schlumberger; Riches et al.). Among tumors reported to the California Tumor Tissue Registry, they constitute 2.7 percent of all malignant renal tumors (Table II). These estimates are very likely on the high side. In our experience, many of the tumors reported as sarcomas of the kidney represent sarcomatoid renal adenocarcinomas or nephroblastomas.

Malignant tumors of the renal pelvis and ureter combined are only one-fourth to one-fifth as frequent as malignant tumors of the renal parenchyma. Approximately 72 percent are carcinomas of the renal pelvis and 28 percent carcinomas of the ureter (Table III). Renal pelvic and ureteral carcinomas are almost exclusively found in adults, and their incidence increases with advancing age (Graph III).

Table III

RELATIVE FREQUENCY OF MALIGNANT TUMORS OF THE
RENAL PELVIS AND URETER BY RACE AND SEX*
(NOT INCLUDING TUMORS OF UNDETERMINED HISTOLOGIC TYPE)

Race	Carcinoma of Renal Pelvis		Carcinoma of Ureter		Total
	Males	Females	Males	Females	
White	460	269	176	104	1009 (94%)
Black	16	16	2	3	37 (3.4%)
American Indian	1	0	0	0	1 (0.1%)
Chinese	2	0	1	0	3 (0.3%)
Japanese	1	1	1	1	4 (0.4%)
Other	2	0	1	1	4 (0.4%)
Unspecified	2	5	7	1	15 (1.4%)
Subtotal	484	291	188	110	1073
Total	775 (72.2%)		298 (27.8%)		(100%)

*Courtesy of Mr. George Linden, Chief, State of California Department of Public Health, California Tumor Registry, 1942–1969.

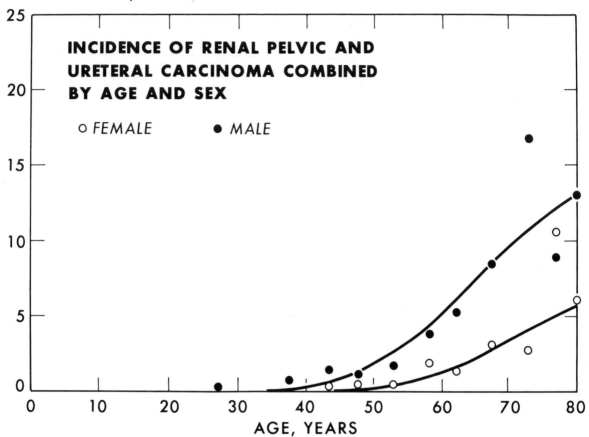

GRAPH III

RATES PER 100,000 POPULATION

INCIDENCE OF RENAL PELVIC AND URETERAL CARCINOMA COMBINED BY AGE AND SEX

○ *FEMALE*   ● *MALE*

AGE, YEARS

Further discussion of the epidemiology of renal, renal pelvic, and ureteral tumors is covered in the section in which the specific tumor is presented.

References

Abrams, H. L., Spiro, R., and Goldstein, N. Metastases in carcinoma: Analysis of 1000 autopsied cases. Cancer 3:74-85, 1950.

Bennington, J. L., and Kradjian, R. M. Renal Carcinoma. Philadelphia: W. B. Saunders Co., 1967.

Case, R. A. M. In: Monographs on Neoplastic Diseases at Various Sites, Vol. V. Tumors of the Kidney and Ureter, p. 8. (Ed.) Riches, E. W. Baltimore: Williams & Wilkins Co.; Edinburgh: E. & S. Livingstone, Ltd., 1964.

Cresson, S. L., and Pilling, G. P. Renal tumors. Pediatr. Clin. North Am. 6:473-490, 1959.

Ledlie, E. M., Mynors, L. S., Draper, G. J., and Gorbach, P. D. Natural history and treatment of Wilms's tumour: An analysis of 335 cases occurring in England and Wales, 1962-6. Brit. Med. J. 4:195-200, 1970.

Lucke, B., and Schlumberger, H. G. Tumors of the Kidney, Renal Pelvis and Ureter, p. 81. Fascicle 30, Atlas of Tumor Pathology. Washington: Armed Forces Institute of Pathology, 1957.

Riches, E. W., Griffiths, I. H., and Thackray, A. C. New growths of the kidney and ureter. Br. J. Urol. 23:297-356, 1951.

Steiner, P. E. Sources, Materials, Racial Composition, Age, Sex, Methods, Comments, and Comparisons with Sedentes, pp. 9-23; Carcinoma of the Kidney, pp. 255-264. In: Cancer: Race and Geography. Baltimore: Williams & Wilkins Co., 1954.

Willis, R. A. Pathology of Tumours, 4th ed. New York: Appleton-Century-Crofts, 1968.

TUMORS OF THE KIDNEY

EMBRYONAL TUMORS

NEPHROBLASTOMA

SYNONYMS AND RELATED TERMS: **Embryonic nephroma**; adenocarcinoma renum congenitum; adenocarcinoma sarcomatodes; adenochondrosarcoma; adenoma carcinomatodes; adenoma myosarcomatosum; adenomyosarcoma; adenomyofibrosarcoma; adenomyosarcoma pericanaliculare striocellulare; adenomyxoma; adenomyxosarcoma; adenosarcoma; adenosarcoma pericanaliculare; alveolar carcinoma; alveolar sarcoma; alveolar round cell sarcoma; angiomyosarcoma; blastomal tumor; blastoma mesoblastica polyvalentia; carcinosarcoma; chondromyosarcoma; cystosarcoma; developmental tumor; dysembryoma; ectomesodermic mixed tumor; embryoma; embryonal adenocarcinoma; embryonal adenomyosarcoma; embryonal carcinoma; embryonal carcinosarcoma; embryonal mixed tumor; embryonal nephroma; embryonal nephrosarcoma; embryonary nephroma; embryonal sarcoma; encephaloid tumor; fibrolipoosteochondroma; fibrosarcoma; fungus haematodes; hamartoblastoma; hypernephroid sarcoma; leiomyoadenosarcoma; leiomyosarcoma; malignant adenoma; malignant embryoma; malignant leiomyoma; malignant nephroma; malignant teratoma; medullary carcinoma; mesenchymal tumor; mesoblastic nephroma; mesoblastic sarcoma; mesodermic mixed tumor; mesothelioma; metanephroma; metanephric hamartoma; mixed tumor; mixed teratoid tumor; myoblastic sarcoma; myochondroadenocarcinoma; myochondroadenosarcoma; myochondrosarcoma; myofibrosarcoma; myoma sarcomatodes renum; myosarcoma; myosarcoma striocellulare; myxosarcoma; myxosarcoma haemmorhagicum; myxosarcoma striocellulare; nephrogenous dysembryoma; nephroma; nephroma embryonale malignum; osteoblastoma; renal blastoma; rhabdomyosarcoma; rhabdomyoangiosarcoma; round cell sarcoma; sarcoma carcinomatosum; sarcoma fusocellulare; small round cell sarcoma; spindle cell sarcoma; striated myosarcoma; striped myosarcoma; teratoma; wolffian adenoma; Wilms' tumor.

DEFINITION. A satisfactory definition of nephroblastoma is hindered by unresolved controversies as to the classification of certain tumors composed entirely of one tissue pattern, but otherwise typical of nephroblastoma. For example, tumors composed entirely of rhabdomyoblastic

....
WHO nomenclature for this system is at present under development and not yet available.

tissue occur occasionally in the infant's or child's kidney, and except for a somewhat higher incidence of bilaterality seem epidemiologically similar to mixed nephroblastomas. It is our view that the traditional definition of nephroblastoma as a mixed renal tumor, composed of metanephric blastema and its recognized stromal and epithelial derivatives at variable stages of differentiation, should be expanded to include as variants those monotypic neoplasms composed predominantly or exclusively of one of the histologic patterns common to typical mixed nephroblastomas of the kidney.

HISTORICAL ASPECTS. Renal tumors undoubtedly representing nephroblastoma, but without microscopic documentation, were reported frequently throughout the nineteenth century, usually under the term ''fungus haematodes'' or ''encephaloid tumor'' of the child's kidney. An example of bilateral nephroblastoma, obtained by John Hunter during the eighteenth century, is on display in the Museum of the Royal College of Surgeons in London, along with microscopic slides of excellent quality. Schuberg's 1861 report, generally overlooked in reviews of the subject, may have been the first to mention microscopic study of a nephroblastoma, but the remarkable histopathologic features of this tumor were not appreciated until Eberth's brief report in 1872. During the next few years, a large amount of literature on the subject accumulated and a lively debate arose concerning the histogenesis of nephroblastoma.

Since the outstanding characteristic of nephroblastoma is diversity of differentiation, including a number of tissues foreign to the normal metanephros, the field was unusually ripe for speculation. Early theories of histogenesis fall into several categories, arranged into progressively earlier stages in ontogeny when the primary abnormality was thought to have occurred:

1. Origin from metanephric blastema (Muus, 1899; Busse, 1899).

2. Inclusions of wolffian body (mesonephros) (Eberth, 1872; Birch-Hirschfeld, 1898).

3. Origin from mesoderm prior to separation of nephrogenic mesenchyme from somites (Wilms, 1899).

4. Origin from totipotential blastomeres prior to differentiation of germ layers (Ribbert, 1892). This represented a change from Ribbert's earlier work on the subject in 1886, wherein he proposed the origin of skeletal muscle in nephroblastoma by metaplasia of metanephric smooth muscle.

These postulated concepts of origin reflect the various theories as to the developmental potentialities of the metanephric blastema. Increasing experience with renal dysplasia, however, led to an awareness that metanephric blastema possesses the capability for differentiation into many tissues not normally found in the metanephros (Bernstein). With the possible exception of striated muscle, all heterotopic tissues seen in nephroblastomas have been described in normal or dysplastic human kidneys. It, therefore, became unnecessary to postulate the inclusion of aberrant embryonic tissues in the kidney in order to account for the tissue elements of nephroblastomas. Except for Masson's neuroepithelial theory of origin for nephroblastoma, there has been virtually unanimous acceptance for many years of the origin of this tumor from metanephric cells possessing embryonal potentialities.

Histogenesis

While most authors have presumed an origin of this tumor from metanephric blastema, there has been surprisingly little written about specific mechanisms of origin. Theoretically, three general mechanisms of development might be proposed:

1. **Development prior to birth while metanephric blastema is still normally present.** Nephroblastomas have been encountered in stillborn infants, but the age distribution curve peaks between three and five years rather than the first year as might be expected for congenital tumors (Muto; Nicholson) (see p. 46). There is, in fact, a paucity of nephroblastomas diagnosed in the first year of life, and many have not appeared until adulthood (Favara et al.; Olsen and Bischoff). It, therefore, seems unlikely that progressive tumor growth characteristically begins during fetal life.

2. **Development from differentiated cells which may under certain circumstances regain embryonic potentialities.** "De-repression" of genetic information in differentiated cell systems can result in reactivation of embryonal characteristics (Frenster and Herstein). If this concept is applied to nephroblastoma, one would have to postulate that the child's kidney cell is more susceptible to "de-repression" than that of the adult to account for the age distribution curve of nephroblastoma. Experimental production of this tumor in animals is usually possible only in the very young (p. 45).

3. **Development from cells with persistent embryonal potentialities.** Despite the fact that Cohnheim's "cell rest" theory of

tumor formation has been regarded as obsolete by modern workers (Willis), and clearly does not pertain to most human neoplasms, there is considerable evidence in support of his concept when its application is restricted to a few tumors, including nephroblastoma.

That nodular foci of blastema might occasionally persist in the human kidney was first suggested by the observations of Potter (1961), who depicted incidentally encountered microscopic nodules resembling nephroblastomas in infant kidneys. She concluded that had these infants survived, they would have developed nephroblastomas. Shanklin and Sotelo-Avila described two additional specimens, coining for them the term "nephroblastoma-in-situ." Bove and associates, in a review of 1895 pediatric autopsies, found such foci in five cases, which they termed "nodular renal blastema." This incidence of 1 to 379 cases was far greater than one would expect from the known frequency of incidentally encountered early nephroblastomas. Three additional cases were found when the authors systematically reviewed tissue from six cases of trisomy 18. Of particular interest was their discovery of small dysplastic lesions with a similar appearance and location as nodular renal blastema in 8 of 46 kidneys containing clinically diagnosed nephroblastomas. Potter (1972) has summarized data from 15 cases of persistent blastema, which she views as "incipient Wilms' tumors." Our previously unpublished observations indicate that this phenomenon occurs even more frequently than the available literature would suggest. A systematic search of available renal sections from 2452 consecutive pediatric necropsies uncovered 12 examples, giving an incidence of 1 in 204 children. Among 1035 infants in this series who were under three months of age, the frequency was even greater. Nine had one or more nodules of persistent blastema—an incidence of 1 in 115 in young infants. It seems likely that a prospective study, with more comprehensive sampling of renal tissue, would yield an even higher figure.

In addition to the examples of persistent blastema found during the study of their incidence, we have encountered 11 specimens during the course of our routine review of pediatric necropsy and surgical material, giving a total of 23 personally studied examples of persistent blastema. Two were in nephrectomy specimens, the remainder being incidental necropsy findings. The blastematous foci were multifocal in 16 instances, of which 14 were probably and 12 definitely bilateral. Associated malformations were encountered in 15 infants, including 8 with genitourinary anomalies. A high incidence of associated malformations was also observed by Bove and associates, which is of interest since nephroblastoma shows a statistically significant association with certain malformations, including those of the genitourinary tract (Miller et al.). The multiplicity and bilaterality of these foci of persistent blastema are significant in view of the occurrence of multicentric and bilateral nephroblastomas.

Persistent blastema has a characteristic appearance and distribution, as illustrated in figures 20 through 24. It is almost invariably found at the periphery of the renal lobules, just beneath the renal capsule (figs. 20, 21), or in the centers of the columns of Bertin (fig. 20-C). Such foci may occur in the peripelvic region, because of the normal reflection of the cortex and renal capsule into the renal sinus (fig. 20-A). The blastematous foci are distinctly nodular, and are sharply demarcated from the adjacent

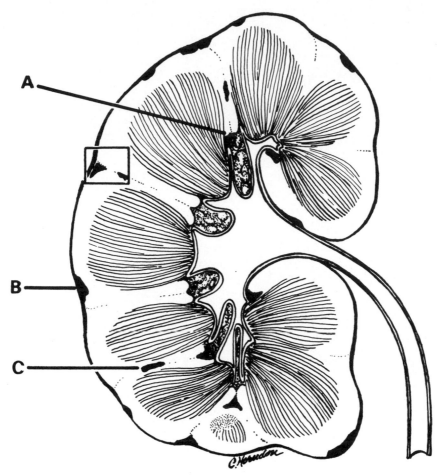

Figure 20
SITES OF PERSISTENT NEPHROGENIC BLASTEMA
This diagram illustrates the sites where persistent nephrogenic blastema is found. Usually it is located in the immediate subcapsular region (B), including that portion reflected into the renal sinus (A). However, the midportion of the columns of Bertin (C), representing the periphery of the embryonic renal lobe, additionally may contain blastematous nodules.

cortex. In serial sections, we have been unable to trace continuity of nephronic elements into the blastematous nodules. Occasionally, persistent blastema forms an almost continuous layer around the surface of the entire kidney (fig. 21), but in most cases it takes the form of scattered, minute foci which are easily overlooked. Varying degrees of epithelial differentiation occur within these islands (fig. 23), and rarely are sufficiently complete to justify the term adenoma (fig. 24). Stromal differentiation

into fibrous tissue is less commonly seen. With increasing age of the infant, there is a distinct tendency for the degree of differentiation to increase. All specimens in this series were from infants under the age of seven months.

Since the rate of occurrence of persistent blastema is far greater than expected if all were early nephroblastomas, it seems clear that most are destined for another fate, one of which is probably spontaneous disappearance. However, there is evidence

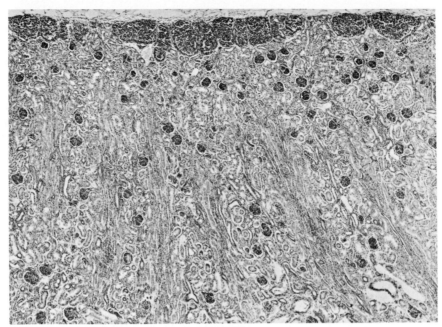

Figure 21
NODULES OF RENAL BLASTEMA
(Figures 21—23 from same case)
Multiple, partially confluent nodules of blastema were found beneath the renal capsule of a 3½ month old infant girl in whom the kidneys were grossly normal. X37.

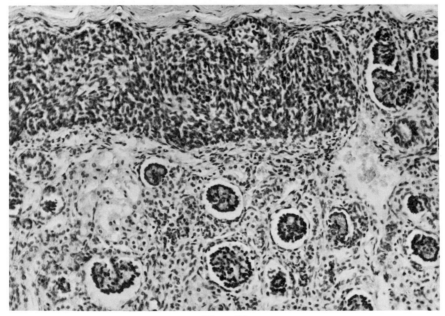

Figure 22
UNDIFFERENTIATED BLASTEMA
(Figures 21—23 from same case)
This nodule is composed of undifferentiated blastema and shows a characteristically sharp demarcation from the adjacent renal cortex. The kidneys were grossly normal in this 2 month old infant girl. X100.

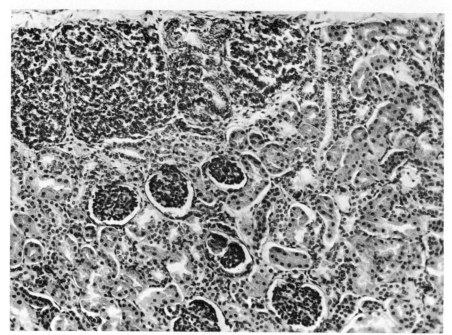

Figure 23
PERSISTENT BLASTEMA
(Figures 21—23 from same case)
Two adjacent nodules of persistent blastema are illustrated; the nodule on the right shows evidence of epithelial differentiation. X110.

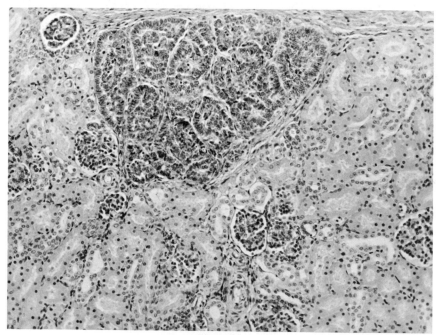

Figure 24
DIFFERENTIATED BLASTEMA
This microscopic nodule from a 4½ month old infant girl is similar in size and position to persistent blastema and shows nearly total epithelial differentiation. X110. (Courtesy of Dr. Benjamin H. Landing, Los Angeles, Calif.)

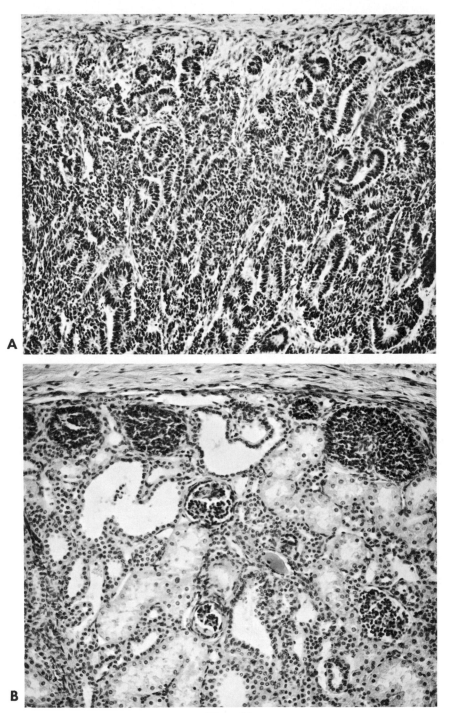

Figure 25
NEPHROBLASTOMA
A. This nephroblastoma, 6.5 cm. in diameter, was removed from the right kidney of a 4 month old infant girl. X100. B. Multiple subcapsular foci of persistent blastema are diffusely scattered over the surface of the kidney beyond the edges of the tumor. X110. (Courtesy of Dr. Nathan B. Friedman, Los Angeles, Calif.)

that these foci of persistent blastema are related to the pathogenesis of nephroblastoma. Bove and associates observed such foci in the kidneys of 17 percent of 46 cases of nephroblastoma, and one of us (JBB) has frequently observed this association (fig. 25). In the National Wilms' Tumor Study, 16 of the first 132 cases reviewed, for which sections of kidney were available (12 percent), contained separate foci of persistent blastema. Many examples of multicentric nephroblastoma have been reported in which numerous subcapsular tumors of varying size were distributed over the kidney surface (Bodian and Rigby; Hedrén; Miller et al.; Liban and Kozenitzky; Weigert). Rarely, the tumor takes the form of diffuse subcapsular growth, as illustrated by Allen and in figures 26 and 27. A variation on this theme is the phenomenon of bilateral **nephroblastomatosis** (Hou and Holman; Paul; Vlachos and Tsakraklides). In this condition, the kidneys are bilaterally and diffusely enlarged to several times their normal size, retaining original reniform contours. In some cases, persistent blastema is a prominent feature, while in others, the tissue is predominantly differentiated. Figure 28, from a previously reported case of the Beckwith-Wiedemann, or Exomphalos-Macroglossia-Gigantism (EMG) syndrome, illustrates a typical example of diffuse renal hyperplasia (Beckwith, 1969). This syndrome, in association with nephroblastoma, has been observed at least four times (Beckwith, 1969; Kelker et al.; Reddy et al.) and seems closely related to the syndrome of hemihypertrophy with visceral neoplasia (Fraumeni et al., 1967). It would be worthwhile to systematically search kidneys from cases of hemihypertrophy, sporadic aniridia, and other conditions associated with increased risk of nephroblastoma in order to determine the incidence of persistent blastema (see p. 33).

It is apparent that metanephric blastema may persist in visible form into the postnatal period, is frequently multicentric and bilateral, and occasionally may be diffusely distributed throughout the kidney. This phenomenon is frequently coexistent with nephroblastoma, and in all likelihood represents a major source for this tumor.

Cohnheim postulated that embryonal rests arose from accidental sequestration of undifferentiated cells during oncogenesis. Potter (1972) has proposed that persistent nephrogenic blastema in the human is the result of ampullary failure, a deficiency of organizer effect at the ends of branches of the ureteric buds. This view of persistent blastema as an error of metanephric differentiation is of interest, since there is a significant correlation of nephroblastomas with genitourinary malformations.

The postulate that abnormal persistence of blastema serves as the nidus for subsequent malignant transformation leaves unanswered the central question as to how such malignant activation might occur. There is evidence that genetic influences may play a role. Knudson and Strong present a strong argument for the pathogenesis of nephroblastoma being a two-mutational event (p. 49). They further note that their genetic data are equally consistent with vertical transmission of viral DNA. Other environmental stimuli acting on susceptible cells must be considered, especially in light of the experimental results to be presented. At the present time, in the human, there is no direct evidence bearing on this vital issue, with the possible exception of the demonstration by Smith and associates of a small virus in long term cultures of a human

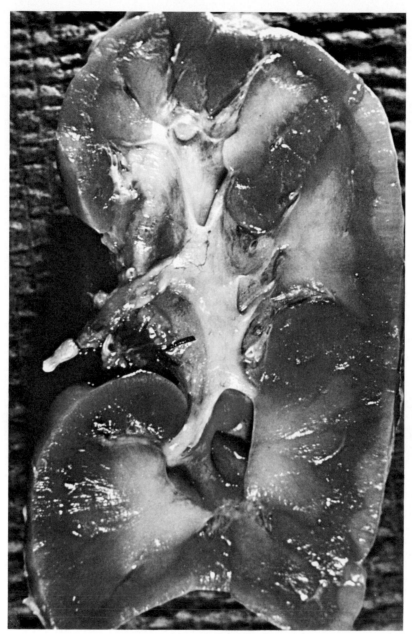

Figure 26
NEPHROBLASTOMA
(Figures 26 and 27 from same case)

This nephrectomy specimen shows diffuse subcapsular tumor formation identical in distribution to that of persistent blastema. An encapsulated nephroblastoma was shelled out of the defect in the lower pole. (Courtesy of Dr. Seth L. Haber, Santa Clara, Calif.)

nephroblastoma. The same workers, however, failed to find evidence of viruses in eight other specimens. Peller, on the basis of indirect evidence, implicated transplacental passage of oncogenic stimuli in the pathogenesis of several childhood tumors, including nephroblastoma.

Ultrastructural and histochemical studies have as yet afforded little additional insight into the pathogenesis of nephroblastoma, but have emphasized the similarities of this tumor to normal metanephric blastema (figs. 29, 30; Balsaver et al.; Imbert and Nezelof; Ito and Johnson; Tannenbaum; Tremblay).

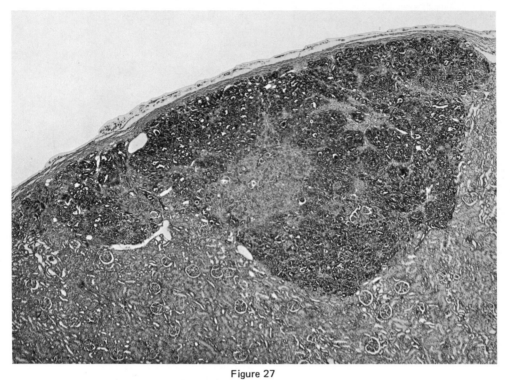

Figure 27
NEPHROBLASTOMA
(Figures 26 and 27 from same case)
This is a typical field from the subcapsular region of the same specimen as seen in figure 26. X31.
(Courtesy of Dr. Seth L. Haber, Santa Clara, Calif.)

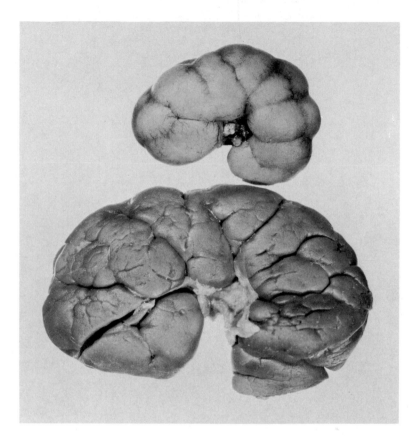

Figure 28
HYPERPLASTIC NEPHROMEGALY
Compare this hyperplastic nephromegaly from a newborn girl to the normal neonatal kidney (top). (Fig. 1 from Beckwith, J. B. Macroglossia, omphalocele, adrenal cytomegaly, gigantism, and hyperplastic visceromegaly. Birth Defects: Original Article Series 5:188-196, 1969.)

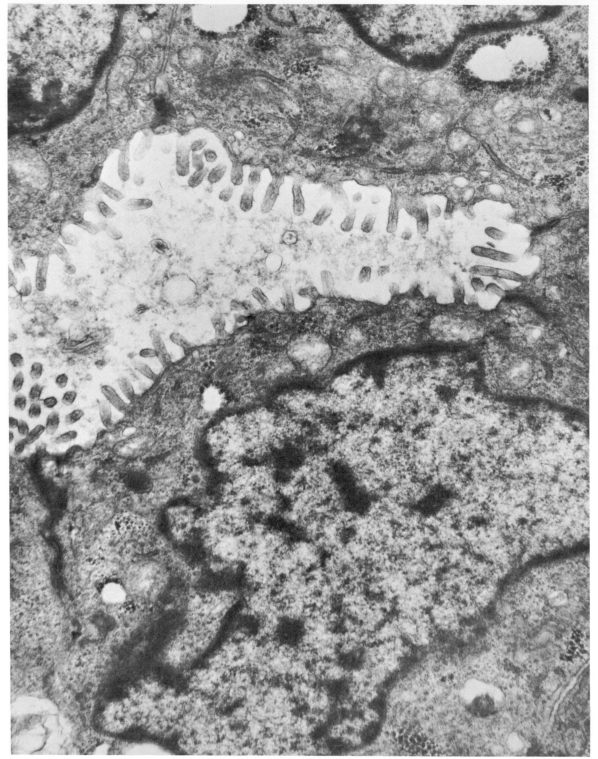

Figure 29
NEPHROBLASTOMA
An electron micrograph of differentiated nephroblastoma reveals epithelial cells with well developed microvilli. X18,000. (Courtesy of Dr. Warren W. Johnson, Memphis, Tenn.)

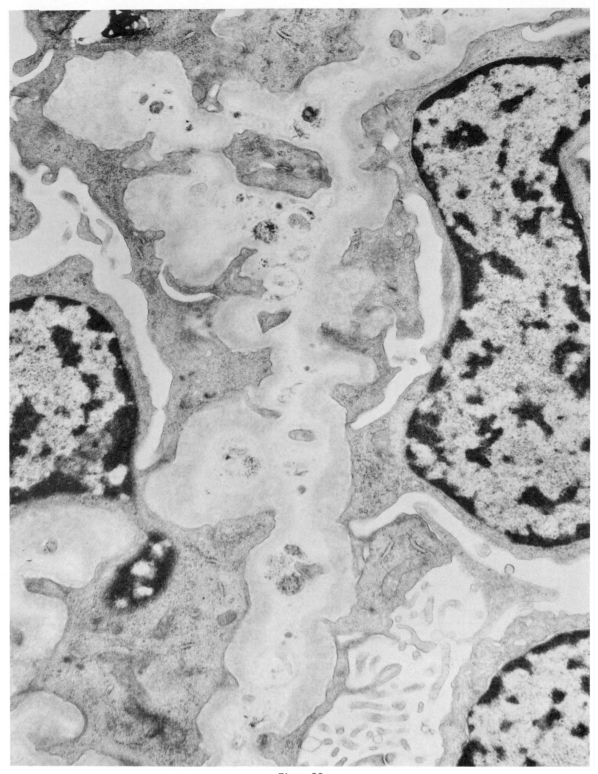

Figure 30
NEPHROBLASTOMA

A portion of pseudoglomerulus in a nephroblastoma shows a scalloped basement membrane near the center, lined on both sides by epithelial cells. X10,800. (Fig. 16 from Johnson, W. W. Ultrastructure of Wilms' tumor. 1. Epithelial cell. J. Natl. Cancer Inst. 42:77-99, 1969.)

Comparative Pathology

The literature on nephroblastomas in animals is confused by application of variable and often controversial criteria for the diagnosis. Some of the tumors reported in animal models to be discussed are supported by excellent and entirely acceptable descriptions and illustrations. Others, however, should be accepted with reservation until better descriptive material becomes available.

Spontaneous Nephroblastomas in Animals

Remarkable variations in the incidence of nephroblastoma occur within the animal kingdom, and often between closely related species. This tumor is fairly frequently encountered in the rabbit and occasionally in the rat, but is exceedingly rare in mice and Syrian hamsters, and apparently has never been reported in the guinea pig (Guerin et al.; Oberling; Hottendorf and Ingraham). Among domestic animals, we are aware of only a single reported nephroblastoma in a cat and several in dogs (Fitts; Coleman et al.). Farm animals are more frequently afflicted with this tumor, particularly the pig. Since Feldman's 1928 classic report of the pathologic appearances of these neoplasms in young pigs, a large number of reports have been published. It is now clear that nephroblastoma is the most frequently encountered malignant tumor of the pig. In a recent survey by Magaki and associates, 205 histologically confirmed nephroblastomas were encountered among 4,718,600 slaughtered swine. Of these, 93 came from six Iowa abbatoirs where 471,254 pigs were studied, an incidence of approximately 20 per 100,000. Ninety-three percent of specimens were obtained from swine under one year of age. Similar tumors have also been reported in

the horse, cow, and sheep (Nyka; Walker; Feldman, 1932, 1933).

Spontaneous nephroblastomas in chickens are reported rather frequently, but are rare in other avian species (Guerin et al.; Helmboldt and Jortner). We know of no acceptable reports in reptiles, but they have been reported in the South African toad *(Xenopus laavis)* and the fire-bellied newt *(Cynops pyrrhogaster)* (Elkan; Zwart). At least two specimens are known to have occurred in the fish mesonephros, the steelhead trout *(Salmo gairdneri),* and the striped bass *(Roccus saxatilis)* (Lucké and Schlumberger; Helmboldt and Wyand).

Experimentally Induced Nephroblastomas

Chemical Agents. Relatively few agents are known to produce nephroblastomas in contrast to the large number capable of inducing renal adenocarcinomas. Interpretation of the relevant literature is particularly difficult due to varied criteria used by different investigators for the diagnosis of nephroblastoma.

N-nitroso Compounds. Dimethylnitrosamine has frequently been reported as producing tumors with a mixed structure suggestive of nephroblastoma in the rat (Magee and Barnes; Riopelle and Jasmin, 1963). However, several recent investigations have indicated that these neoplasms are probably composed only of stromal elements, and that the epithelial components are atrophic or regenerating preexisting portions of nephrons (Hard and Butler; Riopelle and Jasmin, 1969). Tumors in rats produced by a closely related compound, nitroso-methyl urea, were studied in detail by Thomas and associates, who utilized electron microscopy, histochemistry, and autoradiographic technics to demonstrate that most, if not all tubular elements in the tumor were mature nephric elements. Occasionally, undifferentiated epithelial cells were found;

however, it was not possible to determine whether these were neoplastic or represented postinjury hyperplasia. Until more convincing evidence becomes available, it seems unwise to classify the tumors produced by N-nitroso compounds as nephroblastomas, and the term "stromal nephroma" is preferable (Riopelle and Jasmin, 1969).

Urethane. Vesselinovitch and Mihailovich reported nephroblastomas in newborn rats treated with urethane. Guerin and associates observed a single nephroblastoma in a rat treated with this agent at an unspecified age.

Cycasin. Nephroblastomas in the rat have been reported after subcutaneous injection of cycasin, a compound found in the nut of the plant *Cycas circanalis,* in the newborn animal, or after feeding the aglycone, methylazoxymethanol (Hirono et al.; Laqueur). The tumors thus induced have been transplanted successfully, often with retention of a mixed nature for many passages, but with a pronounced tendency toward rejection of grafts by recipients of opposite sex to the donor. Mugera, and Mugera and Nelerito fed flour from nuts of the palmlike plant, *Encephalartos hildebrandtii*, to rat weanlings and successfully induced nephroblastomas. The suspected oncogenic factor in this diet was cycasin.

Dimethylbenzanthracene. Jasmin and Riopelle administered 7, 12-dimethylbenzanthracene by gastric tube to young rats, with induction of nephroblastomas in 14 percent of ovariectomized animals, but none in intact animals. Their photomicrograph leaves no doubt that the resultant tumors are nephroblastomas.

It is probable that this list will be expanded when more experimental models are extended to fetal or neonatal animals, since age is a major determinant of susceptibility to induction of nephroblastomas in all cases studied to date.

Infectious Agents. Nephroblastomas are induced in young chickens with the BAI strain A avian myeloblastosis agent. Ishiguro and associates and Heine and coworkers described the morphogenesis of these tumors in detail in a classical series of papers. They observed that the position of early tumors in the kidney corresponded to that of persistent undifferentiated tissue, and concluded the latter was necessary for successful tumor induction.

The mesenchymal neoplasms of renal medullary or corticomedullary junction induced in newborn rats and hamsters exposed to polyoma virus are probably not true nephroblastomas (Ham et al.; Stanton and Otsuka). Grafts of embryonic kidney cells transformed by SV 40 or Adenovirus type 7 occasionally have been reported to produce nephroblastomas in appropriately treated rats and hamsters (Guerin et al.).

Physical Agents. A few nephroblastomas in rats have been reported following radiation (Berdjis; Maisin et al.). Guerin and associates observed a nephroblastoma in a hamster following urethane treatment associated with radiation, but the relative roles of the two treatment methods is unclear.

Transplantation of Nephrogenic Blastema. A promising model for experimental production of nephroblastomas is that of transplanting metanephric blastema removed from 12 to 15-day mouse fetuses into testes of adult mice of the same strain (Javadpour and Bush). Sixty-seven and a half percent of such transplants resulted in neoplasms, some resembling renal carcinoma and others nephroblastoma. Induction of both tumor types was prevented by actinomycin D or vincristine treatment. However, a more recent study has suggested that the transplant produces only a temporary delay in maturation of the metanephric blastema, rather than true neoplasms (Mount et al.).

Relation to Congenital Mesoblastic Nephroma

In 1967, Bolande and associates delineated an apparently specific clinicopathologic entity which they called congenital mesoblastic nephroma of infancy. The distinctive characteristics of these tumors are: (1) Occurrence usually during the first few months of life; (2) characteristic histologic appearances; and (3) usually benign clinical behavior. The mesoblastic nephroma is composed primarily of spindle cells resembling fibroblasts, smooth muscle cells, or both. Other elements may be present within these tumors, including cartilage, skeletal muscle, hematopoietic cells, and vascular elements. Abnormal epithelial cells may also be present, but usually it is impossible to prove that these are part of the tumor instead of entrapped nephrons. A distinctive feature of these lesions is their interface with adjacent tissue structures, which is usually irregular and characterized by interdigitations of tumor with normal renal parenchyma. The appearance is that of diffuse growth within the kidney rather than the usual expansile, locally compressive type of growth. Extension through the renal capsule may occur; however, complete excision appears to be adequate therapy. All these tumors cannot be regarded as benign because in one instance the tumor extended to one margin of resection and later there was a massive recurrence (Fu and Kay). Bolande's view is that these tumors are a cytodifferentiated variant of nephroblastoma, a view supported by tissue culture observations from

such tumors (Bolande; Crocker and Vernier). Large regions resembling congenital mesoblastic nephroma may be seen in otherwise typical nephroblastomas, suggesting that some nephroblastomas might have arisen in lesions that previously were congenital mesoblastic nephromas (Bolande; Beckwith).

Other workers take issue with the above concept, and view this type of lesion as being entirely unrelated to nephroblastoma. Terms such as fetal renal hamartoma, leiomyomatous hamartoma, and fibroma reflect the various concepts of the nature of this tumor (Wigger; Bogdan et al.; Hamanaka et al.). It is impossible at the present time to resolve this issue, which is largely nosologic rather than representing widely divergent histogenetic concepts.

It has been observed that at the outset of nephrogenesis the metanephric blastema is predominantly stromagenic in activity (Potter, 1972). It seems possible that congenital mesoblastic nephroma represents the result of neoplastic induction in the embryonic metanephros during this stage of development, with subsequent growth of tumor and kidney occurring together but at differing rates. This suggestion is consistent with the predominantly stromal composition of these tumors, their almost invariably antenatal onset (Bolande), the relatively diffuse growth pattern within the kidney (Bolande; Garcia-Bunuel and Brandes), and with our observation that this type of tumor is often found in the medullary region of the kidney where early stromagenic activity is most pronounced.

Epidemiology

Age
Nephroblastomas have been encountered in fetuses and in the aged, although

some reported cases in adults are undoubtedly anaplastic renal adenocarcinoma (Klapproth). Despite this wide age distribution, it is clear that nephroblastoma is characteristically a tumor of young children. In the Alameda County, California Cancer Registry records for the years 1960–1969, the age adjusted incidence rate was about 0.2 in males and females. The age at diagnosis of 210 cases of histologically confirmed nephroblastoma, excluding mesoblastic nephroma, diagnosed since 1968 and followed by the National Wilms' Tumor Study is presented in Graph IV. These data have the advantages of reflecting contemporary conditions of health care delivery and diagnostic

methods. The diagnoses of these tumors have been confirmed histologically by one of the authors (JBB). The peak incidence of nephroblastoma occurs during the second year of life, with 50 percent of cases diagnosed before the third birthday, and 75 percent before the age of five years. As was noted in a recent series of 335 nephroblastomas, when cases are grouped into those diagnosed under two years, from two to four years, and over four years, the number of patients in each group will be approximately equal (Ledlie et al.). Preliminary data from the National Wilms' Tumor Study (Table IV) suggest that nephroblastomas diagnosed in older children tend to be more advanced, and thus may have

GRAPH IV

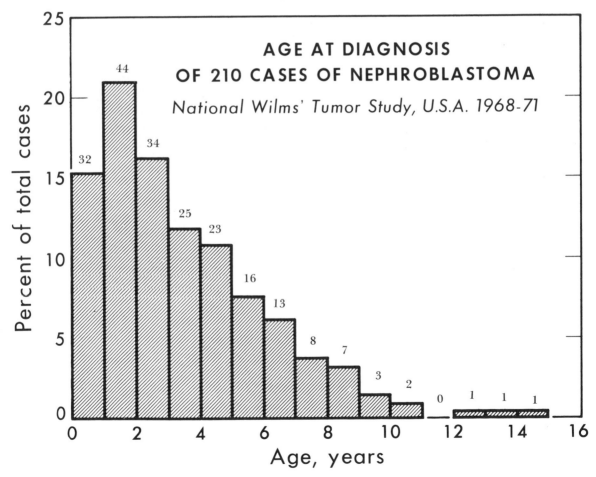

been present for a relatively longer period of time prior to diagnosis than those occurring at a younger age.

Cochran and Froggatt first noted that bilateral and familial nephroblastomas occur at a younger age than nephroblastomas in general. This finding was recently confirmed by Knudson and Strong, and extended to include nephroblastomas associated with aniridia, but not hemihypertrophy, suggesting that there are epidemiologic subgroups among patients with nephroblastoma with different ages of onset and differing pathogenic mechanisms.

Table IV

AGE AT DIAGNOSIS OF 177 CASES OF NEPHROBLASTOMA, RELATED TO EXTENT OF CLINICAL DISEASE

Clinical Group	Mean Age (Months)	Number of Cases
I	28	65
II, III	38	80
IV	68	32

Group I: Tumor limited to kidney.
Groups II, III: Tumor extends beyond kidney but limited to abdomen. No hematogenous metastases.
Group IV: Hematogenous metastases.

From D'Angio, G. J., Beckwith, J. B., Bishop, H. C., Breslow, N., Evans, A. E., Goodwin, W. E., King, L. R., Pickett, L. K., Sinks, L. F., Sutow, W. W., and Wolff, J. A. Childhood Cancer. The National Wilms' Tumor Study: A Progress Report, pp. 627-636. In: Proceedings of the VII National Cancer Conference. Philadelphia: J. B. Lippincott Company, 1972.

Sex

Nephroblastoma occurs with equal frequency in males and females. Among 215 patients with nephroblastoma in the National Wilms' Tumor Study for which data are presently available, 110 were female and 105, male. In the 317 cases recorded in the California Tumor Registry 1942–1969, 163 were males and 154, females (Table II), and in another large study of 440 cases by Miller and associates, there were 223 males and 217 females. The only large series of nephroblastomas in which the sex ratio was not equal is that reported for 335 cases, with a male to female ratio of 1.2 to 1 (Ledlie et al.).

It is interesting to note that in a series of cases of hemihypertrophy with associated Wilms' tumor, there was a marked preponderance of females: 24 females and only nine males (Knudson and Strong).

Geographic and Racial Distribution

Nephroblastomas occur with about the same frequency in all countries for which adequate data are available, although there are minor variations between regions (Davies). A recent monograph on cancer incidence in five continents disclosed no areas with a particularly high rate of occurrence (Doll et al.). In a registry of malignant tumors of children in Louisiana, 37 of 289 malignant tumors in Black children were nephroblastomas while in the same region there were only 12 nephroblastomas among 238 malignant tumors in White children (Davies). The racial background of 185 children with nephroblastoma recorded in the National Wilms' Tumor Study at present is: 161 White, 20 Black, 3 Mexican, and 1 Japanese. Virag and Modan noted an incidence of 0.7 nephroblastomas per 100,000 Israeli Jews and 1.7 per 100,000 among Israeli Arabs. The relative frequency of nephroblastoma among Whites, Blacks, American Indians, Chinese, and Japanese recorded in the California Tumor Registry from 1942–1969 is shown in Table II.

Despite minor variations in the frequency of nephroblastoma in different racial groups, there is no evidence at present to suggest that racial or geographic factors exert important influences in its occurrence. Indeed, it has been suggested that, since the incidence in all areas studied is so nearly the same, nephroblastoma should be considered an index tumor in geographic studies of other childhood tumors (Innis).

Heredity

A recent review of familial nephroblastomas included 25 families in which more than one nephroblastoma has been confirmed and 19 families in which two or more siblings were affected (Knudson and Strong). In several families, the genetic history suggests an autosomal dominant mode of inheritance. The genetics of nephroblastoma are rendered even more complex by the possibility that one may inherit a predisposition toward nephroblastoma without developing overt tumors. This possibility is suggested by the fact that nodular masses of nephrogenic blastema histologically identical to nephroblastoma are occasionally found incidentally in autopsy material (figs. 21–24) and are not infrequently encountered in association with nephroblastomas (figs. 25–27; Bove et al.). It is our experience (Beckwith and Perrin) that the nodular masses of nephrogenic blastema occur in about one percent of infant postmortems, which is approximately 100 times the expected incidence of nephroblastoma based on the estimate that a nephroblastoma develops in approximately one per 10,000 live births (Cochran and Froggatt).

Evidence that a propensity for retained nephrogenic blastema may be inherited, rests on observations made in one family, when the first offspring, who died at two days, was found to have multiple nephrogenic rests in his normal-sized kidneys (Liban and Kozenitzky). A stillborn sibling born three years later had bilaterally enlarged kidneys with widespread masses of nodular renal blastema, a condition referred to by the authors as nephroblastomatosis.

We do not know whether nephrogenic rests are precursors of nephroblastoma or merely associated with this tumor. If there is a genetic influence, as these cases suggest, it may operate to predispose to the development of the rests as well as nephroblastoma or to the development of nephrogenic rests, and subsequently influence transformation to nephroblastoma. Cochran and Froggatt observed that instances of familial nephroblastoma and bilateral nephroblastoma tend to occur at an earlier age than sporadic unilateral disease. This has been recently confirmed by Knudson and Strong who used these observations to develop an ingenious mathematical model which supports the hypothesis that nephroblastomas are the result of two separate mutational events.

According to this hypothesis, the first mutation may be prezygotic or postzygotic and the second mutation is always postzygotic. If the first mutation is prezygotic, the resulting tumor is hereditary; if the first mutation is postzygotic, then the tumor is nonhereditary. The two-event mutation model predicts that a fraction of nephroblastomas are hereditary (38 percent), occur at an early age, and may be bilateral, while the remaining fraction (62 percent) are nonhereditary, occur at a later age, and are unilateral; among carriers of the prezygotic mutation, 37 percent will not develop nephroblastoma while 63 percent will develop nephroblastoma with a ratio of unilateral to bilateral tumors of 3 to 1 (Knudson and Strong). The association of nephroblastoma with aniridia, hemihypertrophy, and genitourinary abnormalities is consistent with the model.

In view of the currently high cure rates

for both unilateral and bilateral nephroblastoma, verification of this hypothesis may be possible, although a large percentage of cured individuals may be rendered infertile by tumor therapy.

It is intriguing to speculate that persistence of nephrogenic rests may be a manifestation of a prezygotic mutation, and that transformation to nephroblastoma represents the second event in the two-step process.

Gestational Factors

The characteristic early onset of nephroblastoma suggests that gestational influences play a role in the pathogenesis of this tumor. However, the largest study to date does not support this theory. MacMahon and Newill, in a study of birth characteristics including maternal age, birth order, history of previous stillbirths, twinning, and birth weight, found no statistically significant relation to the likelihood of developing nephroblastoma. This study, based on death certificates, was limited to lethal nephroblastomas and, therefore, contains an inherent bias. Since nephroblastomas in the young infant have a higher cure rate than those diagnosed in older children, a study of lethal nephroblastomas is likely to include more tumors arising in older children and would be less likely to reveal gestational influences which one would expect to be operational in tumors of the very young.

In five categories of childhood malignant tumors, MacMahon and Newill observed that the proportion of infants with a birth weight over 8½ pounds (18.8 percent) was greater in those infants with nephroblastoma, and Irving reported in her series that there was a tendency for higher than average birth weight in infants with nephroblastoma.

Maternal radiation has not been related to an increased risk of nephroblastoma. Although the reason is not apparent, neonatal nephroblastomas are associated with a statistically significant increase in maternal hydramnios (Favara et al.). Peller has postulated on theoretical grounds that transplacental carcinogens might be implicated in the genesis of nephroblastoma.

Association with Other Conditions

Nephroblastoma is a part of several syndromic malformations. Following the initial discovery of a high incidence of **sporadic aniridia** among a series of patients with nephroblastoma (Miller et al.; Fraumeni and Glass), an additional 30 cases have come to light (Knudson and Strong). The risk of development of nephroblastoma in a child with sporadic aniridia is approximately 33 percent (Fraumeni and Glass). Other abnormalities associated with nephroblastoma include microcephaly, developmental retardation, malformed ears, genitourinary anomalies, and recently reported lumbosacral spina bifida, with lipoma and meningocele (Haicken and Miller). When nephroblastomas occur in a child with aniridia, the tumor is almost always diagnosed before three years of age and appears to have a particularly unfavorable prognosis (Knudson and Strong). Partial deletion of the short arm of chromosome 18 was detected in a recent case of aniridia with nephroblastoma, using computer analysis of chromosome banding preparations (Ladda et al.) Further investigation of this finding is important.

Another condition associated with nephroblastoma is **hemihypertrophy** in which the asymmetry may involve a portion, or an entire side of the body, or may be crossed, with portions of each side of the body involved (fig. 31; Fraumeni et al.,

1967). There is no association between laterality of the tumor and the side of the body involved by hemihypertrophy. There are more instances of nephroblastoma and hemihypertrophy among females than males (Knudson and Strong). The reasons for this disparity are not known. The age at diagnosis is no different for patients with nephroblastoma and hemihypertrophy than for patients with nephroblastomas in general. Adrenal adenocarcinoma and hepatoblastomas are also associated with hemihypertrophy. Meadows and associates have recently reported the case of three infants with nephroblastoma, born to a mother with congenital hemihypertrophy.

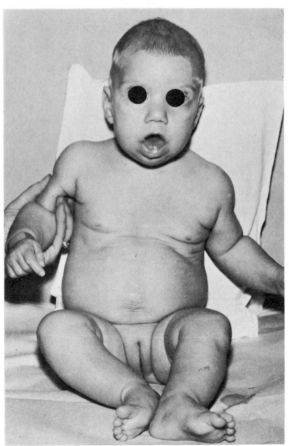

Figure 31

The syndrome of macroglossia, omphalocele, gigantism, adrenal cytomegaly, and visceromegaly (E.M.G. or Beckwith-Wiedemann syndrome) is closely related to the hemihypertrophy-visceral neoplasia syndrome, and has been associated with nephroblastoma in four known instances (Beckwith, 1969; Filippi and McKusick; Irving; Kelker et al.; Reddy et al.). This association is of particular interest because of the florid proliferation of nephrogenic blastema that sometimes occurs as part of this entity (Beckwith, 1969). The relationship of nephrogenic blastema to the genesis of nephroblastoma is discussed further on page 38.

Recently, another association has emerged between nephroblastoma and **pseudohermaphroditism with glomerulonephritis and nephrotic syndrome** (Drash et al.; Denys et al.; Spear et al.). Among the four reported cases, two nephroblastomas were discovered as incidental postmortem findings; three patients had normal karyotypes, while one had an XX/XY mosaic pattern. To date, this condition has not been recognized as being familial, but there is one report of nephrotic syndrome with nephroblastoma in siblings (Zunin and Soave). There have been two isolated instances of nephroblastoma and nephrotic syndrome (Lines; Smith) and three reports of nephroblastoma in infants with intersex anomalies (Angström; Raubitschek; Stump and Garrett).

Figure 31
INFANT WITH BECKWITH'S SYNDROME
This 6 month old infant with Beckwith's syndrome had a large tongue, gigantism, an umbilical scar from repair of an omphalocele, and evidence of obesity. (Fig. 7 from Beckwith, J. B. Macroglossia, omphalocele, adrenal cytomegaly, gigantism, and hyperplastic visceromegaly. Birth Defects: Original Article Series 5:188-196, 1969.)

A relationship between nephroblastoma and **hamartomas, renal anomalies, cryptorchidism,** and **hypospadias** is less certain. Each of these lesions occurred with a frequency greater than that expected on the basis of chance in a study of associated malformations in a large collection of nephroblastomas (Miller et al.). Renal anomalies, in particular, associated with nephroblastoma have been the subject of many case reports and reviews. Such renal anomalies include horseshoe kidney, unilateral agenesis, renal dysplasia, duplication anomalies, and ectopia. However, a recent review of a large series of childhood tumors disclosed no significant relationship of urinary anomalies to nephroblastoma (Berry et al.). While hamartomas, renal anomalies, cryptorchidism, and hypospadias may possibly be associated with an increased frequency of nephroblastoma, the association is at best weak and has not yet been shown to be statistically significant.

Chromosomal Disorders

Chromosomal disorders are infrequently reported with nephroblastoma. One case with trisomy 18 has been mentioned twice in the literature (Mingazzini; Geiser and Schindler). This disorder is of interest because of the apparently high frequency of associated nephrogenic rests (Beckwith and Perrin; Bove et al.). It is likely that early death of most infants with trisomy 18 masks a significant association with nephroblastoma.

Clinical Pathologic Features

CLINICAL FEATURES. The presenting symptoms of nephroblastoma usually occur after the lesion has reached considerable size. An abdominal mass is the primary presenting sign in over 90 percent of cases

(Snyder et al.). Other frequent abnormalities apparent at the time of clinical presentation are hypertension, 0—60 percent; abdominal pain, 20—30 percent; anorexia, nausea, and vomiting, 15 percent; fever, 10—20 percent; and constipation and gross hematuria, 5—10 percent. Occasionally, venous obstruction can produce leg edema or sudden appearance of a varicocele. Metastatic disease is present in about 25 percent of cases at the time of diagnosis, and may produce symptoms referable to the site of metastases.

The preoperative investigation of children with abdominal masses is primarily radiographic (Cope et al.). Plain abdominal radiographs are of limited value in the differential diagnosis, demonstrating opacification in the retroperitoneum and frequent displacement of organs by the mass (Cope et al.). Calcification is uncommon in nephroblastomas, occurring in fewer than 5 percent of cases, although in one series of 49 cases, calcification was visible in six (14 percent) (Perez et al.). This is in distinct contrast to neuroblastomas, which often demonstrate finely stippled calcification. Intravenous pyelography is of great value in the differential diagnosis, although in a small proportion of cases, even with increased dosage of contrast material, the kidney is nonfunctioning. Distortion and displacement of the caliceal system is usually apparent, and discrimination from extrarenal masses or from hydronephrosis is usually facilitated (fig. 32). Especially with lesions of the renal poles, however, there may be difficulty in distinguishing the lesion from a perirenal neoplasm. Excretory pyelography should be included as a routine part of the preoperative investigation, since it will establish the functional and anatomic integrity of the opposite kidney. The frequent association of

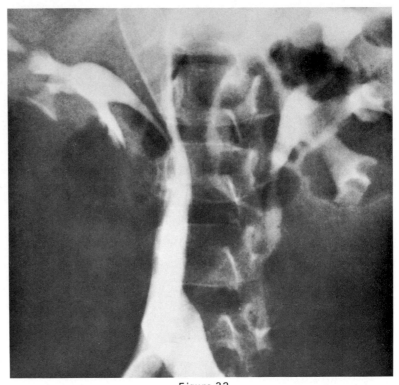

Figure 32
NEPHROBLASTOMA
(Figures 32 and 33 from same case)
A combined intravenous pyelogram and inferior vena cavagram of a 4 year old girl shows a large lower pole mass in the right kidney, compressing and deforming the calices, ureter, and vena cava. (Courtesy of Dr. Howard Ricketts, St. Louis, Mo.)

Figure 32

nephroblastoma with renal malformations, plus the occurrence of bilateral nephroblastomas, makes this point vitally important. Retrograde pyelography is technically difficult and carries the potential for rupturing the tumor (Snyder et al.).

A number of recent articles have emphasized the value of selective renal arteriography as an adjunct to the diagnosis of renal neoplasms (Clark et al.; Cremin and Kaschula; Hidai et al.). In addition to permitting visualization of tumors in pyelographically nonfunctional kidneys, arteriography can increase the preoperative detection of bilateral tumors, and is helpful in following the response to therapy when initial nephrectomy is not performed. Characteristically, the arteriogram shows poor vascularity, without the vascular pooling, tumor stains, and arteriovenous shunting usually seen in renal adeno-

carcinoma. Despite poor vascularity, nearly all cases will have some neoformation of vessels, having a fine wavy or zigzag pattern in contrast to the appearances in hydronephrosis (fig. 33).

The usefulness of scanning with a variety of isotopes has been demonstrated (Samuels), especially in the preoperative detection of hepatic metastases, and in the discrimination of left renal tumors from splenomegaly. Ultrasonic tomography, retroperitoneal pneumography, and nephrotomography are also of potential value (Hünig; Emmett).

Several ancillary laboratory methods may be useful in the diagnosis and management of nephroblastoma. Perhaps the most promising of these is the determination of erythropoietin levels in urine and plasma. In a series of 12 patients with nephroblastoma, 11 had elevated levels, all but

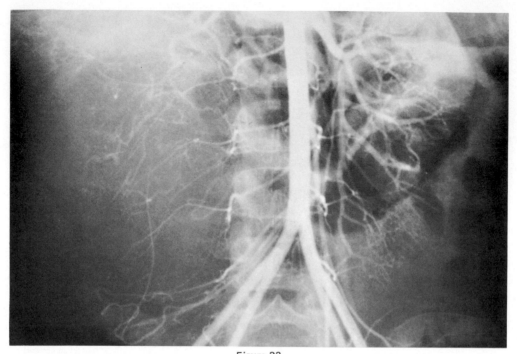

Figure 33
NEPHROBLASTOMA
(Figures 32 and 33 from same case)

This aortogram with renal arteriogram reveals typical tortuous vessels of a tumor. Nephroblastomas characteristically are much less vascular than renal carcinomas, and thus are usually readily distinguished by arteriography. (Courtesy of Dr. Howard Ricketts, St. Louis, Mo.)

one dropping to normal after nephrectomy (Murphy et al., 1972). During subsequent follow-up, there is an apparently excellent correlation of erythropoietin levels with the presence of recurrent or persistent tumor. Polycythemia is virtually never seen with nephroblastoma, and was not seen in any of 37 patients in whom erythropoietin levels were increased (Murphy et al.,1972).

It is possible that some instances of hypertension seen in patients with nephroblastoma are due to renal radiation; however, hypertension is a well documented presenting sign in some cases of nephroblastoma. Ganguly and associates recently reported that hypertension in nephroblastoma is associated with increased renin levels in plasma and tumor, but not in adjacent renal cortex. Bowie stains of the tumor, which was of typical mixed histologic appearance, were negative. Subsequent study of this patient revealed that the circulating substance was a high molecular weight structure, apparently a polypeptide prohormone activated by acidification and warming to 32 degrees centigrade (Day and Luetscher). Powars and his coworkers described a mucin-like substance in smears of blood, bone marrow, and direct tumor imprints of three children with nephroblastoma. This material is precipitated in granular form and clearly visible with Wright's stain (fig. 34), periodic acid-Schiff stain, or methods for acid mucopolysaccharide, and decreased markedly by hyaluronidase. Further work is needed to establish the value of this material as an aid to diagnosis and management. Serum acid phosphatase may be increased and one child exhibited marked parahydroxyphenyllactic aciduria, but ascorbic acid deficiency was not ruled out as a possible cause for the defect in tyrosine metabolism (Kumar and Gupta; Greer et al.). Ectopic hormone secretion by nephroblastoma is apparently rare, although at least one instance of an ACTH producing tumor has been reported (Cummins and Cohen).

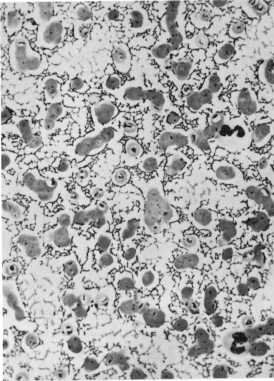

Figure 34
NEPHROBLASTOMA
This peripheral blood smear from a patient with nephroblastoma shows characteristic precipitate. The larger globular pale staining structures are erythrocytes; two neutrophilic leukocytes are included. Wright-Giemsa stain. (Fig. 3 from Powars, D. R., Allerton, S. E., Beierle, J., and Butler, B. B. Wilms' tumor clinical correlation with circulating mucin in three cases. Cancer 29:1597-1605, 1972.)

Exfoliative cytologic examination is of potential value in detection of metastatic disease, because malignant cells are frequently seen in pleural or peritoneal effusions associated with metastatic nephroblastoma. Only rarely, however, are they found in the urine (Hajdu).

Needle biopsy is rarely indicated and has obvious hazards, but occasionally will be deemed necessary when extensive metastases are present and the patient's condition does not permit laparotomy (Snyder et al.).

GROSS FEATURES. Unilateral nephroblastomas show no marked predilection for either kidney, although many series show a slight preponderance of left renal nephroblastomas; 55 percent of unilateral nephroblastomas entered on the National Wilms' Tumor Study to date were left-sided. Extrarenal nephroblastomas were extremely rare (fig. 35) and it is generally presumed that they arise from displaced remnants of metanephric blastema or from extrusion of tumor arising at the surface of the kidney (Bhajekar et al.; Thompson et al.). However, this explanation would not readily account for a nephroblastoma possibly arising in the mediastinum (Moyson et al.). The reported incidence of bilateral primary tumors varies considerably. Among the first 484 nephroblastomas entered on the National Wilms' Tumor Study, 27 (5.8 percent) were bilateral at the time of original diagnosis. This is probably the most accurate estimate available. On occasion, multifocal involvement of a kidney is seen, either in the form of multiple nodules of varying size, or as a diffuse subcapsular neoplastic "cap" (figs. 26, 27, 36).

Most nephroblastomas, because of their remote position within the abdomen, attain relatively large size before being detected. Among 258 nephroblastomas randomly chosen or followed on the National Wilms' Tumor Study between November, 1969

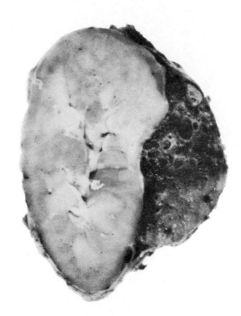

Figure 35
EXTRARENAL NEPHROBLASTOMA
This illustrates an extrarenal nephroblastoma located completely outside the kidney and separated from the renal cortex by a thickened renal capsule. (Fig. 138 from Bodian, M., and Rigby, E. The Pathology of Nephroblastoma. In: Monographs on Neoplastic Disease at Various Sites, Vol. V. Tumours of the Kidney and Ureter. (Ed.) Riches, E. W. Baltimore: Williams & Wilkins Co.; London: E. & S. Livingstone, Ltd., 1964.)

Figure 35

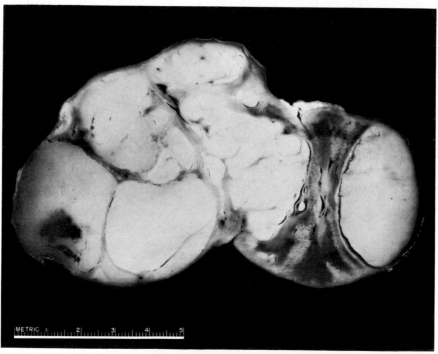

Figure 36
MULTICENTRIC NEPHROBLASTOMA
Multiple separate tumor nodules were present in a 2 year old boy, in addition to numerous foci of persistent nodular blastema at the cortical surface. There was no evidence of tumor in the opposite kidney after an 8-year follow-up.

and June, 1973, the median tumor diameter was 12 cm., and the median weight of tumor and kidney was 540 gm. Because the tumors are usually large and the child's kidney is relatively small, the latter is typically a compressed shell around the tumor, and it is rarely possible to determine whether the tumor arose from the cortex or medulla. Our experience with small and multicentric tumors, however, indicates that they are probably cortical in origin. A pseudocapsule composed of compressed renal tissue, renal capsule, and adjacent perirenal tissue is usually a prominent feature, although tumor often penetrates to the surface of this pseudocapsule (figs. 37,

38). On section, the typical nephroblastoma is soft, gray or tan, and bulges markedly above the cut surface of the kidney (fig. 39), and it is apparent why many early accounts referred to them as "encephaloid tumors." The pale color contrasts with the usually red to purple of neuroblastomas. Instead of the usual uniform gray to tan, soft, uniform appearance, one may encounter a variegated pattern due to focal hemorrhage or necrosis. However, this is less frequently seen than in neuroblastomas. Some tumors with considerable stromal differentiation may have a tougher texture, and hemorrhage or necrosis may alter the appearance. Occa-

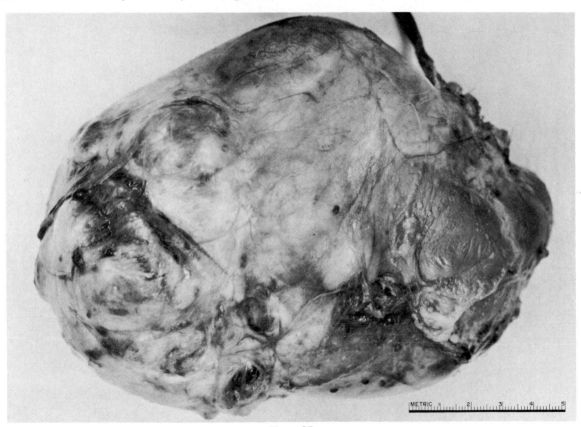

Figure 37
NEPHROBLASTOMA
A typical tumor capsule is seen in this external view of a nephroblastoma.

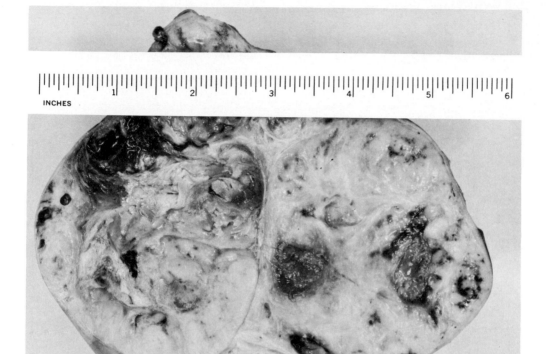

Figure 38
NEPHROBLASTOMA

Two large confluent lobules of tumor might indicate a multicentric origin, although this is equivocal. Note the formation of a tumor capsule by attenuated kidney tissue. Focal hemorrhage and necrosis are apparent.

Figure 39
NEPHROBLASTOMA

On section, this relatively small tumor shows the pale, bulging appearance that is typical of most nephroblastomas. (Courtesy of the Armed Forces Institute of Pathology, Washington, D. C.)

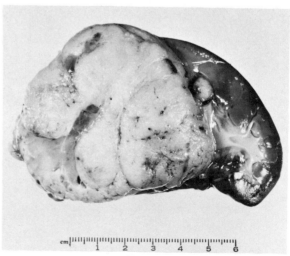

Figure 39

sionally, marked cystic change within the tumor may lead to misinterpretation as a polycystic kidney (fig. 40). Calcification is quite uncommon, occurring in from 3 to 14 percent in various reports (Marsden and Steward; Perez et al.).

The junction between tumor and kidney is usually sharp, with compressed renal tissue forming a pseudocapsule. However, infiltrative margins are often grossly apparent. The pelvis is compressed and attenuated, and may be infiltrated by tumor. Occasionally, metastatic foci of tumor are present in the ureter and even the urinary bladder (Taykurt). Local spread into the perirenal soft tissue, the renal vein, and hilar nodes is frequent, and significantly

alters the prognosis, so these sites require careful examination both grossly and microscopically.

Based upon the degree of gross extension of the tumor, the National Wilms' Tumor Study has proposed the following clinical and pathologic grouping of patients, based upon their status at the time of diagnosis.

Group I: Tumor limited to kidney and completely resected

Group II: Tumor extends beyond kidney but apparently completely resected

Group III: Tumor extends beyond kidney; gross tumor remains in abdomen

Group IV: Hematogenous metastases present

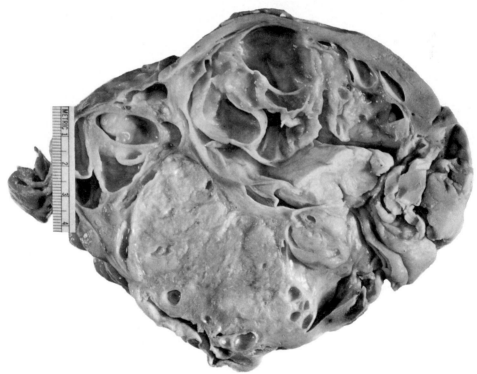

Figure 40
NEPHROBLASTOMA
This tumor, which contains many large cysts, may be confused at operation with polycystic kidneys. A narrow rim of renal tissue is identifiable near the top of the photograph. (Fig. 74 from Lucké, B., and Schlumberger, H. G. Tumors of the Kidney, Renal Pelvis and Ureter. Fascicle 30, Atlas of Tumor Pathology, First Series. Washington: Armed Forces Institute of Pathology, 1957.)

HISTOPATHOLOGIC FEATURES. The microscopic appearances of nephroblastoma are protean. Typically, there is an admixture of three components—epithelial, stromal, and blastematous (figs. 41, 42), although any one of these may be predominant. Gradual transitions of blastemal regions into both epithelial and stromal tissues are often observed. The blastemal elements are composed of closely packed, slightly ovoid cells with scanty cytoplasm (fig. 43), and when these predominate, differentiation of nephroblastoma from other small cell tumors of childhood may be difficult. Usually, however, the blastemal elements are subdivided by stromal

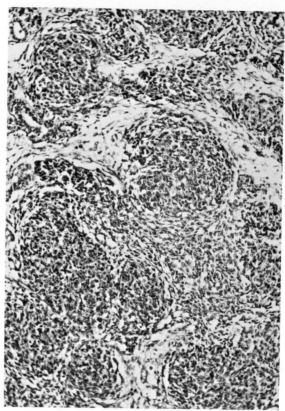

Figure 42
NEPHROBLASTOMA
This higher magnification of a nephroblastoma shows blastema separated by narrow stromal septa and slight tubular differentiation. X100.

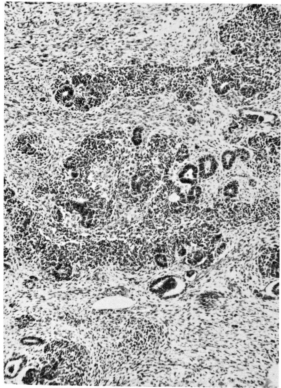

Figure 41
NEPHROBLASTOMA
This illustrates the typical mixed appearance of a nephroblastoma. Islands of blastema are shown as closely packed, small, darkly stained cells, as well as epithelial structures and a spindle cell stroma. X70.

tissues into circumscribed nodules, or into a trabecular pattern (fig. 44). Within the blastematous nodules, tubular formation is often discernible. This is usually randomly distributed within the blastematous trabeculae, being central, eccentric, or marginal. Occasionally, however, a tumor will present relatively consistent orientation of epithelial differentiation around the periphery of the blastema, as shown in figure 45. The appearance of the blastematous foci may be altered by several changes. One, which we have observed only rarely, and have not seen mentioned in the literature, is an apparently degenerative change, characterized by enlarged cells, usually within the

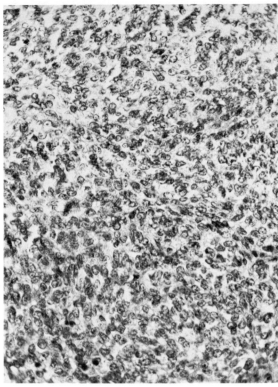

Figure 43
NEPHROBLASTOMA
When this pattern of blastema is predominant, it may cause confusion with other small cell tumors of childhood. X265.

Figure 43

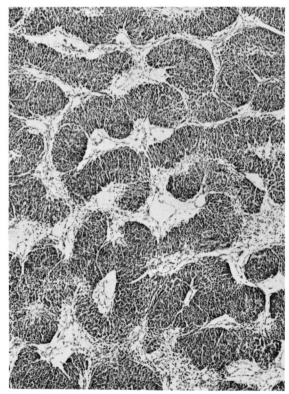

Figure 44

Figure 44
NEPHROBLASTOMA
This trabecular arrangement of blastema shows well differentiated stromal septa, but no epithelial elements. X42.

central regions of blastematous islands, having an abundance of granular, acidophilic cytoplasm. This "oncocytoid" change is illustrated in plate I-A. Another uncommon pattern is produced by the appearance within blastematous nodules of thin-walled cysts mimicking dilated lymphatics (fig. 46). On occasion, a papilliferous formation of blastema within larger cystic spaces is presented (fig. 47).

Figure 45
NEPHROBLASTOMA
Epithelial formation is more prevalent at the periphery of blastemic zones in this specimen. Sometimes tubules are predominantly central, but more often they are randomly oriented. X50.

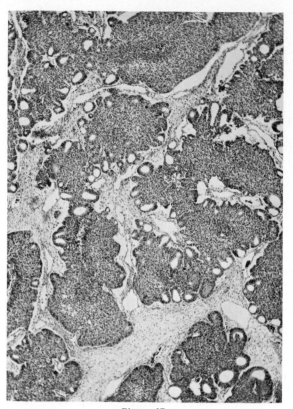

Figure 45

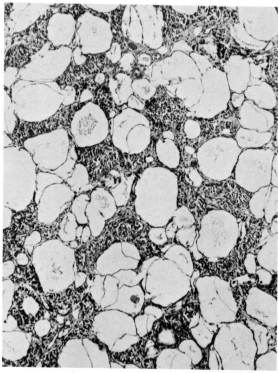

Figure 46
NEPHROBLASTOMA
Thin-walled cysts within the blastemic regions of the tumor resemble the cavities in a lymphangioma. X70.

Figure 47
NEPHROBLASTOMA
This tumor illustrates a papillary intracystic growth pattern. X42.

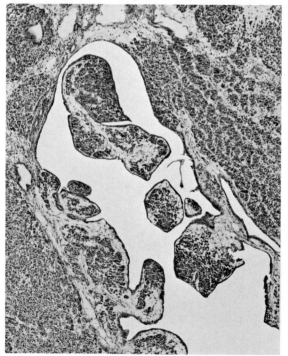

Figure 47

Epithelial differentiation may be faintly apparent (fig. 48) or predominantly tubular (figs. 49—52), mimicking various stages in fetal nephronic differentiation. Sometimes, the epithelium is papillary in large regions. Commonly, glomeruloid differentiation is apparent, although these structures are not usually vascularized (pl. I-B). In addition to mimicry of normal metanephrogenesis, epithelial elements in nephroblastomas may show differentiation into cell forms not seen in normal human kidneys. Keratinizing squamous epithelium is encountered

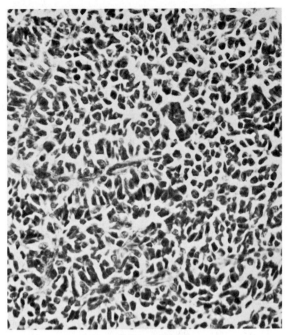

Figure 48

Figure 48
NEPHROBLASTOMA
Early epithelial differentiation is observed within the blastemic zone of this nephroblastoma. X265.

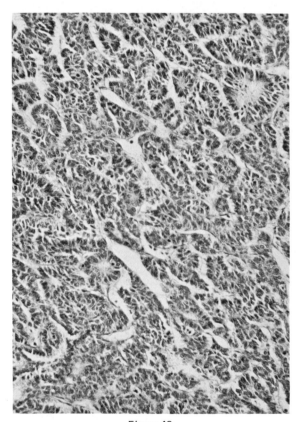

Figure 49
NEPHROBLASTOMA
A clearly defined tubular pattern was present in the entire tumor. X145.

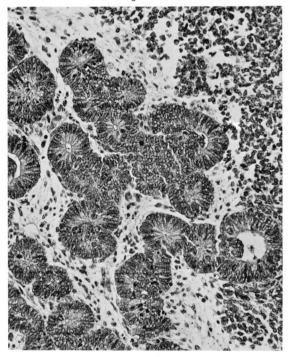

Figure 50
NEPHROBLASTOMA
Well formed embryonal tubules are surrounded by fibrous tumor stroma, and a blastemic region is visible in one corner. X165.

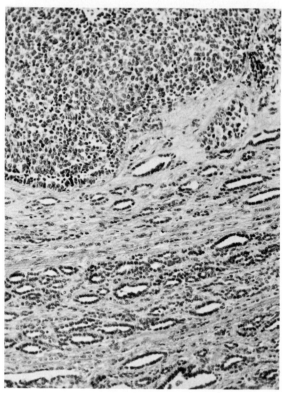

Figure 51

Figure 51
NEPHROBLASTOMA
Highly differentiated, benign-appearing epithelium and stroma are adjacent to a blastemic zone. X165.

Figure 52
NEPHROBLASTOMA
Most of this neoplasm consists of well defined, but embryonal tubular epithelium. The stroma, however, is more prominent than in the tumor illustrated in figure 49. X70.

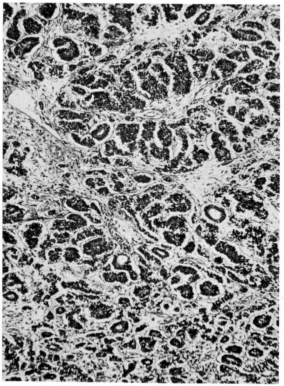

Figure 52

in dysplastic kidneys (pl. I-C). Mucinous epithelium, also uncommon, was viewed by Hou and Azzopardi as a derivative of collecting tubules (fig. 53). Argentaffin cells were also found by Hou and Azzopardi.

Epithelial differentiation in nephroblastomas may assume "basaloid" features, with an epithelioid outline around blastemal trabeculae (fig. 54) or narrow serpentine anastomosing cord patterns (fig. 55).

Figure 53
NEPHROBLASTOMA
Mucinous epithelium is observed in this nephroblastoma. X115.

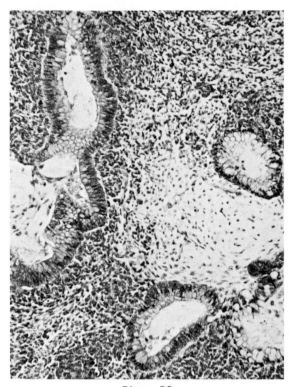

Figure 53

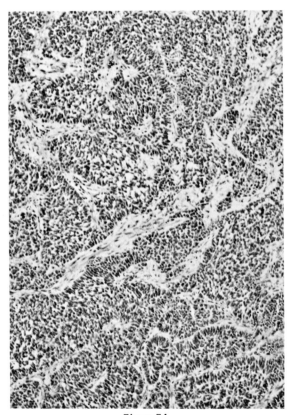

Figure 54
NEPHROBLASTOMA
The "basaloid" pattern shown here is produced by epithelial outlining of blastemic zones. X90.

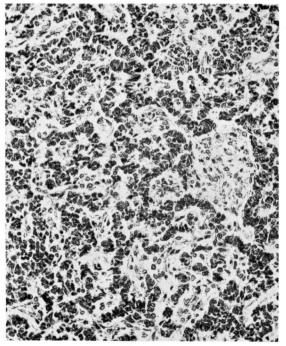

Figure 55
NEPHROBLASTOMA
This is a cylindromatous "basaloid" variant. X145.

Stromal constituents of nephroblastoma usually include fibroblastic and myxoid regions. Smooth muscle may be a prominent feature, as may dense populations of spindle cells that cannot readily be classified (fig. 56). A frequent component of nephroblastomas is skeletal muscle (figs. 57, 58). This characteristically shows moderate differentiation, with narrow myofibers possessing central nuclei and exceptionally well defined cross striations. However, anaplastic skeletal muscle may be seen mimicking pleomorphic rhabdomyosarcoma of soft tissues (figs. 59, 60). When the tumor is composed exclusively of myogenous elements, controversy exists as to its proper classification. As mentioned previously, we view these and other monotypic lesions of the kidney, composed of

cell types identical to those of nephroblastomas, as "monotypic nephroblastomas." Other stromal constituents of nephroblastoma include cartilage, which is usually well differentiated but may be anaplastic (pl. I-D). Fat cells may be present (fig. 61), and a few examples of osteoid have been described in the literature (Bannayan et al.; Bodian and Rigby). Elastic fibers are variably present, and a lymphoid tissue is rarely seen (Wilms).

Neural elements were emphasized by Masson and by DeMuylder (see p. 32). Using the Bodian silver method, Hou and Azzopardi found positive reactions in 6 of 26 specimens, postulating they may be derivatives of the enterochromaffin system. Ganglion cells were described by Busse and depicted by Bannayan and associates.

Uncommonly, one finds markedly anaplastic elements within nephroblastomas that defy classification. Representative fields are shown in figures 62 through 65.

The appearance of metastatic lesions is extremely variable, and often shows a marked difference in relative proportions of the various tissue types present in the primary tumor.

Radiation alters the appearance, and in radiated tumors differentiated stromal elements usually predominate (fig. 66; Bannayan et al.).

Ultrastructural Studies

See section on histogenesis on page 39.

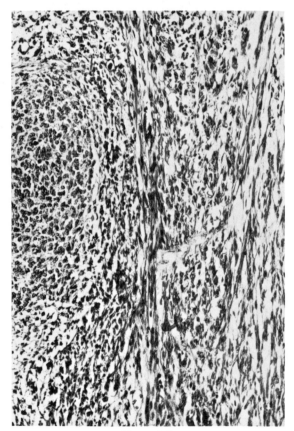

Figure 56

Figure 56
NEPHROBLASTOMA
This nephroblastoma reveals an undifferentiated stromal pattern. X130.

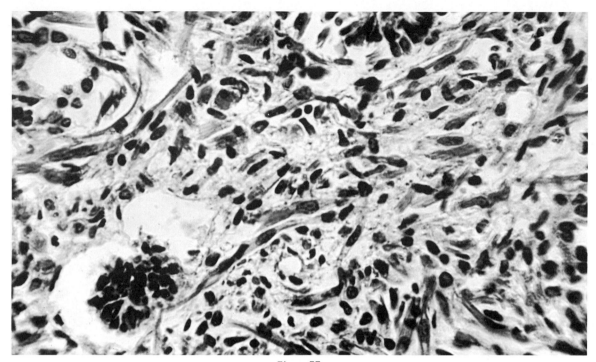

Figure 57
NEPHROBLASTOMA
(Figures 57 and 58 from same case)
Skeletal muscle differentiation is clearly apparent, together with two poorly formed tubules. X270. (Fig. 76 from Lucke', B., and Schlumberger, H. G. Tumors of the Kidney, Renal Pelvis and Ureter. Fascicle 30, Atlas of Tumor Pathology, First Series. Washington: Armed Forces Institute of Pathology, 1957.)

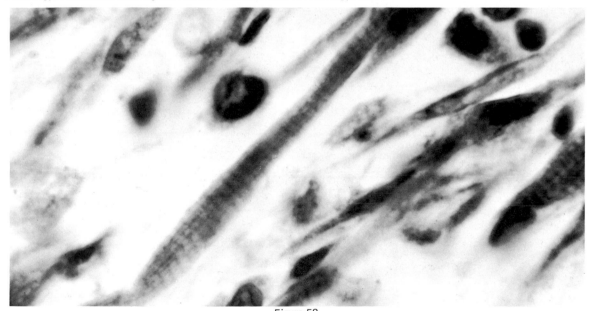

Figure 58
NEPHROBLASTOMA
(Figures 57 and 58 from same case)
Higher magnification of figure 57 shows characteristic cross striations. X2200. (Fig. 77 from Lucke', B., and Schlumberger, H. G. Tumors of the Kidney, Renal Pelvis and Ureter. Fascicle 30, Atlas of Tumor Pathology, First Series. Washington: Armed Forces Institute of Pathology, 1957.)

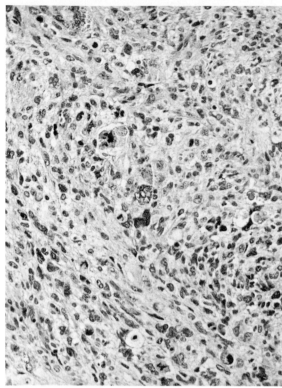

Figure 59

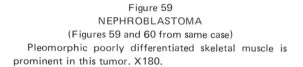

Figure 59
NEPHROBLASTOMA
(Figures 59 and 60 from same case)
Pleomorphic poorly differentiated skeletal muscle is prominent in this tumor. X180.

Figure 60
NEPHROBLASTOMA
(Figures 59 and 60 from same case)
Abnormal mitotic figures may be observed in this higher magnification of the tumor in figure 59. X485.

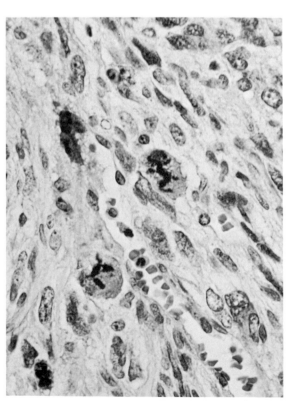

Figure 60

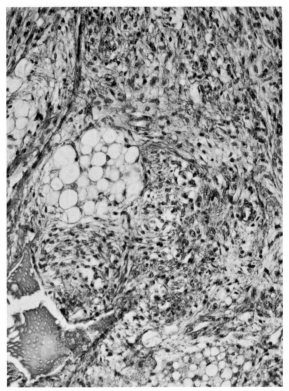

Figure 61

Figure 61
NEPHROBLASTOMA
Several islands, probably representing fat cells, are apparent in this tumor. X180.

Figure 62
NEPHROBLASTOMA
An anaplastic region is evident in this otherwise typical nephroblastoma. Classification is difficult when the entire tumor presents only this pattern. X145.

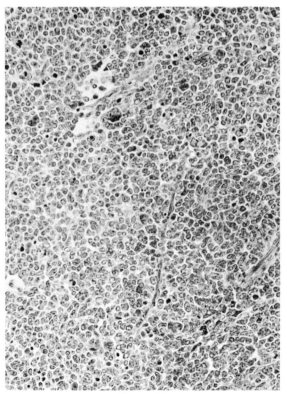

Figure 62

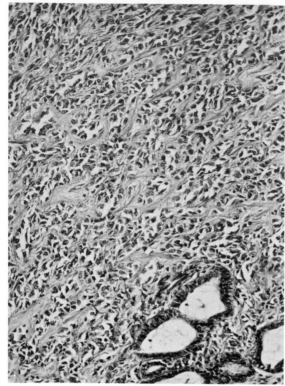

Figure 63

Figure 63
NEPHROBLASTOMA
This anaplastic region surrounds embryonal tubular elements. Without the latter elements, such a specimen might be mistaken for anaplastic sarcoma or renal carcinoma. X165.

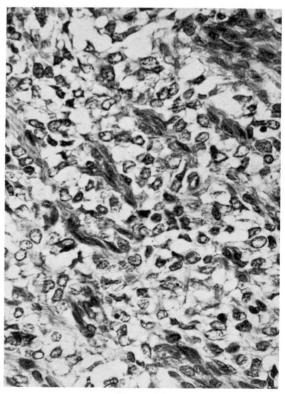

Figure 64
NEPHROBLASTOMA
This illustrates another anaplastic variant of nephroblastoma. X305.

Figure 64

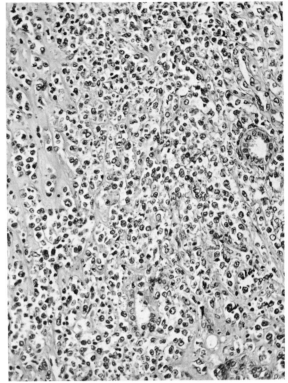

Figure 65

Figure 65
NEPHROBLASTOMA
These undifferentiated cells are of variable size with hyalinizing stroma. The tubule may be a preexistent renal tubule, but the presence of several less well defined tubular structures suggests it may be a differentiated component of the tumor. X180.

Figure 66
NEPHROBLASTOMA
Predominantly well differentiated stroma and glomeruloid regions are seen in this tumor, which received 2500 rads prior to surgical removal. Blastema is virtually absent. X50.

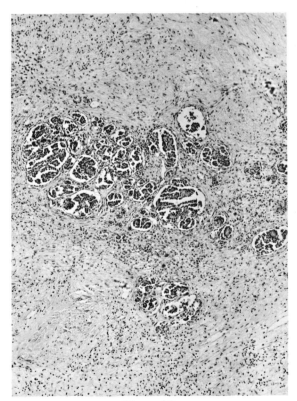

Figure 66

PLATE I

NEPHROBLASTOMA

A.   This "oncocytoid" appearance within blastematous zones may be a degenerative change. X320.

B.   Well defined glomerular differentiation is apparent in this nephroblastoma. X100.

C.   A squamous nest is seen within the fibromyomatous stroma of this nephroblastoma. X115.

D.   This is a nodule of anaplastic cartilage. X70.

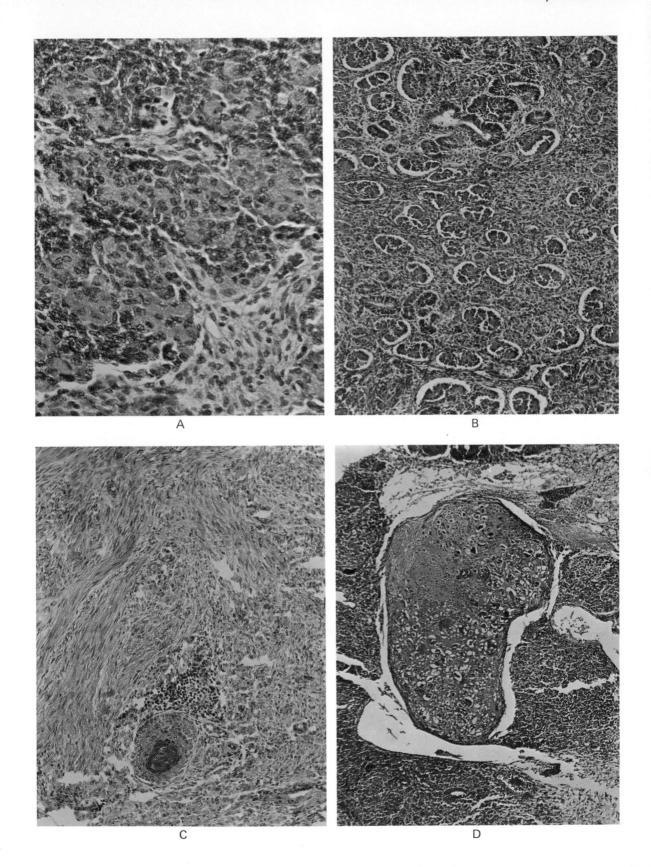

A

B

C

D

PLATE I

Classification

Because of the diversity of microscopic patterns presented by nephroblastomas, several attempts to classify these tumors on histologic grounds and to correlate them with their biologic behavior have been reported. Bodian and Rigby were able to define seven patterns, designated A through G, respectively. Most of their specimens were of the "mixed mesenchymal-blastemal" (F) or "massive blastemal" (G) types; only a few of the patients survived. On the other hand, specimens composed of predominantly epithelial or differentiated mesenchymal elements resulted in a more favorable outcome for the patient. Hardwick and Stowens devised a relatively complex classification into six types, based primarily on resemblances to the normal or developing kidney. These were further subclassified into A or B variants, depending upon the predominance of differentiated or undifferentiated components within the tumor. They observed an apparently more favorable outcome among patients with tumors when differentiated tubular and glomeruloid structures predominated. Perez and associates presented a grouping into four stages, also based on the predominance of differentiated or undifferentiated elements, and similarly found better survival in patients with the predominantly glomerular or tubular tumors. Jereb and Sandstedt produced a simple classification of three types, based upon the degree of differentiation of the least mature element in the neoplasm, and also found better survival among those patients with higher degrees of differentiation. All the above series are based upon rather small numbers of cases, especially in the highly differentiated groups. Each study is based upon collections spanning many decades, with marked variation in modes of therapy.

One of the major aims of the National Wilms' Tumor Study is to develop an objective histologic classification of nephroblastoma based upon a large cohort of similarly treated cases. This unique opportunity should shed considerable light upon the relationship of the histopathologic features to prognosis.

Natural History and Patterns of Metastasis

Local extension through the external tumor capsule significantly worsens the prognosis, but is usually a late occurrence. Involvement of intrarenal blood vessels and lymphatics is frequently encountered, and preliminary data from the National Wilms' Tumor Study indicate a somewhat lower frequency of patients free of disease at one year when such involvement is present. Extension by way of the renal vein into the inferior vena cava may propagate into the right atrium (Murphy et al., 1973). The incidence of involvement of renal hilar and paraaortic lymph nodes is uncertain, but sufficiently frequent to justify routine surgical exploration of regional nodes at the time of nephrectomy. Martin and Reyes found involved nodes in 7 of 20 patients in whom complete periaortic node dissection was carried out, none of whom had known hematogenous metastases at the time of operation. Perez and associates noted positive nodes in 10 of 43 cases. The renal pelvis is often infiltrated by tumor, and polypoid tumor nodules may fill the pelvis and ureter. Occasionally, bladder implants also are encountered (Watkins).

Metastases most often are found in the lungs, where they may be situated in the perihilar or parenchymal regions, but most often they are predominantly subpleural, and frequently pedunculated (fig. 67). The distribution of metastatic disease was reviewed by Bannayan and associates, who found that 43 of 55 patients with metastatic nephroblastoma had lung involvement. In 23 patients, the tumors had metastasized to the liver. Other sites commonly involved were mediastinal nodes, adrenal glands, the diaphragm, and the retroperitoneum. Involvement of the opposite kidney is often interpreted as a separate primary tumor, although this point remains controversial.

Bone is rarely involved, in contrast to neuroblastoma. Most large series include fewer than 5 percent of cases with skeletal involvement. Among unusual metastatic sites that have been reported are the thyroid gland, orbit (fig. 68), mandible, testis, nasopharynx, tonsil and parotid gland, bone marrow, and brain (Hardwick and Stowens; Apple; Marsden and Steward; Doykos; Dew; Rao; Movassaghi et al.; Bannayan et al.; Howard).

Metastatic disease usually presents within two years after diagnosis of the primary tumor and is exceptional thereafter. However, a few recurrences from 5 to 8 years after nephrectomy have been documented (Cassady et al.; Haas and Jackson; Williams). Collins found that only 2 of 422 cases recurred beyond his theoretical "period of risk," which is a time interval

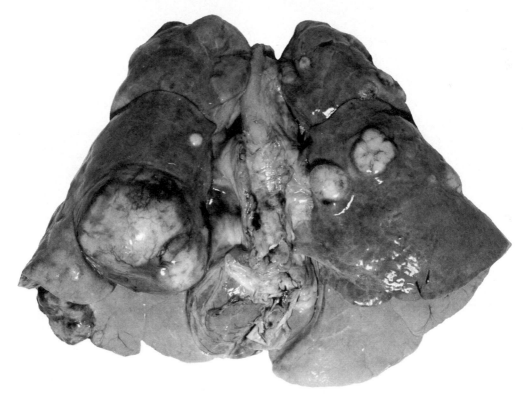

Figure 67
METASTATIC NEPHROBLASTOMA IN LUNGS
Multiple subpleural nodules, which may be pedunculated, are present. Additional metastases were scattered throughout the lung parenchyma. (Courtesy of Dr. Sidney Farber, Boston, Mass.; also fig. 69 from Lucke', B., and Schlumberger, H. G. Tumors of the Kidney, Renal Pelvis and Ureter. Fascicle 30, Atlas of Tumor Pathology, First Series. Washington: Armed Forces Institute of Pathology, 1957.)

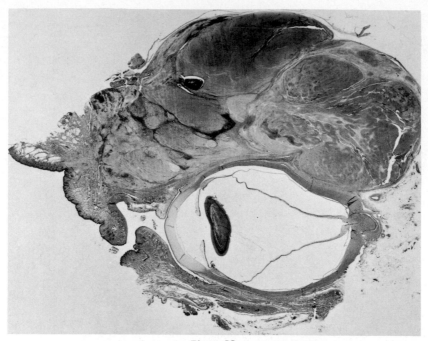

Figure 68
METASTATIC NEPHROBLASTOMA TO ORBIT
Orbital exenteration revealed this tumor to be compressing, but not infiltrating the globe. X2. (Courtesy of Dr. Joseph B. Crawford, San Francisco, Calif.)

following diagnosis equal to the age of the child at diagnosis, plus nine months. However, Platt and Linden found a disease free interval of two years to be as reliable an indicator of cure as Collins' risk period. Of particular note is the relatively high frequency of cures following therapy for pulmonary and hepatic metastases (Howard; Kilman et al.).

The histologic appearances of metastases are as variable as those of the primary tumors, although epithelial, blastemal, and stromal elements are all usually present (fig. 69). Frequently in metastases there is a larger proportion of poorly differentiated elements.

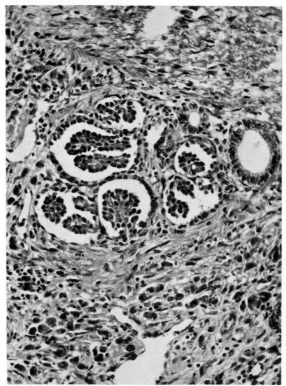

Figure 69
NEPHROBLASTOMA
Metastasis to the liver shows well defined stromal and glomeruloid structures. X180.

Figure 69

Treatment

Remarkable advances in the treatment of nephroblastoma have been achieved through the combined use of surgery, radiation therapy, and chemotherapy. Survival figures exceeding 80 percent are now being reported from many centers (D'Angio).

The surgical approach to nephroblastoma is through a wide anterior transperitoneal incision, which may be extended to a thoracoabdominal approach when necessary (Snyder et al.; Sullivan et al.). The advantages of this approach over a flank incision include the ability to inspect the contralateral kidney for tumor, and the remainder of the abdomen for extension or metastases. The opposite kidney should routinely be examined on both the anterior and posterior surfaces. Hilar and periaortic lymph node dissection should be carried out unless there are obvious metastases elsewhere, since gross impressions concerning nodal involvement are frequently erroneous (Hilton and Keeling; Martin and Reyes). The tumor margins, and any residual tumor, should be marked with clips to guide postoperative radiotherapy. When extensive metastases, large tumor size, or poor condition of the patient make initial nephrectomy unwise, preoperative radiation and chemotherapy are often utilized, and the resultant tumor regression usually makes subsequent nephrectomy feasible.

When the tumor extends beyond the kidney, radiotherapy to the tumor bed and to any involved areas is customary, the dose being graduated according to the age of the patient and other factors (D'Angio).

The National Wilms' Tumor Study is currently involved in a study of the necessity for radiation of the tumor bed for group I tumors, in the hope that this can be omitted for tumors localized to kidney and completely resected.

The optimal chemotherapy for nephroblastoma is still being defined. Since the pioneering work of Farber and his colleagues, actinomycin D has been widely recognized as an effective adjunct to nephroblastoma therapy, capable of markedly improving the cure rate over figures obtained prior to its introduction (Soper; Sullivan et al.). This agent is usually administered in the form of intermittent courses for 15 months, although individualization of dose and length of course are often necessary. More recently, vincristine sulfate (Oncovin) has become recognized as a useful adjunct to therapy (D'Angio; Sullivan et al.). It produces complete regression of metastases in many patients, although this is usually temporary unless given in conjunction with radiotherapy. The National Wilms' Tumor Study is currently exploring the relative efficiency of actinomycin D or vincristine sulfate given alone as compared to combination therapy.

Cyclophosphamide (Cytoxan) has been found to be moderately effective against nephroblastoma, and may be considered an alternative form of therapy for children whose tumor is resistant to the drugs already mentioned (Finklestein et al.).

Preliminary results in patients with nephroblastoma given adriamycin are also encouraging (D'Angio).

When pulmonary or hepatic metastases are either solitary or limited to one side, surgical removal has been demonstrated to be feasible and potentially curative (Wedemeyer et al.). However, if hepatic lobectomy is performed, chemotherapy and radiation should be withheld until liver regeneration is complete (Filler et al.).

Treatment of bilateral nephroblastomas presents particular problems. However, a relatively high cure rate has been observed in some series. For example, Ragab and associates reported cures in 3 of 5 children with bilateral nephroblastomas. The therapy is necessarily highly individualized and depends upon the nature and extent of tumor in the two kidneys, as well as upon the presence of extension or remote metastases. When the extent of tumor involvement is asymmetrical, removal of the more severely affected kidney, and partial nephrectomy on the other side, is often feasible. Sometimes bilateral partial nephrectomies are indicated. It has been shown that if 15 to 35 percent of original renal tissue remains, a normal life is possible (Ragab et al.). Bilateral complete nephrectomy with renal transplantation has been used for diffuse or extensive renal involvement (DeLorimier et al.). However, radiation and chemotherapy to both kidneys before nephrectomy may be more effective (Ragab et al.).

Prognosis

Dramatic improvement in the prognosis for patients with nephroblastoma has occurred in the past few decades with the introduction of multimodal therapy as outlined above. The proportion of cured patients has increased from fewer than 20 percent prior to 1930 to about 50 percent by 1950, with the introduction of radiotherapy. Recent reports indicate overall cure rates in the range of 80 percent (D'Angio; Marsden and Steward; Wedemeyer et al.; Williams). Fraumeni and associates (1972) found 433 fewer deaths from renal cancer in American children between 1960 and 1967 than would have been predicted from the death rate between 1950 and 1959.

Age of Patient at Diagnosis

Several series have demonstrated a tendency toward higher cure rates for tumors diagnosed under two years of age, although others have found little effect of age on outcome (Sukarochana and Kiesewetter; Fleming and Johnson; Perez et al.). Williams noted a more favorable outcome for younger patients treated since, but not before 1944. Clearly, the effect of age on prognosis is far less dramatic than for neuroblastoma. It is essential that in evaluating this variable, congenital mesoblastic nephromas be excluded, and also that results in the various age categories be corrected for extent of disease at the time of diagnosis. The National Wilms' Tumor Study has shown that the mean age for group I tumors is considerably lower than for groups II, III, and IV (see epidemiology of tumors of the upper urinary tract on page 46).

Sex

Although an effect of the patient's sex on outcome has not been documented, Fraumeni and associates (1972) found, in their review of death certificates of children who died of renal cancer, that the recent reduction in mortality appears to be greater in boys than in girls. There is no apparent explanation for this difference.

Tumor Size

While Garcia and associates found a tumor size in excess of 550 ml. to be an adverse prognostic indicator, Jereb and Sandstedt found no effect of tumor size upon outcome, except for a more favorable prognosis for the few specimens under 5 cm. in diameter.

Extent of Disease at Diagnosis

Capsular permeation, nodal involvement, venous extension, and distant metastases significantly worsen the outlook for nephroblastoma; this is well documented by Perez and coworkers. However, numerous cures have been documented when any, or all these adverse factors were present. Hematuria, considered a grave prognostic indicator by Gross and Neuhauser, was found by Williams and by Marsden and Steward to exert no influence on eventual outcome.

CONGENITAL MESOBLASTIC NEPHROMA

SYNONYMS AND RELATED TERMS: Congenital Wilms' tumor; fetal hamartoma; fibroid hamartoma; fibroma; fibromyoma; fibromyomatous hamartoma; fibrosarcoma; hamartoma (leiomyomatous type); leiomyoma; leiomyomatous hamartoma; leiomyosarcoma; mesenchymal hamartoma; rhabdomyoma; spindle cell sarcoma; stromagenic nephroma.

HISTORICAL ASPECTS. Although examples of this tumor have been included both in reported series and individual case reports of nephroblastomas, Bolande and associates in 1967 delineated this as a specific and characteristic type of neoplasm. They proposed the term "congenital mesoblastic nephroma," and viewed these lesions as a differentiated variant of nephroblastoma. Subsequently, there has been lively debate surrounding the classification and nomenclature of these tumors. Some investigators have contended that they are purely stromal in nature and hence should be viewed as stromal hamartomas (Bogdan et al.; Favara et al.; Wigger). The histogenetic aspects of this issue are discussed under histogenesis on page 46. A comprehensive review by Bolande in 1973 should also be consulted. Of interest is the characteristic relationship to age. With rare exceptions, these lesions have been diagnosed in the early months of life, and most have apparently been present at birth. However, Bogdan and associates found one such tumor in a 10 year old girl, and Block and associates reported one in a woman aged 31 years.

GROSS FEATURES. All cases of congenital mesoblastic nephroma reported to date have been unilateral. The tumor varied from 0.8 cm. to 14 cm. in diameter, with a mean of 6.2 cm. in the series of Bogdan and associates. The tumor typically presents a vague unencapsulated junction with uninvolved kidney (fig. 70) and often extends beyond the renal capsule (fig. 71). The appearances on section resemble a leiomyoma of the uterus, with a tough, uniform, finely trabeculated surface (fig. 70). Cystic change is sometimes prominent, and hemorrhage may occur, although necrosis is not commonly found. The lack of sharp encapsulation and diffuse growth pattern distinguish this entity from leiomyomas of the adult kidney (Wigger).

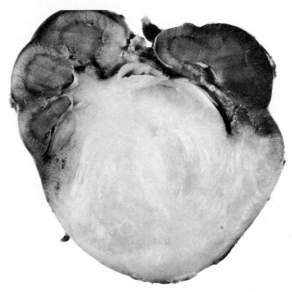

Figure 70
CONGENITAL MESOBLASTIC NEPHROMA
An indistinct margin is visible between the tumor and the kidney, with an apparent fibromyomatous pattern on the sectioned surface.

MICROSCOPIC FEATURES. The predominant pattern is produced by interlacing sheets of variably mature connective tissue cells (figs. 72, 73). These may be either fibroblasts (Bolande; Bolande et al.) or smooth muscle cells as demonstrated by Favara and coworkers' ultrastructural study, and are conveniently termed fibromyomatous for simplicity of description.

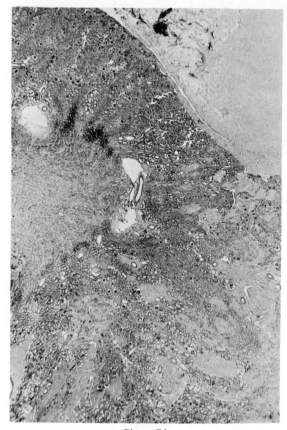

Figure 71
CONGENITAL MESOBLASTIC NEPHROMA
(Figures 71 and 72 from same case)
Permeation of the perirenal fat is not a malignant sign,
but emphasizes the need for wide resection. X10.

Occasionally, there may also be skeletal muscle, myxoid regions reminiscent of embryonic mesenchyme, or cartilage, although the latter is often in the form of dysplastic elements in the adjacent kidney (fig. 73; Bogdan et al.; Bolande; Bolande et al.; Wigger). Clusters of vascular structures occasionally impart an angiomatous appearance, and extramedullary hematopoiesis has also been found within the tumors (Bolande; Bolande et al.). Well differentiated tubular and glomeruloid structures are scattered through the tumor and have variously been viewed as entrapped, pos-

sibly dysplastic nephrons or as a differentiated component of the tumor (figs. 72, 73).

An essential characteristic of congenital mesoblastic nephroma is its growth pattern. Small bundles of fibromyomatous cells are diffusely interspersed with adjacent kidney, usually without producing compression of renal tissue (figs. 72, 73). This diffuse growth pattern, seeming to fit comfortably into the adjacent renal parenchyma, is one of the primary reasons most investigators view this tumor as arising early in development, growing as the kidney differentiates.

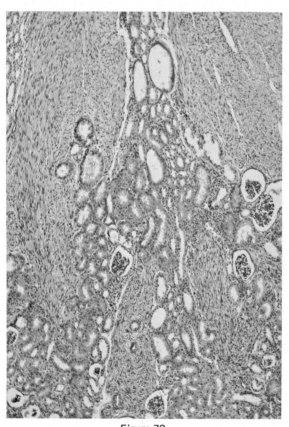

Figure 72
CONGENITAL MESOBLASTIC NEPHROMA
(Figures 71 and 72 from same case)
The growth pattern in this tumor shows a diffuse intermingling with the renal parenchyma at the periphery of the lesion. X70.

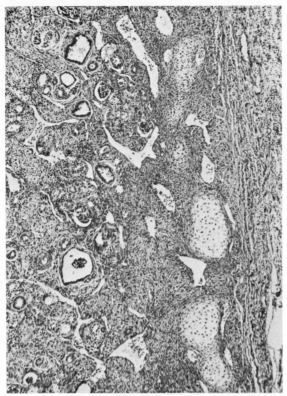

Figure 73
CONGENITAL MESOBLASTIC NEPHROMA
There is fibromyomatous proliferation, with several islands of presumably dysplastic cartilage, in this congenital mesoblastic nephroma. X70.

An interesting and hitherto unpublished observation has been the presence of a prominent lymphoid infiltrate at the margins of the lesion in many specimens.

Mitotic figures may be fairly numerous, and small islands of rather dense cellularity may be present without apparently altering the outcome (Bolande; Bolande et al.; Wigger). However, when the entire tumor is relatively undifferentiated, there is an understandable tendency to view the lesion with correspondingly greater concern. A precise dividing line remains to be drawn between congenital mesoblastic nephroma on the one hand and sarcomatous nephroblastoma on the other.

CLINICAL FEATURES, TREATMENT, AND PROGNOSIS. The characteristically early age of onset has already been mentioned. Rarely, there is a history of rapid recent growth. Clinically, the features are otherwise similar to those of nephroblastoma, except that an association with syndromes such as hemihypertrophy or aniridia has apparently not yet been established.

The clinical benignity of almost all such tumors has been repeatedly emphasized (Beckwith, 1970; Bogdan et al.; Bolande; Bolande et al.). However, two recent reports of recurrence following nephrectomy have appeared (Fu and Kay; Walker and Richard). In the latter report, the tumor proved lethal in spite of radiation therapy. On the other hand, instances of scoliosis and one lethal result from attempted chemotherapy and radiation of a patient with mesoblastic nephroma has also been reported (Beckwith, 1970).

It would appear that the majority of patients will do well without further therapy if there is complete removal of the tumor with adequate margins of uninvolved tissue.

SOLITARY MULTILOCULAR CYST OF THE KIDNEY (SEGMENTAL CYSTIC DISEASE)

SYNONYMS AND RELATED TERMS: Multilocular cystic nephroma; polycystic nephroma; differentiated nephroblastoma; lymphangioma; papillary cystadenoma.

The solitary multilocular cyst of the kidney is an apparently uncommon, benign renal tumor which may or may not be neoplastic. It is included here pending better definition of its nature because: (1) It is strongly held by some authorities to be a renal neoplasm; (2) it has an embryonic histologic appearance; and (3) it is easily confused clinically, radiologically, and pathologically with other renal neoplasms, particularly nephroblastoma.

This tumor was probably first reported by Edmunds in 1892, although the term he used was cystadenoma. Since that time, at least 40 additional cases have been reported under a variety of histologic terms which reflect the uncertainty of its histogenesis (Aterman et al.). While this tumor generally has been considered rare, the increasing numbers of reports suggest it is being more widely recognized and may be more common than is generally appreciated. In a number of instances, multilocular cysts of the kidney have been erroneously reported as examples of polycystic kidney, nephroblastoma, or lymphangioma. Since relatively few well documented cases of multicystic renal disease have been reported, and none of the large studies of renal tumors include this entity, our knowledge of its epidemiology is sketchy.

While subject to revision, Aterman and associates suggest the following criteria which characterize the solitary multilocular cyst of the kidney:

1. The cyst should be unilateral.
2. It should be solitary.
3. It should be multilocular.
4. The locules should not communicate with one another.
5. The locules should have an epithelial lining.
6. The cyst should not communicate with the pelvis.
7. The remaining kidney should be normal.
8. No fully developed nephrons or portions of nephrons should be present in the septa of the cystic lesion.

In reports of multilocular cyst of the kidney, the age range is from newborn infants to 70 years. Approximately one-half the cysts have been found in young children (fig. 74) and the remainder in adults (fig. 75), with few cases having been reported in adolescents or young adults. Among the children, more cysts have been observed in males than in females, while the reverse has been true for adults. Since the numbers of cases are not large, these observations may not be statistically significant. Various theories have been advanced on the pathogenesis of solitary multilocular cysts of the kidney. These have been reviewed by Boggs and Kimmelstiel and Aterman and associates. The three most likely alternatives are that this lesion represents: (1) A benign neoplasm arising from metanephric blastema, perhaps analogous to mesoblastic nephroma which it resembles; (2) nephroblastoma which has undergone benign differentiation (Fowler); or (3) a developmental abnormality, i.e., cystic disease of the kidney (Johnson et al.; Potter, 1972). Potter refers to this entity as segmental cystic disease, and found eight such cases among 12,000 autopsies from 110,000 live births at the University of Chicago Lying-in Hospital.

The association of this lesion with nephroblastoma has been advanced as evidence that multilocular cystic disease of the kidney is a neoplasm. However, considering the relatively high frequency of nonneoplastic congenital urinary tract abnormalities associated with nephroblastoma, it is not a convincing argument.

CLINICAL FEATURES. The most common presenting feature of multilocular cyst of the kidney is an abdominal or renal mass found on routine physical examination. Less frequently reported symptoms are hematuria and hypertension.

Because of the difficulty in distinguishing this tumor clinically and radiologically from nephroblastoma in the pediatric age group, there have been several instances when radiotherapy or actinomycin D treatment was given prior to nephrectomy (Aterman et al.).

GROSS FEATURES. All cases of multilocular cystic renal disease have been unilateral. The majority of the tumors have been relatively large; even in children, most tumors have been between 5 and 10 cm. in greatest diameter. The tumor frequently extends beyond the renal capsule as a bulging bosselated mass. The cut surfaces reveal a well circumscribed multilocular tumor composed of cysts, ranging from several millimeters up to 4 cm. in greatest diameter, filled with clear colorless to

bluish fluid. The fibrous septae between the cysts and the dense capsule or pseudocapsule are usually gray-white (figs. 74, 75). Calcification, hemorrhage, and necrosis are not features of this tumor. The cystic pattern may suggest a nephroblastoma or renal adenocarcinoma; however, the absence of hemorrhage, necrosis, and calcification militates against these possibilities. The gross appearance may also resemble a mesoblastic nephroma; however, the well encapsulated margins of the solitary multilocular cyst distinguish this lesion from a mesoblastic nephroma, which has a poorly circumscribed infiltrative margin.

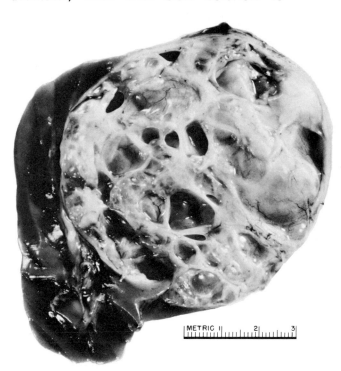

Figure 74

Figure 74
MULTILOCULAR CYST OF KIDNEY
This is a multilocular cyst of the kidney from a 28 month old girl. The mass is composed of gray-white fibrous partitions separating fluid-filled cysts ranging up to 1.5 cm. in diameter. The tumor is encapsulated and compresses the surrounding renal parenchyma. (Fig. 1B from Johnson, D. E., Ayala, A. G., Medellin, H., and Wilbur, J. Multilocular renal cystic disease in children. J. Urol. 109:101-103, 1973.)

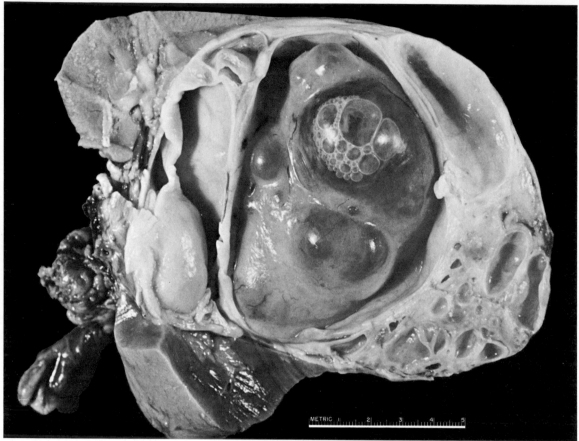

Figure 75
MULTILOCULAR CYST OF KIDNEY IN AN ADULT
(Figures 75–77 from same case)

This multilocular cyst of the kidney was found in a 46 year old woman, who presented with a right upper quadrant mass and hypertension. Renal arteriography revealed a cystic tumor. Grossly, the tumor was well circumscribed and partially encapsulated. Individual cysts contained clear colorless fluid. The patient is well seven years following nephrectomy, although the hypertension persists. (Courtesy of Dr. Seth L. Haber, Santa Clara, Calif.)

MICROSCOPIC FEATURES. The most striking histologic features of this tumor are the large dilated tubules, many dilated to cystic proportions, lined by flattened (fig. 76) or occasionally hobnail type epithelium (fig. 77), and supported by a loose mesenchymal stroma composed of plump spindle cells resembling fibroblasts. In some areas, the stroma may be immature, reminiscent of the loose mesenchymal stroma seen in nephroblastomas; in others, it may be hyalinized and infiltrated by lymphocytes. Scattered throughout the stroma are clusters of small tubules; some have indistinct lumens while others are well defined and contain proteinaceous material. The small tubules are lined by clear cuboidal cells with large vesicular nuclei containing small nucleoli (figs. 76 and 77). Cartilage, skeletal muscle, and adipose tissue are not components of this tumor, although a thin rim of smooth muscle is frequently observed in the tumor capsule.

TREATMENT AND PROGNOSIS. Whatever the genesis of the multilocular cyst of the kidney, it appears to be a benign lesion which may be adequately treated by nephrectomy. However, instances of simple enucleation of the lesion have been described when preservation of renal function is essential (Aterman et al.). We are aware of no reports of recurrence or metastases in well documented examples of this entity.

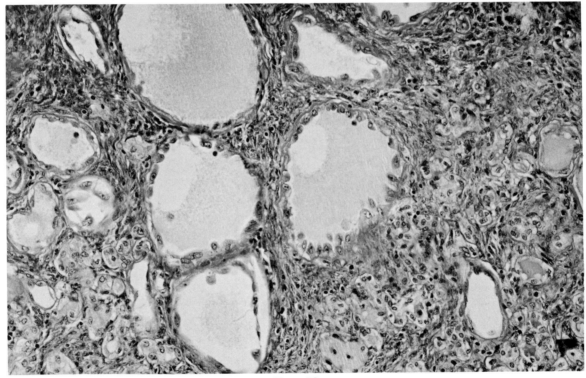

Figure 76
MULTILOCULAR CYST OF KIDNEY IN AN ADULT
(Figures 75–77 from same case)
The histologic appearance of the tumor shown in figure 75 is characterized by large, cystic, dilated tubules containing proteinaceous material and lined by an epithelium which is composed of flattened cuboidal or squamoid cells in some cysts, and hobnailed cells in others. Small tubules are lined by tall, clear cuboidal cells containing large vesicular nuclei. X180. (Courtesy of Dr. Seth L. Haber, Santa Clara, Calif.)

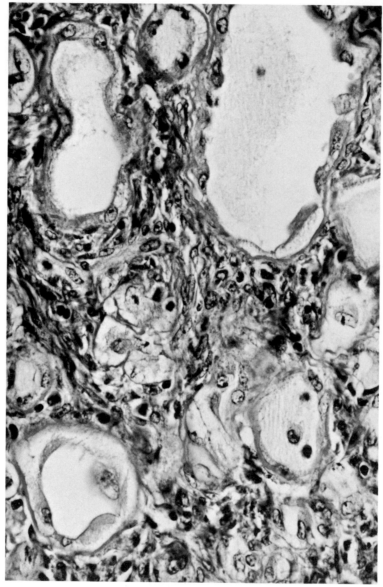

Figure 77
MULTILOCULAR CYST OF KIDNEY IN AN ADULT
(Figures 75—77 from same case)
This higher magnification of figure 76 demonstrates the active appearing spindle-shaped stromal cells of the tumor.
X450. (Courtesy of Dr. Seth L. Haber, Santa Clara, Calif.)

References

Allen, A. C. The Kidney: Medical and Surgical Diseases, 2d ed., p. 710. New York: Grune and Stratton, 1962.

Angström, T. Nephroblastoma in a case of agonadism. Cancer 18:857-862, 1965.

Apple, D. J. Wilms' tumor metastatic to the orbit. Arch. Ophthalmol. 80:480-483, 1968.

Aterman, K., Boustani, P., and Gillis, D. A. Solitary multilocular cyst of the kidney. J. Pediatr. Surg. 8:505-516, 1973.

Balsaver, A. M., Gibley, C. W., Jr., and Tessmer, C. F. Ultrastructural studies in Wilms's tumor. Cancer 22:417-427, 1968.

Bannayan, G. A., Huvos, A. G., and D'Angio, G. J. Effect of irradiation on the maturation of Wilms' tumor. Cancer 27:812-818, 1971.

Beckwith, J. B. Macroglossia, omphalocele, adrenal cytomegaly, gigantism, and hyperplastic visceromegaly. Birth Defects: Original Article Series 5:188-196, 1969.

.... Mesenchymal renal neoplasms of infancy. J. Pediatr. Surg. 5:405-406, 1970.

............, and Perrin, E. V. Nephrogenic Rests: New Light on the Histogenesis of Nephroblastomas. Presented at the Sixth Annual Meeting of the Teratology Society, Corpus Christi, Texas, May 26, 1966.

Berdjis, C. C. Kidney tumors and irradiation pathogenesis of kidney tumors in irradiated rats. Oncologia 16:312-324, 1963.

Bernstein, J. Developmental abnormalities of the renal parenchyma: renal hypoplasia and dysplasia. Pathol. Annu. 3:213-247, 1968.

Berry, C. L., Keeling, J., and Hilton, C. Coincidence of congenital malformation and embryonic tumours of childhood. Arch. Dis. Child. 45:229-231, 1970.

Bhajekar, A. B., Joseph, M., and Bhat, H. S. Unattached nephroblastoma. Br. J. Urol. 36:187-190, 1964.

Birch-Hirschfeld, F. V. Sarcomatöse Drüsengeschwulst der Niere im Kindesalter. Beitr. Pathol. 24:343-362, 1898.

Block, N. L., Grabstald, H. G., and Melamed, M. R. Congenital mesoblastic nephroma (leiomyomatous hamartoma): first adult case. J. Urol. 110:380-383, 1973.

Bodian, M., and Rigby, E. The Pathology of Nephroblastoma, pp. 219-234. In: Monographs on Neoplastic Disease at Various Sites, Vol. V, Tumours of the Kidney and Ureter. (Ed.) Riches, E. W. Baltimore: Williams & Wilkins Co.; Edinburgh: E. & S. Livingstone, Ltd., 1964.

Bogdan, R., Taylor, D. E. M., and Mostofi, F. K. Leiomyomatous hamartoma of the kidney. A clinical and pathologic analysis of 20 cases from the kidney tumor registry. Cancer 31:462-467, 1973.

Boggs, L. K., and Kimmelstiel, P. Benign multilocular cystic nephroma: Report of two cases of so-called multilocular cyst of the kidney. J. Urol. 76:530-541, 1956.

Bolande, R. P. Congenital mesoblastic nephroma of infancy. Perspect. Pediatr. Pathol. 1:227-250, 1973.

............, Brough, A. J., and Izant, R. J., Jr. Congenital mesoblastic nephroma of infancy. A report of eight cases and the relationship to Wilms' tumor. Pediatrics 40:272-278, 1967.

Bove, K. E., Koffler, H., and McAdams, A. J. Nodular renal blastema: definition and possible significance. Cancer 24:323-332, 1969.

Busse, O. Ueber Bau, Entwickelung und Eintheilung der Nieren-Geschwülste. Virchows Arch. (Pathol. Anat.) 157:346-372, 1899.

Cassady, J. R., Tefft, M., Filler, R. M., Jaffe, N., and Hellman, S. Considerations in the radiation therapy of Wilms' tumor. Cancer 32:598-608, 1973.

Clark, R. E., Moss, A. A., DeLorimier, A. A., and Palubinskas, A. J. Arteriography of Wilms' tumor. Am. J. Roentgenol. Radium Ther. Nucl. Med. 113:476-490, 1971.

Cochran, W., and Froggatt, P. Bilateral nephroblastoma in two sisters. J. Urol. 97:216-220, 1967.

Cohnheim, J. Lectures on General Pathology. Handbook for Practitioners and Students. Translated from 2d German ed. by McKee, A. B. London: New Sydenham Society, 1889.

Coleman, G. L., Gralla, E. J., Knirsch, A. K., and Stebbins, R. B. Canine embryonal nephroma: A case report. Am. J. Vet. Res. 31:1315-1320, 1970.

Collins, V. P. The treatment of Wilms's tumor. Cancer 11:89-94, 1958.

Cope, J. R., Roylance, J., and Gordon, I. R. The radiological features of Wilms' tumour. Clin. Radiol. 23:331-339, 1972.

Cremin, B. J., and Kaschula, R. O. Arteriography in Wilms' tumour—the results of 13 cases and comparison to renal dysplasia. Br. J. Radiol. 45:415-422, 1972.

Crocker, J. F., and Vernier, R. L. Congenital nephroma of infancy: Induction of renal structures by organ culture. J. Pediatr. 80:69-73, 1972.

Cummins, G. E., and Cohen, D. Cushing's syndrome secondary to ACTH—secreting Wilms' tumor. J. Pediatr. Surg. 9:535-539, 1974.

D'Angio, G. J., Beckwith, J. B., Bishop, H. C., Breslow, N., Evans, A. E., Goodwin, W. E., King, L. R., Pickett, L. K., Sinks, L. F., Sutow, W. W., and Wolff, J. A. Childhood Cancer. The National Wilms' Tumor Study: A Progress Report, pp. 627-636. In: Proceedings of the VII National Cancer Conference. Philadelphia: J. B. Lippincott Company, 1972.

.........., Management of children with Wilms' tumor. Cancer 30:1528-1533, 1972.

Davies, J. N. P. Some Variations in Childhood Cancers Throughout the World, pp. 13-36. In: Recent Results in Cancer Research No. 13. New York: Springer-Verlag, 1968.

Day, R. P., and Luetscher, J. A. Big renin: A possible prohormone in kidney and plasma of a patient with Wilms' tumor. J. Clin. Endocrinal. Metab. 38:923-926, 1974.

DeLorimier, A. A., Belzer, F. O., Kountz, S. L., Kushner, J. H. Simultaneous bilateral nephrectomy and renal allotransplantation for bilateral Wilms' tumor. Surgery 64:850-855, 1968.

DeMuylder, C. G. Neurogenesis observed in a mixed Grawitz-Wilms' tumor. Arch. Pathol. 44:451-458, 1947.

Denys, P., Malvaux, P., Van Den Berghe, H., Tanghe, W., and Proesmans, W. Association d'un syndrome anatomo-pathologique de pseudohermaphrodadisme masculin, d'une tumeur de Wilms, d'une nephropathie parenchymateuse et d'un mosaicisme XX/XY. Arch. Franc. Pediatr. 24:729-739, 1967.

Dew, H. Sarcomatous tumors of the testicle. Surg. Gynecol. Obstet. 46:447-458, 1928.

Doll, R., Payne, P., and Waterhouse, J. Cancer Incidence in Five Continents, a Technical Report. U.I.C.C. Berlin, Heidelberg, New York: Springer-Verlag, 1966.

Doykos, J. D. Wilms' tumor metastatic to mandible and oral mucosa. Report of a case. Oral Surg. 27:220-224, 1969.

Drash, A., Sherman, F., Hartmann, W. H., and Blizzard, R. M. A syndrome of pseudohermaphroditism, Wilms' tumor, hypertension, and degenerative renal disease. J. Pediatr. 76:585-593, 1970.

Eberth, C. J. Myoma sarcomatodes renum. Virchows Arch. (Pathol. Anat.) 55:518-520, 1872.

Edmunds, W. Cystic adenoma of the kidney. Trans. Path. Soc. London 43:89, 1891-92.

Elkan, E. Three different types of tumor in Salientia. Cancer Res. 23:1641-1645, 1963.

Emmett, J. L. Intravenous Nephrotomography in the Differential Diagnosis of Renal Cyst and Tumour, pp. 190-209. In: Monographs on Neoplastic Disease at Various Sites, Vol. V. Tumours of the Kidney and Ureter. (Ed.) Riches, E. W. Baltimore: Williams & Wilkins Co.; London: E. & S. Livingstone, Ltd., 1964.

Farber, S., D'Angio, G. J., Evans, A., and Mitus, A. Clinical studies on actinomycin D with special reference to Wilms' tumor in children. Ann. N. Y. Acad. Sci. 89:421-425, 1960.

Favara, B. E., Johnson, W., and Ito, J. Renal tumors in the neonatal period. Cancer 22:845-855, 1968.

Feldman, W. H. A study of the histopathology of the so-called adenosarcoma of swine. Am. J. Pathol. 4:125-138, 1928.

.... Embryonal nephroma in a sheep. Am. J. Cancer 17:743-747, 1933.

.... Neoplasms of Domesticated Animals. Philadelphia: W. B. Saunders, 1932.

Filippi, G., and McKusick, V. A. The Beckwith-Wiedmann syndrome (the exomphalos-macroglossia-gigantism syndrome). Report of two cases and review of the literature. Medicine 49:279-298, 1970.

Filler, R. M., Tefft, M., Vawter, F., Maddock, C. L., and Mitus, A. Hepatic lobectomy in childhood: effects of x-ray and chemotherapy. J. Pediatr. Surg. 4:31-41, 1969.

Finklestein, J. Z., Hittle, R. E., and Hammond, G. D. Evaluation of a high dose cyclophosphamide regimen in childhood tumors. Cancer 23:1239-1242, 1969.

Fitts, R. H. Bilateral feline embryonal sarcoma. J. Am. Vet. Med. Assoc. 136:616, 1960.

Fleming, I. D., and Johnson, W. W. Clinical and pathologic staging as a guide in the management of Wilms' tumor. Cancer 26:660-665, 1970.

Fowler, M. Differentiated nephroblastoma: solid, cystic or mixed. J. Pathol. 105:215-218, 1971.

Fraumeni, J. F., Jr., and Glass, A. C. Wilms' tumor and congenital aniridia. J.A.M.A. 206:825-828, 1968.

............, Everson, R. B., and Dalager, N. A. Declining mortality from Wilms' tumour in the United States. Lancet 2:48, 1972.

............, Geiser, C. F., and Manning, M. D. Wilms' tumor and congenital hemihypertrophy: Report of five new cases and review of literature. Pediatrics 40:886-899, 1967.

Frenster, J. H., and Herstein, P. R. Gene de-repression. N. Engl. J. Med. 288:1224-1229, 1973.

Fu, Y-S., and Kay, S. Congenital mesoblastic nephroma and its recurrence. Arch. Pathol. 96:66-70, 1973.

Ganguly, A., Gribble, J., Tune, B., Kempson, R., and Leutscher, J. Renin-secreting Wilms' tumor with severe hypertension. Report of a case and brief review of renin-secreting tumors. Ann. Intern. Med. 79:835-837, 1973.

Garcia-Bunuel, R., and Brandes, D. Fetal hamartoma of the kidney: Case report, with ultrastructural cytochemical observations. Johns Hopkins Med. J. 127:213-221, 1970.

Garcia, M., Douglass, C., and Schlosser, J. V. Classification and prognosis in Wilms's tumor. Radiology 80:574-580, 1963.

Geiser, C. F., and Schindler, A. M. Long survival in a male with 18-trisomy syndrome and Wilms' tumor. Pediatrics 44:111-116, 1969.

Greer, M., Hutcheson, C. E., and Williams, C. M. Abnormal urinary excretion of p-hydroxyphenyllactic acid in Wilms' tumor. Clin. Chim. Acta 22:460-462, 1968.

Gross, R. E., and Neuhauser, E. B. D. Treatment of mixed tumors of the kidney in childhood. Pediatrics 6:843-852, 1950.

Guerin, M., Chouroulinkov, I., and Rivieire, M. R. Experimental Kidney Tumors, pp. 199-268. In: The Kidney: Morphology, Biochemistry, Physiology, Vol. II. (Eds.) Rouiller, C., and Muller, A. F. New York and London: Academic Press, 1969.

Haas, L., and Jackson, A. D. Wilms' tumour: lobectomy for pulmonary metastasis; a case report. Br. J. Surg. 48:516-518, 1961.

Haicken, B. N., and Miller, D. R. Simultaneous occurrence of congenital aniridia, hamartoma, and Wilms' tumor. J. Pediatr. 78:497-502, 1971.

Hajdu, S. I. Exfoliative cytology of primary and metastatic Wilms' tumors. Acta Cytol. 15:339-342, 1971.

Ham, A. W., McCullock, E. A., Axelrod, A. A., Siminovitch, L., and Howatson, A. F. The histopathological sequence in viral carcinogenesis in the hamster kidney. J. Natl. Cancer Inst. 24:1113-1129, 1960.

Hamanaka, Y., Okamoto, E., and Ueda, T. Fibroma of the kidney in the newborn. J. Pediatr. Surg. 4:250-255, 1969.

Hard, G. C., and Butler, W. H. Cellular analysis of renal neoplasia: Induction of renal tumors in dietary-conditioned rats by dimethylnitrosamine, with a reappraisal of morphological characteristics. Cancer Res. 30:2796-2805, 1970.

Hardwick, D. F., and Stowens, D. Wilms tumors. J. Urol. 85:903-910, 1961.

Hedrén, G. Zur Kenntnis der Pathologie der Mischgeschwülste der Nieren. Beitr. Pathol. 40:1-107, 1907.

Heine, U., deThé, G., Ishiguro, H., Sommer, J. R., Beard, D., and Beard, J. W. Multiplicity of cell response to the BAI strain A (myeloblastosis) avian tumor virus. II. Nephroblastoma (Wilms' tumor): ultrastructure. J. Natl. Cancer Inst. 29:41-105, 1962.

Helmboldt, C. F., and Jortner, B. S. Histologic patterns of the avian embryonal nephroma. Avian Dis. 10:452-462, 1966.

............, and Wyand, D. S. Nephroblastoma in a striped bass. J. Wildlife Dis. 7:162-165, 1971.

Hidai, H., Fukuoka, H., and Murayama, T. Arteriography of Wilms tumor. J. Urol. 110:347-351, 1973.

Hilton, C., and Keeling, J. W. Staging in relation to treatment of nephroblastoma with actinomycin D. Br. J. Urol. 42:265-269, 1970.

Hirono, I., Laqueur, G. L., and Spatz, M. Transplantability of cycasin-induced tumors in rats, with emphasis on nephroblastomas. J. Natl. Cancer Inst. 40:1011-1025, 1968.

Hottendorf, G. H., and Ingraham, K. J. Spontaneous nephroblastomas in laboratory rats. J. Am. Vet. Med. Assoc. 153:826-829, 1968.

Hou, L. T., and Azzopardi, J. G. Muco-epidermoid metaplasia and argentaffin cells in nephroblastoma. J. Pathol. 93:477-481, 1967.

............, and Holman, R. L. Bilateral nephroblastomatosis in a premature infant. J. Pathol. 82:249-255, 1961.

Howard, R. Actinomycin D in Wilms' tumour: treatment of lung metastases. Arch. Dis. Child. 40:200-202, 1965.

Hünig, R. Ultraschalltomographie am kindlichen Abdomen. Helv. Paediatr. Acta Suppl. 24:3-22, 1970.

Imbert, M. C., and Nezelof, C. Etude histo-enzymologique du nephroblastome. Comparaison avec les activites enzymatiques du rein foetal. Ann. Anat. Pathol. 17:5-20, 1972.

Innis, M. D. Nephroblastoma: Possible index cancer of childhood. Med. J. Aust. 1:18-20, 1972.

Irving, I. M. The "E.M.G." syndrome (exomphalos, macroglossia, gigantism). Prog. Pediatr. Surg. 1:1-61, 1970.

Ishiguro, H., Beard, D., Sommer, J. R., Heine, V., de Thé, G., and Beard, J. W. Multiplicity of cell response to the BA1 strain A (myeloblastosis) avian tumor virus: I. Nephroblastoma (Wilms' tumor): gross and microscopic pathology. J. Natl. Cancer Inst. 29:1-39, 1962.

Ito, J., and Johnson, W. W. Ultrastructure of Wilms' tumor. I. Epithelial cell. J. Natl. Cancer Inst. 42:77-99, 1969.

Jasmin, G., and Riopelle, J. L. Nephroblastomas induced in ovariectomized rats by dimethylbenzanthracene. Cancer Res. 30:321-326, 1970.

Javadpour, N., and Bush, I. M. Induction and treatment of Wilms' tumor by transplantation of renal blastema in a new experimental model. J. Urol. 107:931-937, 1972.

Jereb, B., and Sandstedt, B. Structure and size versus prognosis in nephroblastoma. Cancer 31:1473-1481, 1973.

Johnson, D. E., Ayala, A. G., Medellin, H., and Wilbur, J. Multilocular renal cystic disease in children. J. Urol. 109:101-103, 1973.

Kelker, P. H. (Personal communication)

Kilman, J. W., Kronenberg, M. W., O'Neill, J. A., Jr., and Klassen, K. P. Surgical resection for pulmonary metastases in children. Arch. Surg. 99:158-165, 1969.

Klapproth, H. J. Wilms tumor: a report of 45 cases and an analysis of 1,351 cases reported in the world literature from 1940 to 1958. J. Urol. 81:633-648, 1959.

Knudson, A. G., Jr., and Strong, L. C. Mutation and cancer: A model for Wilms' tumor of the kidney. J. Natl. Cancer Inst. 48:313-324, 1972.

Kumar, M., and Gupta, R. K. Evaluation of serum acid phosphatase study in kidney diseases. J. Indian Med. Assoc. 56:89-94, 1971.

Ladda, R., Atkins, L., Littlefield, J., Neurath, P., and Marimuthu, M. Computer-assisted analysis of chromosomal abnormalities: Detection of a deletion in Aniridia-Wilms' tumor syndrome. Science 185:784-787, 1974.

Laqueur, G. L. Carcinogenic effects of cycad meal and cycasin, methylazoxymethanol glycoside, in rats and effects of cycasin in germ free rats. Fed. Proc. 23:1386-1388, 1964.

Ledlie, E. M., Mynors, L. S., Draper, G. J., and Gorbach, P. D. Natural history and treatment of Wilms's tumour: An analysis of 335 cases occurring in England and Wales, 1962-6. Br. Med. J. 4:195-200, 1970.

Liban, E., and Kozenitzky, I. L. Metanephric hamartomas and nephroblastomatosis in siblings. Cancer 25:885-888, 1970.

Lines, D. R. Nephrotic syndrome and nephroblastoma. Report of a case. J. Pediatr. 72:264-265, 1968.

Lucke, B., and Schlumberger, H. G. Tumors of the Kidney, Renal Pelvis and Ureter. Fascicle 30, Atlas of Tumor Pathology. Washington: Armed Forces Institute of Pathology, 1957.

MacMahon, B., and Newill, V. A. Birth characteristics of children dying of malignant neoplasms. J. Natl. Cancer Inst. 28:231-244, 1962.

Magee, P. N., and Barnes, J. M. Induction of kidney tumours in the rat with dimethylnitrosamine (N-nitrosodimethylamine). J. Pathol. 84:19-31, 1962.

Maisin, J., Maldague, P., Dunjic, A., and Maisin, H. Syndromes mortels et effets tardifs des irradiations totales et subtotales chez le rat. J. Belge Radiol. 40:346-398, 1957.

Marsden, H. B., and Steward, J. K. Recent Results in Cancer Research, Vol. 13. Berlin-Heidelberg-New York: Springer-Verlag, 1968.

Martin, L. W., and Reyes, P. M., Jr. An evaluation of 10 years' experience with retroperitoneal lymph node dissection for Wilms' tumor. J. Pediatr. Surg. 4:683-687, 1969.

Masson, P. The role of the neural crests in the embryonal adenosarcomas of the kidney. Am. J. Cancer 33:1-32, 1938.

Meadows, A. T., Lichtenfeld, J. L., and Koop, C. E. Wilms's tumor in three children of a woman with congenital hemihypertrophy. N. Engl. J. Med. 291:23-24, 1974.

Migaki, G., Nelson, L. W., and Todd, G. C. Prevalence of embryonal nephroma in slaughtered swine. J. Am. Vet. Med. Assoc. 159:441-442, 1971.

Miller, R. W., Fraumeni, J. F., Jr., and Manning, M. D. Association of Wilms's tumor with aniridia, hemihypertrophy and other congenital malformations. N. Engl. J. Med. 270:922-927, 1964.

Mingazzini, E. Tumori renali. Atti. Soc. Ital. Urol. 19:96, 1946.

Mount, B. M., Thelmo, W. L., and Husk, M. A reexamination of the renal blastema graft model for Wilms' tumor production. J. Urol. 111:738-741, 1974.

Movassaghi, N., Leikin, S., and Chandra, R. Wilms' tumor metastasis to uncommon sites. J. Pediatr. 84:416-417, 1974.

Moyson, F., Maurus-Desmarez, R., and Gompel, C. Tumeur de Wilms mediastinale? Acta Chir. Belg. (Suppl.) 2:118-128, 1961.

Mugera, G. M. Induction of kidney tumours in the rats by feeding Encephalartos Hildebrandtii for short periods. Br. J. Cancer 23:755-756, 1969.

..........., and Nderito, P. Tumours of the liver, kidney and lungs in rats fed Encephalartos Hildebrandtii. Br. J. Cancer 22:563-568, 1968.

Murphy, D. A., Rabinovitch, H., Chevalier, L., and Virmani, S. Wilms' tumor in right atrium. Am. J. Dis. Child. 126:210-211, 1973.

Murphy, G. P., Allen, J. E., Staubitz, W., Sinks, L. F., and Mirand, E. A. Erythropoietin levels in patients with Wilms' tumor. Follow-up evaluation. N. Y. State J. Med. 72:487-489, 1972.

Muto, K. Ein Fall von Nierensarkom bei einem siebenmonatlichen Foetus. Gann 34:102-103, 1940.

Muus, N. R. Ueber die embryonalen Mischgeschwülste der Niere. Virchows Arch. (Pathol. Anat.) 155:401-427, 1899.

National Wilms' Tumor Study, U. S. A., 1968-1971.

Nicholson, G. W. An embryonic tumour of the kidney in a foetus. J. Pathol. 34:711-730, 1931.

Nyka, W. Sur une tumeur renale du cheval issue du blasteme metanephrique. Bull. Cancer 17:241-247, 1928.

Oberling, C. Sarcome embryonnaire (adenosarcome) du rein chez un lapin. Bull. Cancer 16:708-710, 1927.

Olsen, B. S., and Bischoff, A. J. Wilms' tumor in an adult. Cancer 25:21-25, 1970.

Paul, F. T. Congenital adenosarcoma of the kidney. Trans. Pathol. Soc. Lond. 37:292-294, 1886.

Peller, S. Statistics and the theory of intrauterine induction of childhood cancer. Am. J. Public Health 51:1583-1589, 1961.

Perez, C. A., Kaiman, H. A., Keith, J., Mill, W. B., Vietti, T. J., and Powers, W. E. Treatment of Wilms' tumor and factors affecting prognosis. Cancer 32:609-617, 1973.

Platt, B. B., and Linden, G. Wilms's tumor—a comparison of 2 criteria for survival. Cancer 17:1573-1578, 1964.

Potter, E. L. Normal and Abnormal Development of the Kidney. Chicago: Year Book Medical Publishers, 1972.

.... Pathology of the Fetus and Infant, 2d ed. Chicago: Year Book Medical Publishers, 1961.

Powars, D. R., Allerton, S. E., Beierle, J., and Butler, B. B. Wilms' tumor clinical correlation with circulating mucin in three cases. Cancer 29:1597-1605, 1972.

Ragab, A. H., Vietti, T. J., Crist, W., Perez, C., and McAllister, W. Bilateral Wilms' tumor. A review. Cancer 30:983-988, 1972.

Rao, P. B. A metastatic Wilms' tumour in the nasopharynx. J. Laryngol. Otol. 83:381-386, 1969.

Raubitschek, H. Uber eine bösartige Nierengeschwulste bei einem kindlichen Hermaphroditen. Frank. Z. Pathol. 10:206-218, 1912.

Reddy, J. K., Schimke, N., Chang, C. H. J., Svoboda, D. J., Slaven, J., and Therou, L. Beckwith-Wiedemann syndrome. Wilms' tumor, cardiac hamartoma, persistent visceromegaly, and glomeruloneogenesis in a 2-year-old boy. Arch. Pathol. 94:523-532, 1972.

Ribbert, H. Beiträge zur Kenntniss der Rhabdomyome. Virchows Arch. (Pathol. Anat.) 130:249-278, 1892.

Riopelle, J. L., and Jasmin, G. Discussion sur la nature des tumeurs renales induites chez le rat par le dimethylnitrosamine. Rev. Can. Biol. 22:365-381, 1963.

..........., and Jasmin, G. Nature, classification, and nomenclature of kidney tumors induced in the rat by dimethylnitrosamine. J. Natl. Cancer Inst. 42:643-662, 1969.

Samuels, L. D. Scans in children with renal tumors. J. Urol. 107:127-132, 1972.

Schuberg, Von W. Einige Mittheilungen. 3. Beobachtung von Carcinoma renis dextri et vesicae urinaria. Virchows Arch. (Pathol. Anat.) 21:291-305, 1861.

Shanklin, D. R., and Sotelo-Avila, C. In situ tumors in fetuses, newborns, and young infants. Biol. Neonate 14:286-316, 1969.

Smith, J. W., Pinkel, D., and Dabrowski, S. Detection of a small virus in a cultivated human Wilms' tumor. Cancer 24:527-531, 1969.

Smith, N. J. Glomerulonephritis, Wilms's tumor and horseshoe kidney in an infant. Arch. Pathol. 42:549-554, 1946.

Snyder, W. H., Hastings, T. N., and Polloc, W. F. Wilms' Tumor: Embryoma of the Kidney, pp. 1024-1037. In: Pediatric Surgery, 2d ed., Vol. 2. (Eds.) Mustard, W. T., Ravitch, M. M., Snyder, W. H., Welch, K. J., and Benson, C. D. Chicago: Year Book Medical Publishers, 1969.

Soper, R. T. Management of recurrent or metastatic Wilms' tumor. Surgery 50:555-559, 1961.

Spear, G. S., Hyde, T. P., Gruppo, R. A., and Slusser, R. Pseudohermaphroditism, glomerulonephritis with the nephrotic syndrome, and Wilms' tumor in infancy. J. Pediatr. 79:677-681, 1971.

Stanton, M. F., and Otsuka, H. Morphology of the oncogenic response of hamsters to polyoma virus infection. J. Natl. Cancer Inst. 31:365-409, 1963.

Stump, T. A., and Garrett, R. A. Bilateral Wilms's tumor in a male pseudohermaphrodite. J. Urol. 72:1146-1152, 1954.

Sukarochana, K., and Kiesewetter, W. B. Wilms' tumor: Factors influencing long-term survival. J. Pediatr. 69:747-752, 1966.

Sullivan, M. P., Hussey, D. H., and Ayala, A. G. Wilms' Tumor, pp. 359-383. In: Clinical Pediatric Oncology. (Eds.) Sutow, W. W., Vietti, T. J., and Fernbach, D. J. St. Louis: C. V. Mosby Co., 1973.

Tannenbaum, M. Ultrastructural pathology of human renal cell tumors. Pathol. Annu. 6:249-277, 1971.

Taykurt, A. Wilms tumor at lower end of the ureter extending to the bladder: case report. J. Urol. 107:142-143, 1972.

Thomas, C., Wessel, W., and Citoler, P. Histochemische, elektronenmikroskopische und autoradiographische Untersuchungen an experimentell erzeugten Nephroblastomen. Beitr. Pathol. 145:68-82, 1972.

Thompson, M. R., Emmanuel, I. G., Campbell, M. S., and Zachary, R. B. Extrarenal Wilms' tumors. J. Pediatr. Surg. 8:37-41, 1973.

Tremblay, M. Ultrastructure of a Wilms' tumour and myogenesis. J. Pathol. 105:269-277, 1971.

Vesselinovitch, S. D., and Mihailovich, N. The development of neurogenic neoplasms, embryonal kidney tumors, Harderian gland adenomas, Anitschkow cell sarcomas of the heart, and other neoplasms in urethan-treated newborn rats. Cancer Res. 28:888-897, 1968.

Virag, I., and Modan, B. Epidemiologic aspects of neoplastic diseases in Israeli immigrant population. II. Malignant neoplasms in childhood. Cancer 23:137-141, 1969.

Vlachos, J., and Tsakraklides, V. A case of renal dysplasia and its relation to "Bilateral Nephroblastomatosis." J. Pathol. 95:560-562, 1968.

Walker, D., and Richard, G. A. Fetal hamartoma of the kidney: Recurrence and death of patient. J. Urol. 110:352-353, 1973.

Walker, R. Embryonal nephroma in a calf. J. Am. Vet. Med. Assoc. 102:7-10, 1943.

Watkins, J. P. Wilms' tumor with ureteral metastases extending into the bladder. J. Urol. 77:593-596, 1957.

Wedemeyer, P. P., White, J. G., Nesbit, M. E., Aust, J. B., Leonard, A. S., D'Angio, G. J., and Krivit, W. Resection of metastases in Wilms' tumor: A report of three cases cured of pulmonary and hepatic metastases. Pediatrics 41:446-451, 1963.

Weigert, C. Adenocarcinoma renum congenitum. Virchows Arch. (Pathol. Anat.) 67:492-500, 1876.

Wigger, H. J. Fetal hamartoma of kidney. A benign, symptomatic, congenital tumor, not a form of Wilms' tumor. Am. J. Clin. Pathol. 51:323-337, 1969.

Williams, D. I. Nephroblastoma: Clinical Picture and Diagnosis, pp. 235-254. In: Monographs on Neoplastic Disease at Various Sites, Vol. V. Tumours of the Kidney and Ureter. (Ed.) Riches, E. W. Baltimore: Williams & Wilkins Co.; Edinburgh: E. & S. Livingstone, Ltd., 1964.

Willis, R. A. Pathology of Tumours, 4th ed. New York: Appleton-Century-Crofts, 1968.

Wilms, M. Die Mischgeschwülste der Niere, pp. 5-90. In: Die Mischgeschwülste. Leipzig: A. Georgi, 1899.

Zunin, C., and Soave, F. Association of nephrotic syndrome and nephroblastoma in siblings. Ann. Paediatr. (Basel) 203:29-38, 1964.

Zwart, P. A nephroblastoma in a fire-bellied newt, Cynops pyrrhogaster. Cancer Res. 30:2691-2694, 1970.

RENAL ADENOCARCINOMA

SYNONYMS AND RELATED TERMS: Hyper-nephroma; Grawitz tumor; metanephroma; malignant nephroma; alveolar carcinoma; clear cell carcinoma; dark cell adenocarcinoma; granular cell carcinoma; renal cell carcinoma.

DEFINITION. Renal adenocarcinoma is a carcinoma which arises from the proximal convoluted tubular epithelial cells. Since the nephron is of mesodermal origin, the use of **adenocarcinoma** has occasionally been challenged. Despite its germ layer origin, the proximal convoluted tubule is morphologically and functionally epithelial and its malignant counterpart is best described by the term renal adenocarcinoma. Because of the extremely variable histologic structures seen in this tumor, the adenomatous pattern at times may be difficult to identify.

Difficulty in recognizing the adenomatous pattern has been a longstanding problem for pathologists. The earliest reports in the literature described this tumor as a sarcoma and as a lipoma of the kidney (König; Grawitz). Distinguishing between a sarcomatoid renal adenocarcinoma and true sarcomas of the kidney is at times still a troublesome problem for pathologists.

PATHOGENESIS

Historical Aspects

By now the historical aspects concerning the controversy over the histogenesis of renal adenocarcinoma are well known. They are reviewed in detail elsewhere and are only briefly summarized here (Bennington and Kradjian).

In 1883, Grawitz, who was influenced by the Cohnheim **cell-rest** theory of neoplasia and who had observed occasional rests of ectopic adrenal tissue in the renal cortex, concluded that adenocarcinomas of the kidney, then regarded as lipomas, arose from such adrenal rests. Ten years later, Sudeck became the first to propose that renal adenocarcinomas arose from cells of the renal tubules. While many pathologists supported Sudeck's observations, bitter controversy persisted for nearly 70 years until Oberling and associates demonstrated electron microscopically the striking similarity between cells of the proximal convoluted tubules and renal adenocarcinoma.

Histogenesis

The observations of Oberling have been confirmed and extended to renal tumors of the rat (Seljelid and Ericsson; Tannenbaum; Seljelid). Spontaneously occurring renal adenomas, as well as renal adenomas and adenocarcinomas induced in the rat by dimethylnitrosamine and by lead compounds, show the characteristic fine structures seen in the proximal convoluted tubules in the rat which are similar to those seen in man (Bernstein; Hard and Butler, 1971; Mao and Molnar).

The terms **Grawitz tumor** and **hyper-nephroma** perpetuate the long held misconception of the histogenetic origin of adenocarcinoma of the renal parenchyma and, while well entrenched in the medical literature and vocabulary, are best abandoned. Descriptive terms such as **clear cell carcinoma, dark cell carcinoma, malignant nephroma, alveolar carcinoma, and metanephroma** are generally inadequate and have nothing to recommend them. The term **renal adenocarcinoma** is preferable. It is sufficiently descriptive and is consistent with the now well established concept of an origin from cells of the renal tubule.

The electron microscopic features of the various anatomic structures of the nephron are described on page 6 and those of the renal adenocarcinoma on page 156. A characteristic structure, found on the surface of the cells in the renal adenocarcinoma and cells of the proximal convoluted tubule but not elsewhere in the nephron, is the presence of tightly packed microvilli forming a brush border. Immunofluorescent studies using antibodies to brush border antigens (specific for cells of the proximal convoluted tubule) and to Tamm-Horsfall antigen (specific for cells of the distal convoluted tubule and loop of Henle) reveal that cells comprising renal adenocarcinomas and so-called renal adenomas react uniformly with brush border antibodies, but not with antibodies to Tamm-Horsfall antigen (Wallace and Nairn). These immunologic studies strengthen the concept that renal adenocarcinomas are derived exclusively from cells of the proximal convoluted tubule, since they contain an antigen found nowhere else in the normal kidney and apparently do not contain antigens found in cells from the distal convoluted tubule and loop of Henle. The possibility that, sometime in the future, tumors or areas of tumors not yet studied may reveal participation by cells of distal or other tubules cannot be excluded, but all current data points to the proximal tubules as the origin for these tumors.

Apitz proposed that the cells of Bowman's capsule participated in the development of renal neoplasms. Very occasionally, the parietal layer of Bowman's capsule undergoes a metaplastic change with replacement of the normal cells by tall, columnar epithelial cells (fig. 78) with a brush border which stains intensely with periodic acid-Schiff stain (Reidbord; Ward).

Frequently, direct continuity can be demonstrated from the proximal tubular epithelium to the metaplastic epithelium of Bowman's capsule (Ward). While epithelial cells of Bowman's capsule have been implicated in the development of renal adenocarcinomas induced in mice by whole body X-radiation, there is no evidence that the normal or metaplastic cells of Bowman's capsule or cells of the glomerulus ever give rise to renal adenocarcinoma in man (Berdjis).

DEVELOPMENT OF RENAL ADENOCARCINOMA AND ITS RELATION TO RENAL ADENOMA. Not long after carcinoma of the kidney was first described, reports began to appear of small, well differentiated glandular tumors of the renal cortex which were regarded as the benign counterpart of the renal adenocarcinoma; these were called **renal adenomas**. Apitz and Newcomb reported approximately 7 percent of individuals over the age of 15 years, examined at autopsy, had such neoplasms. However, investigators soon discovered that if renal adenomas existed, they were difficult to recognize. As early as 1908, Greene and Brooks wrote, "As we grow more familiar with the hypernephromata, most of us are inclined to place among these many or most of the tumors previously considered as adenomata. Thus, two cases of adenomata of the kidney reported by one of us have been subsequently classified as hypernephromata."

Many pathologists shared this cautious approach to the problem of diagnosing the renal adenoma. As Fite remarked, "The similarities between cancerous and noncancerous tumors of the renal cortex are sufficiently great that a description of one is almost a description of the other." But in spite of the lack of any documented cri-

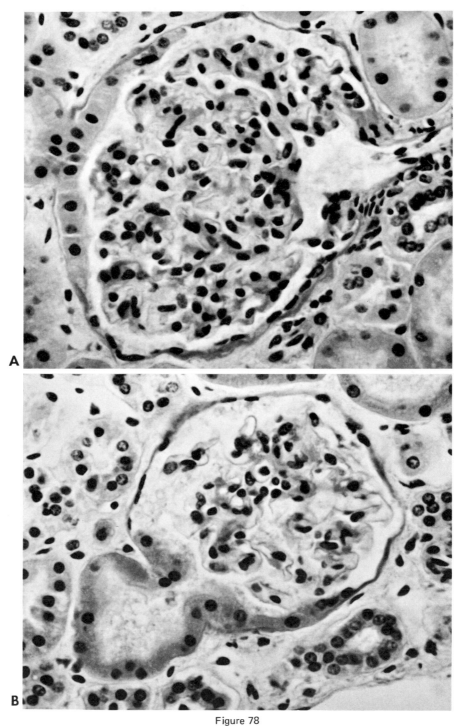

Figure 78
TUBULAR METAPLASIA OF GLOMERULUS
  A. Prominent tubular metaplasia is seen in this capsular epithelium of a glomerulus opposite the vascular pole. Approx.
X400.
  B. Illustrated is a glomerulus with tubular metaplasia of capsular epithelium continuous with normal tubular epithelium.
Approx. X350. (Figs. 1, 3 from Ward, A. M. Tubular metaplasia in Bowman's capsule. J. Clin. Pathol. 23:472-474, 1970.)

teria for the diagnosis of renal adenoma, the concept was popular and became established through constant usage. Later, when Bell published his findings which showed that renal cortical glandular tumors less than 3 cm. in diameter rarely metastasize, these results were accepted as proof of the existence of renal adenoma and size became the *sine qua non* for its diagnosis.

There was almost complete disregard of Bell's other observations; that is, that two tumors less than 2 cm. had metastasized and a large percentage of tumors greater than 10 cm. in diameter had not. The fact that all renal adenocarcinomas sometime in their evolution must measure less than 3 cm. was largely ignored or explained by hypothesizing an origin in a preexisting renal adenoma (Nicholson; deVeer and Hamm; Kozoll and Kirshbaum; Stoerk; Hicks; Long et al.; Newcomb). Unusually large renal tumors without accompanying metastases were frequently reported as benign, therefore proving that renal adenomas did occur (Ellner et al.; Higgins). Thus, the concept of size was adapted to fit the observed clinical or pathologic findings. In the final analysis, however, the real distinguishing feature was the presence or absence of metastases. This circular reasoning developed because without knowing tumor size there are no gross, histologic, histochemical, immunologic, or ultrastructural features yet identified which will reliably distinguish renal adenocarcinoma from so-called adenoma. Reports to the contrary are based on arbitrary distinctions.

The points of similarity between the so-called renal adenoma and renal adenocarcinoma include:

1. Both renal adenoma and adenocarcinoma arise from cells of the proximal convoluted tubule. This has been demon-strated electron microscopically and immunologically (Ericsson et al.; Fisher and Horvat; Pratt-Thomas et al.; Oberling et al.; Seljelid; Seljelid and Ericsson; Wallace and Nairn).

2. There are no light microscopic, histochemical, or electron microscopic features that distinguish one from the other, and any of the histologic patterns seen in renal adenomas may be seen in renal adenocarcinoma (fig. 79)—in humans and experimental animals (Ericsson et al.; Fisher and Horvat; Hard and Butler; Mao and Molnar; Oberling et al.; Pratt-Thomas et al.; Seljelid; Seljelid et al.).

3. Adenomas occur more frequently in kidneys containing a renal adenocarcinoma (Cristol et al.).

4. Both adenoma and adenocarcinoma occur in the same age range (rarely under 30 and then increasing with age), and show the same marked male predominance (2-4/1) (Cristol et al.; Xipell).

5. Both renal adenoma and adenocarcinoma occur with the same increased frequency among tobacco users (Bennington and Laubscher; Bennington et al.).

6. Considering all renal cortical glandular tumors, there is a direct relationship between tumor size and the frequency of metastasis (Bell; McDonald and Priestly).

Willis (1968) has suggested that hyperplastic renal tubules and the cysts in kidneys damaged by scarring give rise to renal adenomas and renal adenocarcinomas. Evidence against this theory, much of which is derived from the experimental production of renal adenocarcinomas, has been reviewed by Bennington and Kradjian. In general, it appears that neither cyst formation nor arterionephrosclerosis are related to the development of renal neoplasms, and they are almost certainly not instrumental in such neoplasia. They are

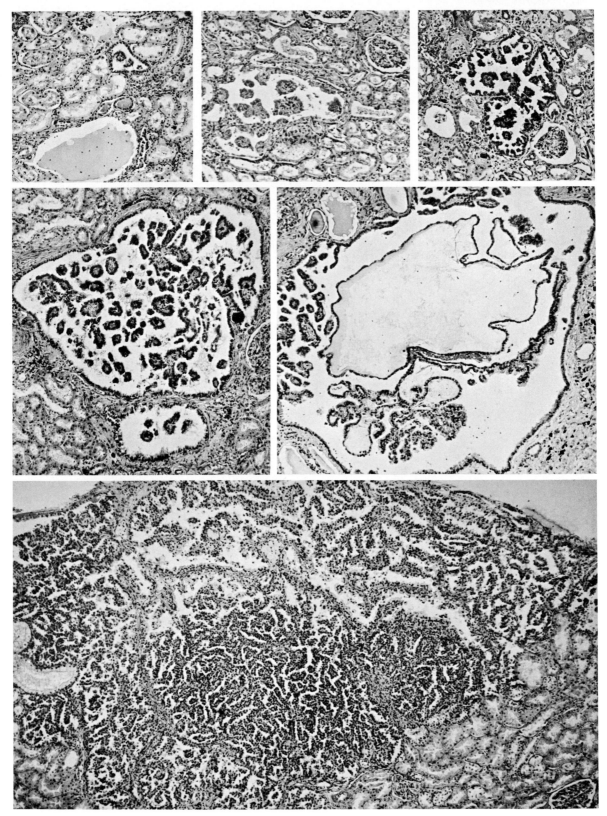

Figure 79
RENAL ADENOMA
The evolution of the so-called renal adenoma from in situ changes of nuclear hyperchromasia and papillary proliferation in a single proximal convoluted tubule, through successively larger tumors, shows increasing complexity. Clear and/or granular cells as well as cystic, trabecular, and papillary patterns are seen in these minute tumors. Each, X50.

probably epiphenomena, as are cataracts, representing only aging changes.

Because there are no morphologic criteria which can be used to distinguish renal adenoma, and because such small cortical glandular tumors can manifest their aggressiveness by perforating their capsule (fig. 80) or metastasizing in spite of benign cytologic pattern, we accept the view first expressed by McDonald and Priestly and

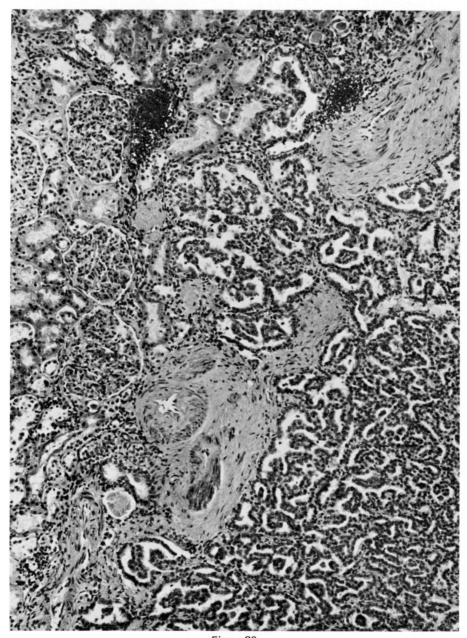

Figure 80
RENAL ADENOMA
A renal adenoma less than 1.5 cm. in diameter shows perforation of the tumor capsule at several points. X130.

now supported by many other authors that the so-called **adenoma** is a small renal adenocarcinoma which has not yet produced metastases (Bennington and Kradjian; Cristol et al.; Evans; Fisher and Horvat).

The small renal cortical glandular tumors, less than 3 cm. in greatest diameter, are almost invariably found incidentally at autopsy, so their classification is of no consequence to the patient. When, rarely, such a tumor is found at surgery, the diagnostic terminology becomes much more important than philosophic or epistomologic distinction. On the one hand, the diagnosis of renal adenoma carries all the authority of a benign disease and does not raise the warning flag that such tumors occasionally metastasize. On the other hand, the diagnosis of renal adenocarcinoma, even with the comment that metastasis is unlikely, carries with it all the overtones of "cancer" for the patient and his family. However, we still feel that it is best to diagnose all such small cortical glandular neoplasms of the kidney as renal adenocarcinoma when found during surgery. The comment that such tumors offer an excellent prognosis but occasionally do metastasize may be added. While we cannot yet predict histologically those tumors that will metastasize, we can hope that raising the possibility of metastasis might help the surgeon to plan the treatment and follow-up for the patient.

The debate whether or not renal adenoma is a benign or malignant tumor may also be of epidemiologic importance. The so-called renal adenoma is many times more frequent than renal adenocarcinoma. If, as we believe, renal adenoma is in fact a small carcinoma, then, even though small renal adenocarcinomas are slow-growing, we may expect that with increasing longev-ity, the incidence of clinically apparent renal adenocarcinoma will rise and that early diagnosis of small cortical glandular tumors will become increasingly important.

Comparative Pathology

Natural Occurrence of Renal Adenocarcinoma in Lower Animals. Among lower animals, both wild and domesticated, adenocarcinoma of the kidney is uncommon. In spite of large numbers of laboratory animals which have been examined as control studies on carcinogenesis, as well as in other various research studies, there are relatively few reports of naturally occurring renal adenocarcinomas in mice, rats, guinea pigs, rabbits, and monkeys, and none in hamsters (Bennington and Kradjian; Guerin et al.). Renal adenocarcinomas have been reported in sheep (fig. 81), cows, pigs, dogs (fig 82), horses, and chickens, as well as in a variety of wild animals including squirrels, marsupials, monkeys (fig. 83), birds, fish, and frogs (fig. 84) (Monlux et al.; Sandison and Anderson; Jabara; Blanchard and Montpellier; Guerin et al.; Lucké).

Experimentally Induced Renal Adenocarcinoma. Renal adenocarcinomas have been produced in experimental animals by chemical, physical, and viral agents. A relatively short time ago there were comparatively few such reports; however, in the past few years the ability of a host of agents to induce renal adenocarcinoma as well as other carcinomas of the urinary tract has been recorded. (See sections on nephroblastoma and renal pelvis and ureteral carcinoma on pp. 44 and 247).

CHEMICAL AGENTS. The first report of an experimentally induced adenocarcinoma by systemic administration of a carcinogen was made in 1939 by Sempronj and Morelli, who used beta-anthraquinoline

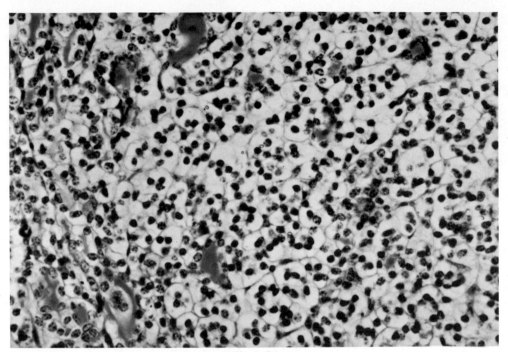

Figure 81
RENAL ADENOCARCINOMA FROM SHEEP
This clear cell renal adenocarcinoma was from a sheep. X520. (Fig. 8 from Sandison, A. T., and Anderson, L. J. Tumors of the kidney in cattle, sheep, and pigs. Cancer 21:727-742, 1968.)

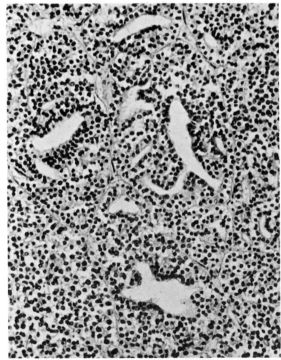

Figure 82
RENAL ADENOCARCINOMA FROM DOG
This clear cell renal adenocarcinoma from a dog shows trabecular and tubular patterns. X180. (Fig. 2 from Jabara, A. G. Three cases of primary malignant neoplasms arising in the canine urinary system. J. Comp. Pathol. 78:335-339, 1968.)

Figure 82

injected subcutaneously in rats. Since then, a wide variety of chemical agents have been used successfully to produce renal tumors which appear to be the counterpart of human renal adenocarcinoma.

Aromatic Hydrocarbons. In addition to beta-anthraquinoline, 4 H-cyclopent (def) phenanthrene has been used in rats and 7,12-dimethylbenz(a)anthracene in rats and mice to produce renal adenocarcinoma. These compounds show no special predilection for the kidney. Their mode of action is not yet known (Bennington and Kradjian; Guerin et al.).

Aromatic Amines and Amides. A number of different aromatic amines and amides have been used to produce renal adenocarcinomas in rats, mice, chickens, and in one instance in a dog (Bennington and Kradjian; Guerin et al.). It is thought that these compounds are not proximate carcinogens but exert their effect as alkylating agents after initial N-hydroxylation and possibly subsequent N-hydroxy esterification or sulfation. Tumor formation which is favored in certain organs, such as kidney and liver, may depend upon the availability of enzymes for activation of

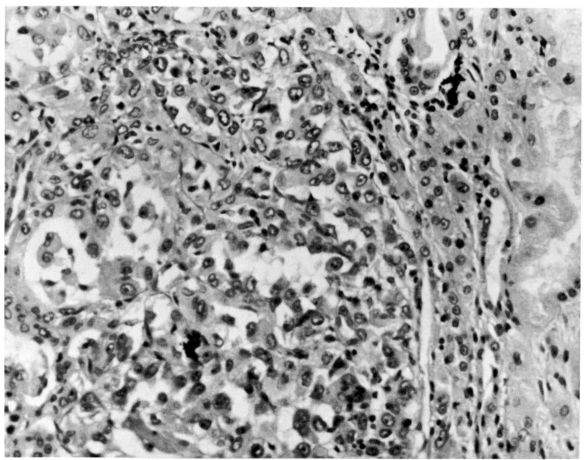

Figure 83
RENAL ADENOCARCINOMA FROM MONKEY
This renal adenocarcinoma from a monkey is composed of poorly formed tubules. Individual cells are large with prominent nuclei and pale eosinophilic cytoplasm; they show moderate pleomorphism. X275. (Courtesy of Dr. H. L. Ratcliffe, Philadelphia, Pa.)

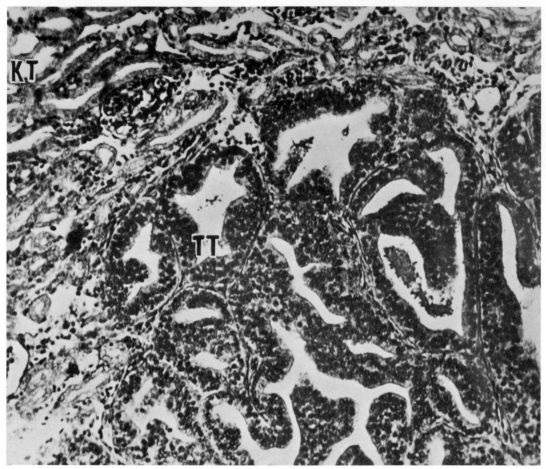

Figure 84
RENAL ADENOCARCINOMA FROM FROG
This renal adenocarcinoma (Lucké renal adenocarcinoma) from a frog is composed of complex, large tumor tubules from a well circumscribed renal cortical nodule. Normal Kidney Tubules (KT). Tumor Tubules (TT). X384. (Fig. 1 from Barch, S. H., Shaver, J. R., and Wilson, G. B. Some aspects of the ultrastructure of cells of the Lucké renal adenocarcinoma. Ann. N. Y. Acad. Sci. 126:188-203, 1965.)

these agents to their carcinogenic form at these sites (Miller and Miller).

Aliphatic Compounds. Urethane (ethyl carbamate) and more frequently the group of N-Nitroso and related compounds have been used to produce renal adenocarcinomas in rats and mice (Guerin et al.; Vesselinovitch and Mihailovich; Bennington and Kradjian; Swann and Magee; Terracini et al.). Dimethylnitrosamine, N-methylnitrosourea, ethyl methanesulphonate, and methylazoxymethanol, and certain antibiotics are chemically related and produce identical renal carcinomas in rats (Magee; Druckrey et al.; Swann and Magee; Spatz; Arison and Feudale; Sternberg et al.)

The acylalkylnitroamides in this group react by heterolysis to a deacylated product which is further degraded in pathways similar to dialkylnitrosamines; that is, hydroxylation to active alkylating agents (Druckrey et al.).

Specific organotropic effects may be related to localized metabolic conversion of an inactive to an active carcinogen as is the case of dimethylnitrosamine by hydroxylation and subsequent demethylation to diazomethane, or in the compound cycasin by deglucosylation to the aglycone, methylazoxymethanol, which is unstable and subsequently demethylated to form diazomethane (Druckrey et al.; Spatz). Similar pathways are likely for the antibiotics Streptozotocin and Daunomycin which contain an aglycone related to methylazoxymethanol and are also capable of producing renal tumors in rats (Arison and Feudale; Sternberg et al.). These studies are relevant in that dimethylnitrosamine is identifiable in tobacco smoke (Johnson; Serfontein and Hurter); and cycasin in the cycad nut from the plant *Cycas circanalis* (Spatz), as well as the palmlike plant, *Encephalartos hildebrandtii*, also of the family *Cyccadaceae* (Mugera and Nderito), which are used as food by natives of Guam and Africa, respectively. The antibiotics Streptozotocin and Daunomycin are employed as cancer chemotherapeutic agents. Both compounds have been used to induce experimental renal adenocarcinomas, but have not been implicated as causing human renal adenocarcinoma (Arison and Feudale; Sternberg et al.).

Aflatoxins. The aflatoxins are admixtures of metabolites produced by the fungus *Aspergillus flavus* and are toxic or carcinogenic to a number of species. Both aflatoxins B1 and B2 contain lactone moieties which are carcinogenic and may function as alkylating agents, although the mechanism of carcinogenesis of these compounds is not well established (Van Duuren). They are found as contaminants in a variety of foodstuffs, and certain of the aflatoxins have a propensity for producing renal adenocarcinomas, renal pelvic carcinomas, and hepatocellular carcinomas in rats (Epstein et al.). Since aflatoxins can contaminate foods ingested by humans, their role in the epidemiology of human renal tumors must be considered.

Hormones. Renal tumors histologically similar to human renal adenocarcinoma and arising in the proximal convoluted tubules have been induced in male and gonadectomized female hamsters by prolonged administration of large doses of estrogens (Kirkman). The uniqueness of this tumor model is indicated by the lack of naturally occurring renal adenocarcinomas in hamsters, resistance of the species to induction of renal tumors by chemical and physical agents which are routinely effective in rats and mice, and inability of estrogen to induce renal adenocarcinomas in other experimental animals. The mode of action and relation to human renal adenocarcinomas is not known. A possible relation is suggested by the observation that exogenous progesterone inhibits the estrogen induction of renal adenocarcinomas in hamsters and also produces some objective evidence of regression in metastatic renal adenocarcinomas in humans with statistically greater benefits for men than women (Bloom).

Lead Compounds. Oral and parenteral administration of certain lead compounds over long periods of time induce renal adenocarcinomas in rats, which are histologically and electron microscopically indistinguishable from the human renal adenocarcinoma (Boyland et al.; Mao and Molnar). However, clinical studies on patients chronically exposed to lead over many years have not demonstrated evidence for a greater frequency of renal adenocarcinomas in individuals with lead exposure than those in the general population (Dingwall-Fordyce and Lane; Radosevic et al.).

PHYSICAL AGENTS. Neoplasms described as renal adenomas and renal adenocarcinomas have been observed in rats and mice after whole body X-radiation and neutron radiation (Bennington and Kradjian; Guerin et al.). Whether or not exposure to comparable doses in man results in the development of renal adenocarcinoma has not yet been determined. To date, there have been no reports of an increased number of renal adenocarcinomas in individuals exposed to atomic explosions or other large doses of radiation. However, there have been instances of renal adenocarcinomas developing in patients many years after the use of thorotrast (a weak alpha emitter) as a radiopaque substance for pyelographic studies (Bennington and Kradjian).

VIRAL AGENTS. Renal adenocarcinomas, histologically similar to those in man that appear to arise in the proximal convoluted tubule, have been produced experimentally in chickens with MH2 reticuloendothelial, ES4 erythroleukemia, TCHF-I erythroblastic, and RPL viruses, and in frogs by the Lucké virus (Lucké; Guerin). In spite of these findings, there has been no evidence to date to support a viral etiology of the human renal adenocarcinoma.

EPIDEMIOLOGY

Age

The age range for patients with renal adenocarcinoma extends from six months to old age (Scotti; Bell). In surveys on the age distribution of patients with renal adenocarcinoma in which the number of patients in each age group of the population has not been standardized to a common base, the peak incidence of this tumor appears to occur at the sixth decade (Bell). Cancer rates per 100,000 population in each age interval, which undoubtedly are more representative of the true incidence of renal adenocarcinoma, taken from the California Alameda County Cancer Registry records (1960–1969) are shown in Graph II. These figures indicate that the incidence of renal adenocarcinoma increases with each passing decade and to a certain extent must be regarded as a progressive process associated with aging.

Incidence figures from large epidemiologic studies with estimated corrections for the inclusion of renal pelvic carcinoma and nephroblastoma are in close agreement with those obtained from the Alameda County Cancer Registry records (Ferber et al.; Morbidity from Cancer in U. S., Public Health Mono. 56; Osborn).

At the time of this writing, fewer than 100 renal adenocarcinomas have been reported in children (Bjelke; Dehner; Palma et al.). Renal adenocarcinoma appears to represent less than 1.5 percent of all renal tumors in children, but represents the majority of renal tumors in adolescents and young adults (Bjelke; Love et al.). From one study reporting the relative frequency of renal adenocarcinoma and nephroblastoma among children and young adults, there were 66 malignant renal tumors. In 63 patients 0 to 9 years, there were 62 nephroblastomas and one renal adenocarcinoma, and in three patients 10 to 19 years, there were two renal adenocarcinomas and one nephroblastoma (Bjelke). Grossly and histologically, renal adenocarcinoma in children is indistinguishable from that of adults (figs. 85, 86).

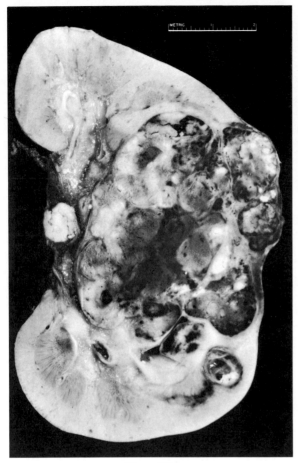

Figure 85
RENAL ADENOCARCINOMA
(Figures 85 and 86 from same case)
This renal adenocarcinoma, which measured 7 cm. in diameter, was removed from the left kidney of a boy aged 8 years, 11 months. Extensive para-aortic lymph node metastases were present at the time of resection.

Figure 86
RENAL ADENOCARCINOMA
(Figures 85 and 86 from same case)
Microscopic features of the renal adenocarcinoma illustrated in figure 85 show (A) solid areas of clear and vacuolated cells with a delicate fibrovascular stroma, X125, and (B) tubular structures formed by cells of the same type as those seen in (A) as well as papillary projections, X320.

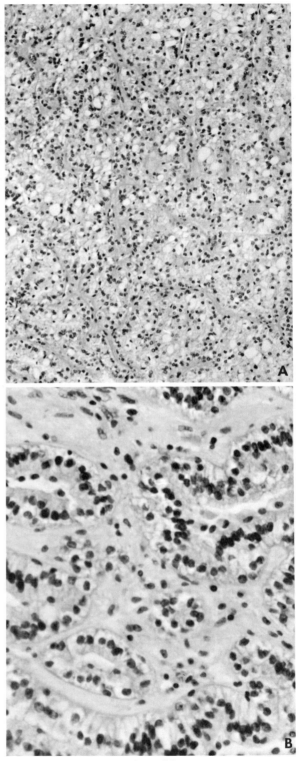

Figure 86

Sex

Renal adenocarcinoma affects more males than females, both in children and in adults (Bjelke; Steiner). Our review of various reported series reveals that about twice as many renal adenocarcinomas are observed in males as in females; however, after adjusting the rates to compensate for more females in the population than males, especially in the older age groups, it is apparent that the true incidence of renal adenocarcinoma is nearly three times as great in males as in females (Graph II; Bennington and Kradjian). While the frequency of occurrence of renal adenocarcinoma rises steadily with each passing decade, the ratio of males to females with renal adenocarcinoma remains fairly constant.

Geographic and Racial Distribution

Steiner reported that in the African Negro, all carcinomas of the kidney appeared to have about the same frequency relative to other cancers as in the United States, although it seemed that they were less frequent compared to other malignant neoplasms in Mexico, Japan, China, and the Philippines. Unfortunately, the proportion of renal adenocarcinomas to other carcinomas of the kidney is not known in these racial groups.

There are no reliable figures comparing the frequency of renal adenocarcinoma in different racial populations, but it is known to occur in Indians, Chinese, Blacks, Japanese, Filipinos, and Malays (Ali and Muir; Breslow and Milmore; Case; Cooray; Quinland and Cuff; Steiner). In his analysis of the frequency of renal adenocarcinoma among patients of different races who were examined at autopsy in the Los Angeles County Hospital, Steiner found no differences for Caucasians, Mexicans, or Blacks.

The data for Japanese, Chinese, and Filipino patients were not sufficient to warrant any conclusions. On a larger scale, the percentage of Caucasian, Black, Chinese, and Japanese persons in male and female populations in California from 1942 through 1969 may be compared to the percentage of malignant renal tumors found in each of these groups (Table II). Black males appear to have a significantly lower incidence of malignant renal tumors than Caucasian males (at the 1 percent confidence level), an incidence comparable to that for Caucasian and Black females. These figures may be biased by nature of the population served by the hospitals reporting to the California Tumor Registry; however, a low frequency of renal carcinoma in the Black male has also been observed by Hajdu and Thomas. In the California survey, as in Steiner's series, the number of malignant renal tumors in persons of Japanese or Chinese ancestry is too small for statistical analysis.

Heredity

In the majority of laboratory animals, renal adenocarcinoma is almost nonexistent. Exceptions to this are a strain of Wistar rats discovered by Eker, with a high frequency of bilateral renal tumors which he interpreted as adenomas, and a strain of laboratory mice in which renal adenocarcinomas were present in both sexes (Claude). A genetic influence has been postulated for both instances. In the rats, the presence of tumor has been attributed to a dominant gene (Eker and Mossige). Ratcliffe reported the occurrence of renal adenocarcinomas in four Rhesus monkeys of the same family. This is an isolated instance, but a striking one considering the relative infrequency of reports of renal adenocarcinoma in monkeys (Kent).

The familial distribution of renal adenocarcinoma in humans was reported by Brinton in which at least one of the parents and 3 of 5 children developed renal adenocarcinoma. There are other instances in which two members of the immediate family had renal adenocarcinoma (Klinger; Mingazzini; Riches, 1963; Rusche). However, cases of this type appear to be quite rare. Riches, 1963, observed only one instance among 130 cases, and if this is indicative of the frequency, such cases may be due merely to chance.

Renal adenocarcinomas have also been linked with certain hereditary diseases. Development in the kidneys of patients with polycystic disease may be a striking occurrence, but the small number of such instances reported up until 1954 is hardly impressive in view of the frequency of polycystic disease in the population (1 in less than 1000 patients) (Bell; Borski and Kimbrough; Johnson; Dalgaard). Renal adenocarcinoma in the horseshoe kidney also appears to be sporadic and not due to any hereditary influence (Blackard and Mellinger). On the other hand, renal adenocarcinomas are common in patients with von Hippel-Lindau disease. Lindau originally considered these lesions to be adenomas, but more recently other authors have established that the majority of these tumors are renal adenocarcinomas (Greene and Rosenthal; Kernohan et al.; Tonning et al.). Von Hippel-Lindau disease is one of a number of related conditions grouped under the heading of phakomatoses. These include tuberous sclerosis, neurofibromatosis, Sturge-Weber syndrome, and ataxia telangiectasia. Because of overlapping clinical manifestations among these conditions, there is a possibility of a common etiologic relationship (Melmon and Rosen). An association with renal adenocarcinoma in these other diseases should be looked for, although none yet has been documented. However, the association of renal angiomyolipomas and the tuberous sclerosis complex is well documented (see p. 204).

Etiologic Factors

Infectious Agents. Oncogenic viruses have been demonstrated in the renal adenocarcinomas of frogs and fowl (Guerin et al.). Since viruses may be carried in the latent state for many years and are often difficult to demonstrate, the possible role of viruses in human renal adenocarcinoma must be considered. However, no viral type inclusions have been demonstrated to date in the human renal adenocarcinoma.

Sex Hormones. The possible role of sex hormones in the development of renal adenocarcinoma is suggested by the observed greater frequency of this tumor in men than women, and the experimental production of renal adenocarcinomas in male hamsters by long term administration of estrogens (Kirkman; Guerin et al.). On the other hand, sex difference in the frequency of various diseases is well known and may be attributed to factors other than the direct influence of sex hormones. While renal adenocarcinomas have been induced in hamsters with estrogens, they have not been produced in this manner in other experimental animals, nor have there been any reports of an increased frequency of renal adenocarcinoma in men undergoing prolonged treatment with estrogens for prostatic carcinoma.

Willis (1968) has suggested that differences in the frequency of this carcinoma in men and women may be due to different rates of exposure to occupational hazards. Potential chemical and physical agents are discussed in the following paragraphs.

Chemical Agents. A number of chemical carcinogens have been used to experimentally induce renal adenocarcinomas in a wide variety of laboratory animals (Bennington and Kradjian; Guerin et al.). None of these agents or industrial chemicals known to induce carcinomas of the bladder, renal pelvis, and ureter have been definitely linked to human renal adenocarcinoma.

Physical Agents. While radiation (x-ray and neutron) has been used to produce renal adenocarcinomas in mice and rats, there is no indication that the frequency of renal adenocarcinoma is increased in individuals exposed to atomic explosions or other high levels of radiation (Guerin et al.). There have been instances of renal adenocarcinoma developing in patients many years after the use of thorotrast, a weak alpha emitter, as a radiopaque substance for pyelographic studies (Alken et al.; Krueckemeyer et al.).

Habits. The greater frequency of urinary tract carcinoma in men than women may possibly be related to personal habits rather than occupational exposure to industrial carcinogens.

Potential sources for consideration include foodstuffs, drugs, and tobacco. The possibilities have been barely explored, yet there is already considerable evidence along this line. There is a strong association between heavy coffee use and carcinoma of the bladder (Cole), phenacetin abuse and carcinoma of the renal pelvis (Bengtsson et al.; Buch et al.), and various forms of tobacco use and carcinomas of the bladder and kidney (Bennington and Laubscher; Wynder et al.).

Smoking, especially cigars and pipes, is predominantly a masculine habit and shows a strong statistical association with adenocarcinoma of the kidney. The estimated increased factors of risk for developing renal adenocarcinoma with various forms of tobacco use are: more than 10 cigarettes a day, 5.1; pipe, 10.3; cigars, 12.9; and chewing tobacco, 4.8 (Bennington and Laubscher). The greater use of tobacco by men and its association with renal adenocarcinoma may account in part for the observed sex differentiation in the frequency of the disease.

CLINICAL FINDINGS

Presenting Signs and Symptoms. The earliest signs and symptoms of renal adenocarcinoma are usually nonurologic in origin, and while they may precede the usual urologic signs by months or years, they rarely call attention to the possibility of a renal adenocarcinoma (Melicow and Uson). Because of the varied and unusual presenting symptoms and laboratory findings in renal adenocarcinoma, the patient may be seen first by specialists other than a urologist and subjected to intensive diagnostic investigation before attention is directed to the kidney.

The presentation of renal adenocarcinoma with "hematuria, pain, and a flank mass" is the triad regarded as the classic mode of presentation. The frequency of this triad of symptoms ranges from 15 to 70 percent of patients with renal adenocarcinoma in different series and is usually evidence of advanced disease with a poor prognosis (Evans et al.; Harvey; Ochsner; Pinals and Krane; Reiss). Among patients presenting with this triad of symptoms, nearly 50 percent already harbor distant metastases.

Hematuria. Hematuria is usually painless and is the most important single sign indicating a malignant renal neoplasm (Lee and Davis). Characteristically, the hematuria of renal adenocarcinoma is gross, although instances of microhematuria do occur.

Hematuria indicates neoplastic invasion of the renal collecting system or intrarenal circulation and is usually a late event (fig. 87). This sign occurs at some stage of the disease in over 50 percent of patients and has been reported as a presenting sign in as few as 6 percent to as many as 83 percent of patients.

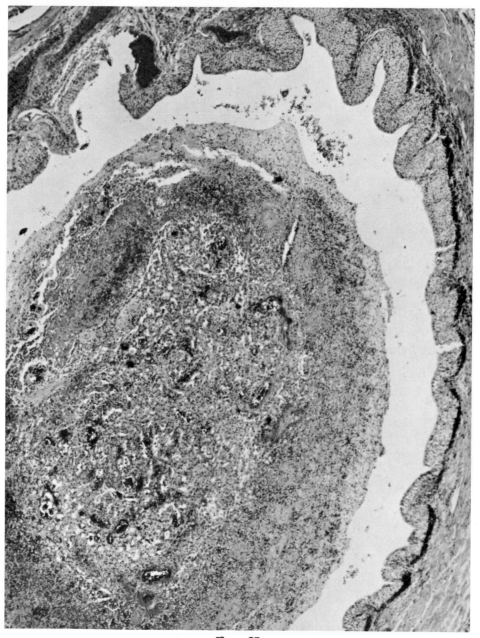

Figure 87
RENAL ADENOCARCINOMA
This renal calix is filled by a renal adenocarcinoma which extended into the renal pelvis. X53.

Pain. Adenocarcinoma of the kidney is clinically silent during its early growth; pain is a late and inconstant symptom, especially in older patients. Estimates of the frequency of clinical pain attributable to renal adenocarcinoma range from fewer than 20 percent to more than 45 percent of patients (Bennington and Kradjian).

Explanations for the genesis of the pain include distension of the renal capsule, secondary to expansion of the tumor, and traction or compression of perinephric structures by a bulky neoplasm.

Renal Mass. The estimates of the frequency of a palpable renal mass in patients with renal adenocarcinoma vary greatly. Reports range from less than 6 percent to over 48 percent of patients (Bennington and Kradjian). Pinals and Krane calculated from reports in the literature that one-third of patients with renal adenocarcinoma present with a palpable mass on initial examination, although detection of a renal adenocarcinoma by incidental discovery of a flank mass in an otherwise asymptomatic patient is rare. A renal tumor sufficiently large to be palpated usually indicates an advanced stage of the disease.

Nonspecific Signs and Symptoms. Because of the late appearance and unreliability of the classic triad of urologic symptoms related to renal adenocarcinoma, it is important to keep in mind the relatively frequent and early nonspecific signs and symptoms in patients with this tumor which include pyrexia, 10 to 20 percent; weight loss, 15 to 30 percent; fatigue, 20 to 40 percent; gastrointestinal complaints (anorexia, nausea, and vomiting), 8 to 14 percent; and neuromuscular abnormalities (neuropathy and myositis), 4 percent (Azzopardi; Bennington and Kradjian; Gordon; Clarke and Goade). These nonspecific signs and symptoms are found singly or in combination, and may be associated with a spectrum of abnormal laboratory and physical findings which are to be discussed.

The basis for the nonspecific systemic manifestations of this disease is unknown and they occur with neoplasms of organs other than the kidneys (Azzopardi).

Physical Findings. The physical findings, other than a flank mass, are relatively infrequent and generally secondary to local extension of the tumor or metastases. Physical manifestations of renal carcinoma secondary to localized metastases include: epistaxsis, hemoptysis, gastrointestinal bleeding and obstruction, headache and psychic disorders, vaginal bleeding, pathologic fractures, pulsating bony masses, soft tissue, thyroid and skin nodules, hepatic vein and vena caval obstruction, acute varicocele, and priapism (Bennington and Kradjian).

Metastases are present in one-third of patients with renal adenocarcinoma at the time of diagnosis, although fewer than 5 percent of patients present with symptoms referable to metastases (Riches, 1963). While such patients have an advanced stage of the disease, the propensity for this tumor to produce a solitary metastasis, in contrast to the characteristically wide distribution of metastases in carcinomas of other organs, should be kept in mind. There have been reports of long survival following nephrectomy and resection of a solitary metastasis (Straus and Scanlon; Riches, 1964).

Hypertension. The frequency of hypertension associated with renal adenocarcinoma is about that expected for the age group in which this tumor is found. In general, it is no greater than for patients without renal disease or with benign renal cysts (Amador et al.; Malament; Melicow and Uson). However, Morlock and Horton studied 144 patients with renal adenocarcinoma and hypertension. Of 46 patients who had preoperative and postoperative blood pressure recorded, 18 became normotensive while 28 had persistent hypertension after nephrectomy. No agent responsible for hypertension in renal adenocarcinoma has yet been demonstrated.

LABORATORY FINDINGS

Erythrocytosis. Renal adenocarcinoma may be associated with erythrocytosis, leukocytosis, and thrombocytosis, alone or in combination. It is estimated that the incidence of polycythemia (a term used in connection with this disease to indicate erythrocytosis with or without elevation of the other blood elements) in patients with renal adenocarcinoma is 1.8 to 6 percent of all cases. Conversely, of patients with polycythemia, 2 to 4 percent have renal adenocarcinoma, and 1 of 3 patients with polycythemia and hematuria will be found to have renal adenocarcinoma (Damon et al.). It is important to note that polycythemia may result from both renal and extrarenal conditions other than carcinoma of the kidney, including renal cysts, polycystic disease of the kidney, pyelonephritis, and hydronephrosis, as well as cerebellar tumors, leiomyomas of the uterus, and hepatocellular carcinomas (Brandt et al.; Murphy et al.; Nixon et al.; Jones et al.; Waldmann et al.; Rothman and Rennard; Lehman et al.). It is frequently stated that the polycythemia associated with renal adenocarcinoma lacks the splenomegaly, thrombocytosis, and leukocytosis of polycythemia rubra vera, but Brandt and associates have shown that this distinction is not always possible. Morphologically, the renal adenocarcinomas associated with polycythemia or erythrocytosis cannot be distinguished from those tumors without these findings.

The erythrocytosis associated with renal adenocarcinoma has in many, but not all cases been associated with an elevation of erythropoietin levels in plasma and other body fluids (Thorling and Ersbak). The kidney is considered a major source of erythropoietin and, therefore, it is not surprising that disease involving the kidney would affect erythropoietin production.

The mechanism by which erythropoietin is elevated in patients with renal adenocarcinoma is unknown, although the various possibilities include: (1) The tumor produces local ischemia which stimulates erythropoietin production; (2) tumor growth mechanically stimulates the erythropoietin apparatus directly; (3) erythropoietin or an erythropoietin-like material is produced by the tumor; and (4) the tumor produces an erythropoietin activator which acts on the existing substrate. Because erythrocytosis associated with renal adenocarcinoma may regress after nephrectomy only to recur coincidentally with the development of metastases, it is apparent that renal ischemia or other effects of the tumor within the kidney are not necessary to produce elevation of erythropoietin (Damon et al.; Frey; Hewlett et al.; Korst et al.; Omland). Demonstrations of high concentrations of erythropoietin in extracts of tumor cells from renal adenocarcinoma indicate that the tumor is actively producing erythropoietin or an erythropoietin-like substance (Hewlett et al.; Thorling and Ersbak).

Anemia. Anemia is much more frequently associated with renal adenocarcinoma than polycythemia. Clarke and Goade reported anemia in 25 percent of patients with this disease. The anemia is usually of the normochromic normocytic type and appears unrelated to hematuria.

Erythrocyte Sedimentation Rate. Erythrocyte sedimentation rate is elevated in nearly two-thirds of patients with renal adenocarcinoma (Olovson). Presumably related are elevations in the levels of haptoglobin, alpha $_1$ and alpha $_2$ globulins, and gamma globulins which are occasionally reported (Böttiger and Ivemark). Abnormalities in serum protein values, in association with anemia and fever in renal adenocarcinoma, have been reported, but the relationship has not been successfully explained (Böttiger et al.; Bowman and Martinez).

Hypercalcemia. Elevated serum calcium levels are frequently found in patients without evidence of bony metastases (O'Grady et al.; Thomson and Karat). Similar occurrences have been reported in carcinomas of other organs, including the lung, ovary, liver, and pancreas, and in transitional cell carcinoma of the renal pelvis (Azzopardi). Patients with hypercalcemia and renal adenocarcinoma may have associated symptoms including polydypsia, polyuria, dysphagia, constipation, muscular weakness, and mental depression.

Explanations for hypercalcemia include: (1) Production of parathormone-like substance; (2) tumor production of a substance which stimulates the parathyroid to produce parathormone; (3) tumor production of vitamin D-like substance; and (4) tumor production of a substance which binds calcium and carries it in the plasma in excessive amounts (Thomson and Karat). Immunologic assays on tumor tissue from patients with renal adenocarcinoma and hypercalcemia have demonstrated substances within the tumor indistinguishable antigenically from parathormone (Goldberg

et al.; Lytton et al.). A fall in the serum calcium to normal levels after nephrectomy has been reported (O'Grady et al.). Tumor-induced hypercalcemia is rapidly progressive and occasionally fatal. In contrast to the more chronic syndrome manifested by parathyroid adenoma, the hypercalcemia of nonmetastatic malignancy is frequently accompanied by hypokalemic alkalosis.

Reversible Hepatic Dysfunction Associated with Renal Adenocarcinoma. Stauffer first reported the syndrome characterized by hepatic dysfunction associated with renal adenocarcinoma. The clinical and biochemical manifestations of hepatic dysfunction syndrome include nontender, nonnodular hepatomegaly without icterus, and at least three of the following: Increased alkaline phosphatase; increased sulfobromophthalein retention; increased serum bilirubin (indirect); hypoprothrombinemia; and increased alpha $_2$ globulin levels by electrophoresis (Utz et al.).

In these patients, histologic examination of the liver reveals nonspecific reactive hepatitis of varying severity characterized by Kupffer cell hyperplasia, mild nonspecific hepatocellular changes with or without fatty change, and portal triaditis (fig. 88). Both the chemical and morphologic features associated with hepatic dysfunction return to normal following nephrectomy. No correlation between the findings and morphologic characteristics of the renal adenocarcinoma has been demonstrated (Walsh and Kissane).

Enzymes. In patients with adenocarcinoma of the kidney, the glycolytic enzymes (LDH, aldolase, and phosphohexoisomerase) are elevated and tend to be higher in patients with metastases (West et al.). While LDH and alkaline phosphatase activity may be elevated in patients with carcinoma of the kidney, elevations are also

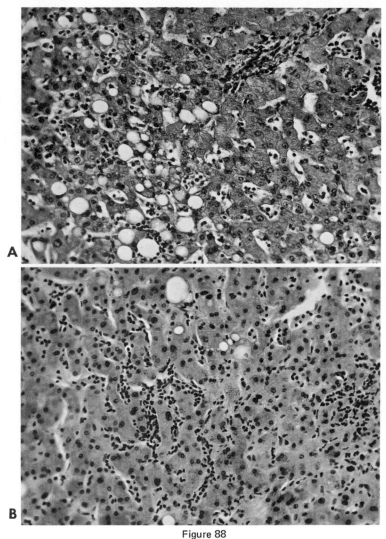

Figure 88

LIVER CHANGE ASSOCIATED WITH RENAL ADENOCARCINOMA

A wedge biopsy of the liver was taken from a 64 year old man with renal adenocarcinoma and reversible hepatic dysfunction. A. There is marked Kupffer cell hyperplasia forming intrasinusoidal clusters. Hemosiderin is present in the Kupffer cells and lipofuscin in the hepatic cells. There is moderate fatty change. X205. B. Elsewhere in the specimen are scattered plasma cells and lymphocytes in the parenchyma as well as Kupffer cell hyperplasia and fatty change. X205. (Figs. 1 and 2 from Utz, D. C., Warren, M. M., Gregg, J. A., Ludwig, A., and Kelalis, P. P. Reversible hepatic dysfunction associated with hypernephroma. Mayo Clin. Proc. 45:161-169, 1970.)

present in normal patients as well as those with nonneoplastic disease of the urinary tract (Amador et al.; Dorfman et al.; Brenner and Gilbert; Wacker et al.).

Amyloidosis. There are occasional reports of amyloidosis in patients with renal adenocarcinoma. Berger and Sinkoff reported a 2.9 percent incidence of amyloid deposits either in the tumor-bearing kidney (fig. 89) or in metastatic sites. The mechanism for the development of amyloid is unknown, although sepsis need not be present. Among the reported instances of amyloidosis in association with carcinoma, 10 to 25 percent involve renal adenocarcinoma (Bogaert et al.; Penman and Thomson).

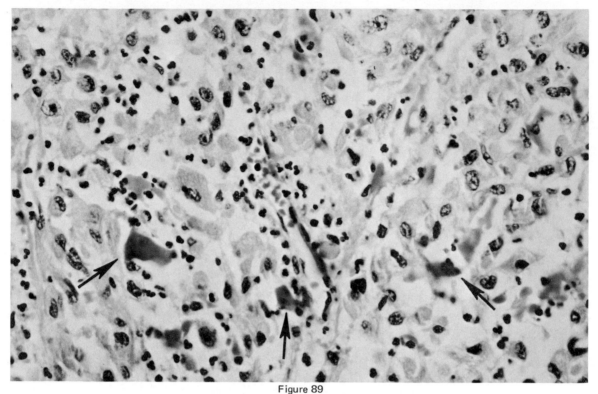

Figure 89

AMYLOID IN RENAL ADENOCARCINOMA

A representative section from an anaplastic renal adenocarcinoma shows deposits of amyloid. The patient, a 69 year old man, had widespread metastases and generalized amyloidosis. X280. (Courtesy of Dr. Louis Komarmy, San Francisco, Calif.)

DIAGNOSTIC TECHNICS

Diagnostic Roentgenography. It is beyond the scope of this fascicle to completely review the many excellent roentgenographic technics which have been developed in the last 10 years for the evaluation of renal masses. Before the development of these technics, diagnosis depended largely upon surgical exploration. With the aid of excretory urography, nephrotomography, retrograde pyelography, aortography, selective renal angiography, selective phlebography, and renal puncture with fluoroscopy, the accuracy of roentgenographic diagnosis of renal masses approaches 95 percent (figs. 90—98; Folin; Halpern).

Because of such excellent results, there has been an increasing tendency to rely completely upon roentgenographic technics to differentiate between the two most common renal masses, i.e., adenocarcinoma and benign cortical cysts, conditions which usually occur in the same age range and may occur in the same patient (1 to 3 percent of cases) (Brannan et al.; Emmett et al.).

Renal adenocarcinoma arising in an otherwise benign cyst does occur, but very rarely (fig. 99; Brannan et al.; Emmett et al.; Melicow and Becker). Necrosis leading to cystic change within an adenocarcinoma, on the other hand, is relatively frequent, but usually is easy to diagnose. Demonstration of an extensive, complex vascular pattern in the rim of a radiolucent mass of the renal cortex is characteristic of a cystic adenocarcinoma. Little or no vascularity is seen in simple cysts of the renal cortex. Differentiation is aided by puncture of the cyst and injection of contrast medium into the lumen under fluoroscopic control (Lang). The lining of a simple cyst is invariably smooth, while that of a carcinoma is made ragged by the remnants of central necrosis (figs. 98, 100). Fluid removed from the cyst prior to the injection of contrast material should be examined cytologically.

Plaine and Hinman showed that in asymptomatic patients with a renal mass, but no clinical or laboratory stigmata of renal carcinoma, the likelihood of renal adenocarcinoma is approximately 5 percent. In this group, the chance of missing a carcinoma by roentgenographic technics is sufficiently low (1 in 200 to 400) that the decision to rely on the roentgenographic diagnosis may be justified, particularly in

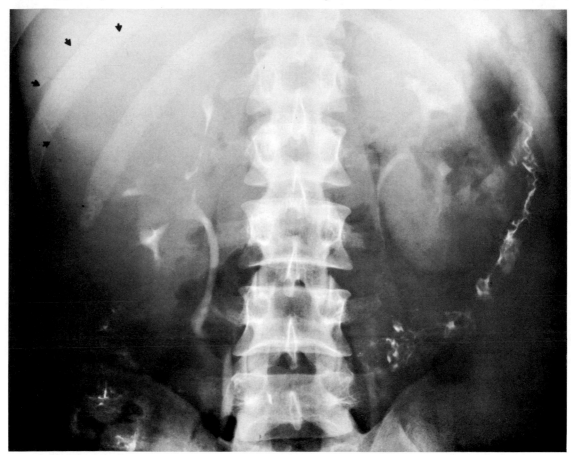

Figure 90
RENAL ADENOCARCINOMA
(Figures 90—92 from same case)
This excretory urogram reveals an enlarged right kidney with caliceal distortion from a parenchymal mass in the superior pole. (Courtesy of Dr. J. S. Ansell, Seattle, Wash.)

older patients in whom the complications of surgical therapy (death or permanent disability) approaches 5 percent. However, in the asymptomatic patient with a renal mass and clinical or laboratory signs of a renal carcinoma, the likelihood of a renal adenocarcinoma is approximately 40 percent. In this latter group, surgical exploration to differentiate between cyst and carcinoma is probably warranted.

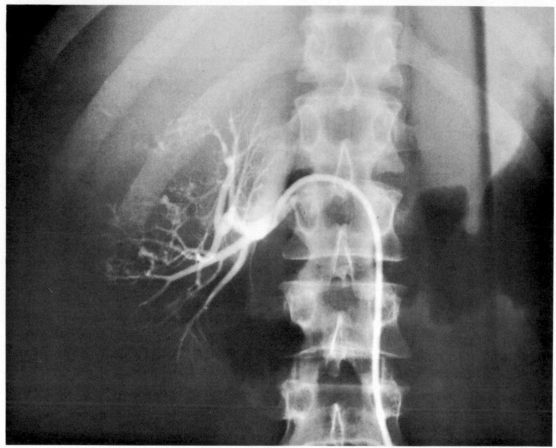

Figure 91
RENAL ADENOCARCINOMA
(Figures 90—92 from same case)

A selective arteriogram of the kidney shown in figure 90 demonstrates an increased vascular supply, irregular branching, and terminal blunting of vessels in a renal adenocarcinoma forming the mass in the superior pole. (Courtesy of Dr. J. S. Ansell, Seattle, Wash.)

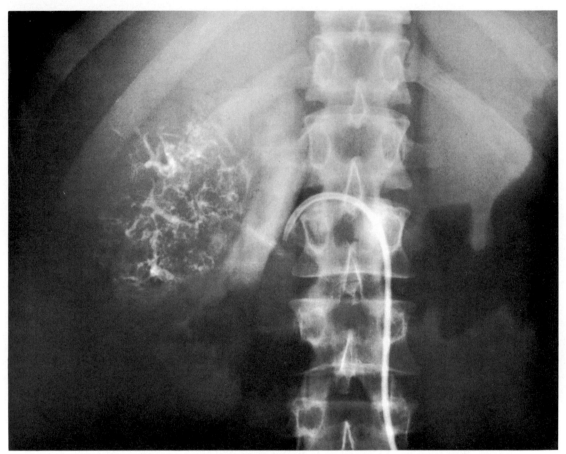

Figure 92
RENAL ADENOCARCINOMA
(Figures 90–92 from same case)
The arteriolar and capillary phase of the arteriogram shown in figure 91 demonstrates a "tumor blush" resulting from hypervascularity. (Courtesy of Dr. J. S. Ansell, Seattle, Wash.)

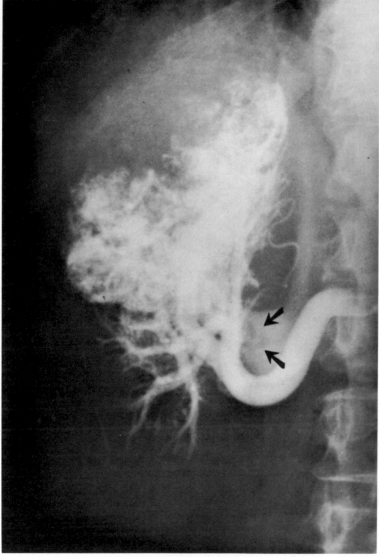

Figure 93
RENAL ADENOCARCINOMA
This is a selective renal arteriogram with contrast material injected immediately after administration of 10 mcg. of epinephrine. Normal renal arteries are constricted by the epinephrine; arteries in the tumor are not affected. Intraluminal tumor in the renal vein is indicated by arrows. (Fig. 1 from Kahn, P. C., Wise, H. M., Jr., and Robbins, A. H. C. Complete angiographic evaluation of renal cancer. J.A.M.A. 204:753-757, 1968.)

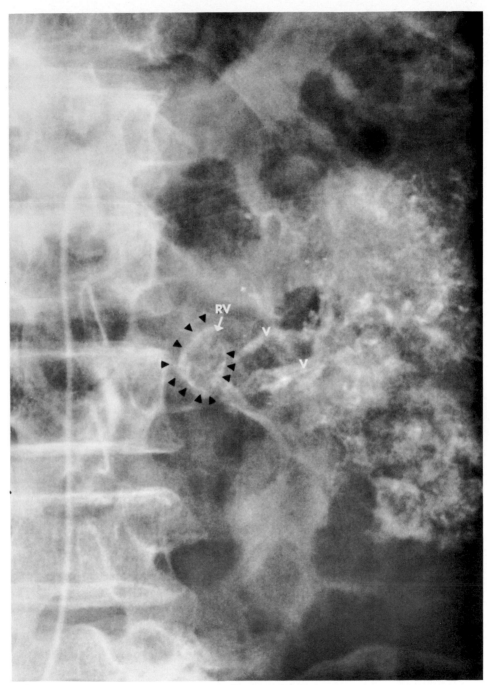

Figure 94
RENAL ADENOCARCINOMA
This selective renal arteriogram demonstrates a richly vascular renal adenocarcinoma in the middle and upper portions of the left kidney, which replaces the renal parenchyma and obstructs the renal vein by a tumor thrombus (arrows). (Courtesy of Dr. Joachim Burhenne, San Francisco, Calif.)

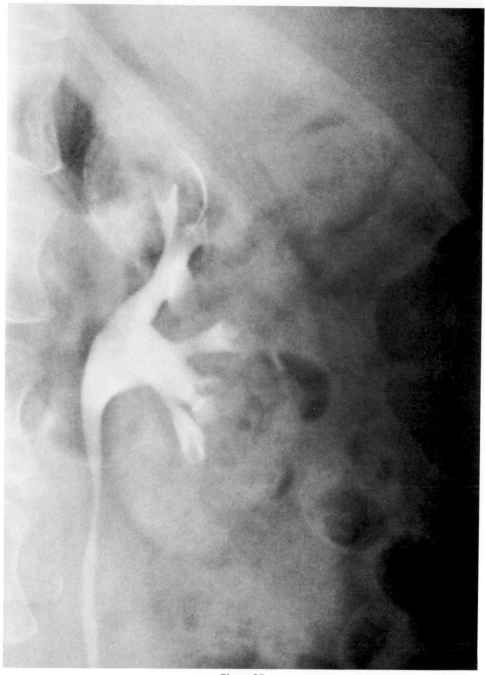

Figure 95
RENAL ADENOCARCINOMA
(Figures 95 and 96 from same case)

Peripheral calcification is present in a renal adenocarcinoma of the superior pole in the left kidney. This excretory urogram reveals no abnormalities of the caliceal system. (Courtesy of Dr. Joachim Burhenne, San Francisco, Calif.)

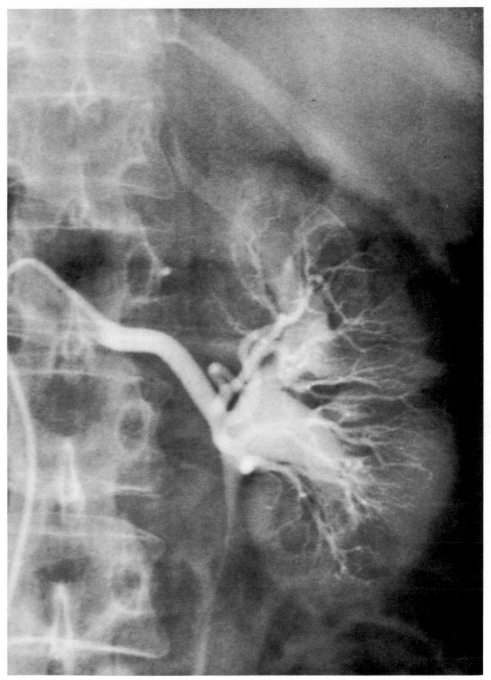

Figure 96
RENAL ADENOCARCINOMA
(Figures 95 and 96 from same case)
A selective arteriogram of the kidney shown in figure 95 demonstrates displacement of vessels around the calcified mass.
(Courtesy of Dr. Joachim Burhenne, San Francisco, Calif.)

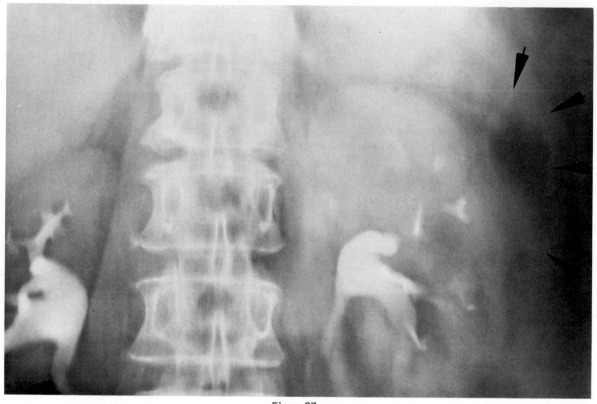

Figure 97
RENAL ADENOCARCINOMA

This nephrotomogram was taken of a patient with renal adenocarcinoma; it demonstrates an eccentric parenchymal mass projecting from the surface of the kidney. (Courtesy of Dr. George Annes, San Francisco, Calif.)

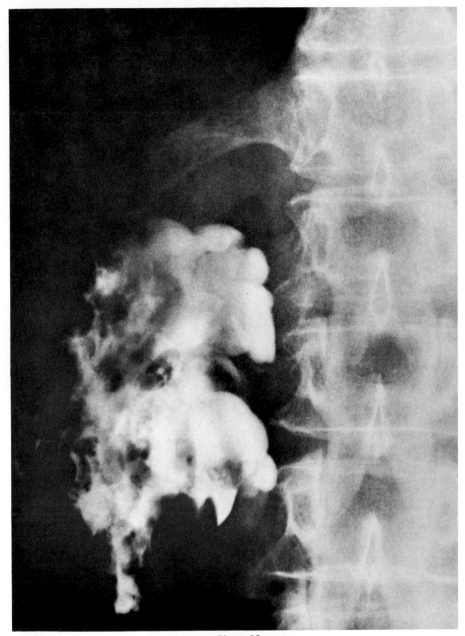

Figure 98
RENAL ADENOCARCINOMA
This roentgenogram shows irregular luminal contours after injection of radiopaque material into the cyst lumen.
(Courtesy of Dr. R. M. Shishido, San Diego, Calif.)

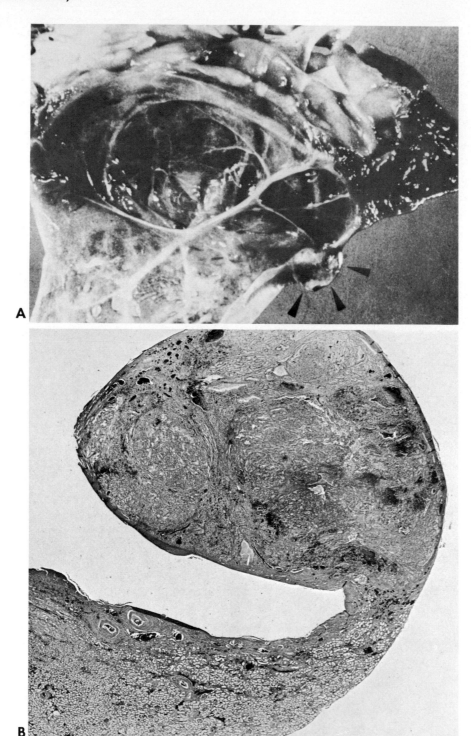

Figure 99
RENAL ADENOCARCINOMA

A. This small renal adenocarcinoma arose in the wall of a simple renal cortical cyst. (Fig. 1 from Weitzner, S. Clear cell carcinoma of the free wall of a simple renal cyst. J. Urol. 106:515-517, 1971.)

B. Histologic appearance of the well localized renal adenocarcinoma demonstrated grossly in A shows it is limited to the cyst wall. X12.

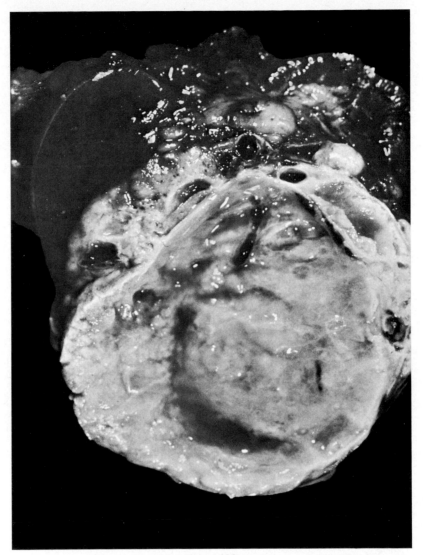

Figure 100
RENAL ADENOCARCINOMA
Note the ragged cyst lining in this cystic renal adenocarcinoma.

Radioisotopic Scan. Radioisotopic scanning is a well established and useful technic used in the diagnosis of renal lesions (Morris et al.). Intravenous injection of 99m Technetium-DMSA (dimercapto succinic acid) or gluconate permits demonstration of the functioning renal parenchyma. It is an accurate and relatively convenient diagnostic procedure. Since the compound is not selectively concentrated in renal cysts and neoplasms, such lesions are visualized as filling defects or "cold spots" in the renal outline of the scintiscan (fig. 101). The diagnostic accuracy of this procedure compares favorably with that of aortography and has the advantage of being relatively painless, safe, and convenient.

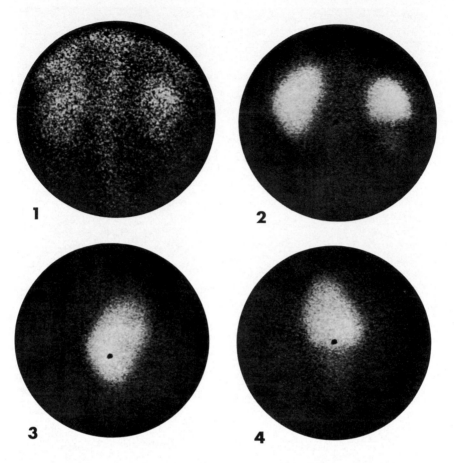

Figure 101
RENAL ADENOCARCINOMA

A scintiscan using technetium 99 gluconate demonstrates a renal adenocarcinoma in the lower pole of the right kidney. The arterial flow phase reveals (1) a nearly equal blood supply to the two kidneys. The parenchymal phase demonstrates (2) a decreased deposition of gluconate in the lower pole of the right kidney; (3) individual views of the normal left kidney; and (4) a cold area in the lower pole of the right kidney. (Courtesy of Dr. James L. McRea, Sydney, Australia.)

Ultrasonic Diagnosis. Ultrasonic scanning may also be of value in the differentiation between renal neoplasms and renal cysts (fig. 102; Kristensen et al.; Schreck and Holmes). Primary advantages are that it is safe, causes no discomfort, and appears to have an accuracy approaching that of radiologic diagnosis in differentiating between cysts and neoplasms. A further advantage is the possibility of being able to identify, on the basis of specific patterns,

those patients with chronic pyelonephritis, nephrosclerosis, glomerulonephritis, renal thrombosis, and renal calculi.

Laboratory Examination. There are no laboratory tests which specifically indicate the presence of a renal adenocarcinoma. Abnormal levels of the globulin fractions, hematuria, erythrocytosis, anemia, elevated erythrocyte sedimentation rate, and the syndrome of reversible hepatic dysfunction have already been discussed. Such findings,

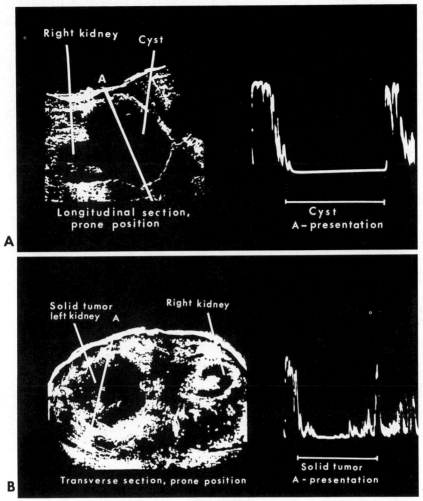

Figure 102
RENAL ADENOCARCINOMA

A. This is a sonogram of a renal cyst, 10 cm. in diameter. The back wall is clearly demarcated. No echo producing structures are present within the cyst.

B. In this sonogram of a renal adenocarcinoma, about 10 cm. in diameter, the contour of the kidney is broken and the caliceal echoes are displaced. The tumor is acoustically homogenous. (Figs. 6 and 8 from Kristensen, J. K., Gammelgaard, P. A., Holm, H. H., and Rasmussen, S. N. Ultrasound in the demonstration of renal masses. Br. J. Urol. 44:517-527, 1972.)

singly or in combination, may direct attention to the presence of a renal adenocarcinoma.

Cytologic Diagnosis. Cytologic examination of exfoliated cells of the urinary tract is often used as an ancillary diagnostic procedure. The most successful application of this technic is in the diagnosis of bladder cancer. Cytologic examination of the urine may occasionally demonstrate carcinomas arising in the renal pelvis and ureter, but is essentially of little value in attempting to establish or rule out the presence of adenocarcinoma of the renal parenchyma (Evans et al.). Umiker was able to make positive diagnoses cytologically only when the renal adenocarcinoma was far advanced. He found malignant cells in the urine of only 4 of 15 patients with known renal adeno-carcinoma; Foot and associates found them in only 5 of 60 such patients, and Evans and associates found them in none of 55 patients.

Urine Enzyme Assays. Assay of urinary enzymes does not appear to contribute importantly as a technic for the diagnosis of tumors of the kidney and bladder. While the urinary levels of lactic dehydrogenase and alkaline phosphatase may be elevated in tumors of the kidney and bladder, they are also found to be elevated in patients with pyelonephritis, glomerulonephritis, malignant hypertension, nephrosclerosis, and in patients with a heavy pyuria (Amador et al.; Dorfman et al.; Wacker et al.; Brenner and Gilbert). In our opinion, the lack of specificity of urinary enzyme determinations greatly limits the usefulness of this technic in the screening for, or diagnosis of tumors of the kidney.

Renal Biopsy. The technic of renal biopsy is well established for the diagnosis or assessment of prognosis in nonneoplastic renal diseases. Because of the possibility of tumor dissemination and hemorrhage, and the ever present possibility of inadvertent damage to other viscera attendant to a renal biopsy, this technic is usually limited to the patient with a likely diagnosis of renal adenocarcinoma who is a poor surgical risk, and when a tissue diagnosis is required before radiation or chemotherapy.

PATHOLOGIC FEATURES

GROSS FEATURES. Renal adenocarcinoma occurs with equal frequency in either kidney (Abeshouse and Weinberg; Griffiths and Thackray; Lucké and Schlumberger). The many conflicting reports ascribing a predilection for upper, middle, and lower portions of the kidney indicate that the distribution is most likely random (Geschickter and Widenhorn; Harvey; Heslin et al.; Judd and Hand; Kozoll and Kirshbaum; Smith and Young). Bilateral tumors are found in 0.5 to 1.5 percent of patients, and multiple tumors in the same kidney in approximately 4.5 percent of patients (Lang; Moertel et al.). Because of the great variation of histologic features in even small renal adenocarcinomas, histologic criteria are of little help in differentiating between metastases to the same or opposite kidney and an independent primary carcinoma.

If one accepts the small cortical glandular neoplasm, "so-called adenoma," as renal adenocarcinoma, then there is a tremendous range in the size of this neoplasm (fig. 79; see p. 94). Unfortunately, there are few series of any size in which the relative frequency of tumor sizes among symptomatic and asymptomatic renal adenocarcinomas is given (Bell; Hajdu and Thomas). In a study of 194 patients by Bell, which seems fairly representative, the distribution of tumor sizes was: less than 3 cm., 23 percent; 3 up to 4 cm., 14 percent; 4 up to 5 cm., 10 percent; 5 up to 6 cm., 10 percent; 6 up to 8 cm., 9 percent; and greater than 10 cm., 44 percent.

In general, the presence and duration of symptoms is directly related to increasing tumor size, although a significant proportion of tumors are silent, especially in elderly patients (Newman and Schulman; Bjornberg; Ostrum and Fetter). In one series in which 22 renal adenocarcinomas were discovered incidentally at the time of diagnostic evaluation for other disease, half of the tumors were already greater than 9 cm. in diameter (Newman and Schulman).

The gross appearance of glandular tumors of the renal cortex is fairly characteristic, irrespective of size. The tumor usually protrudes from the renal cortex as an irregular, bosselated mass which appears yellow to gray and often hemorrhagic beneath the renal capsule (plates II, III, and IV-A). The cut surface typically bulges and has a variegated, lobular appearance. Viable tumor is glistening and pale yellow or orange when there are large amounts of intracellular lipid and gray in sarcomatoid (fig. 121) and lipid-poor areas (plates II-B, III, and IV-A). Necrotic areas are dull gray and opaque, gelatinous, cystic, or fibrous depending upon the stage in the evolution of tumor degeneration (plates II-B, III, and IV; fig. 103). Old and recent hemorrhage is usually evident throughout the tumor and many of the cysts may contain bloody fluid. The degenerative changes appear to be due to the tumor outgrowing its blood supply or invading the delicate stromal vessels of the tumor with resulting hemorrhage and necrosis. Fibrous septa course through the tumor representing replacement of necrotic tumor and may contain foci of calcification (plates III-B and IV). At the periphery of most tumors, the renal parenchyma is compressed, forming a pseudocapsule of condensed connective tissue which merges with the dense fibrous tissue scaffolding of the tumor (pl. IV-B).

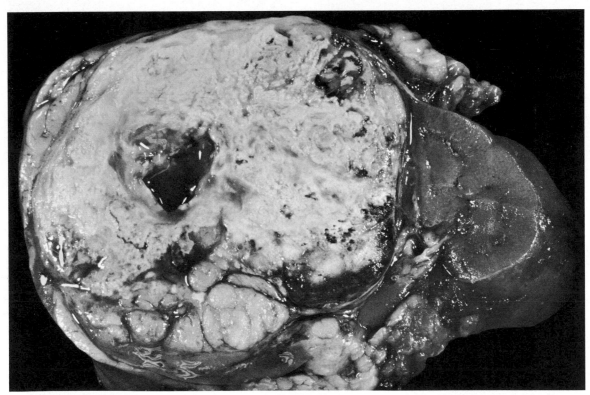

Figure 103
RENAL ADENOCARCINOMA
This renal adenocarcinoma shows extension through the renal capsule into the perirenal fat. Nodules of glistening translucent viable tumor are present at the periphery. Centrally, the tumor is dull gray, opaque, and necrotic with scattered cysts.

HISTOLOGIC FEATURES. Renal adenocarcinoma has many faces. It may be composed of clear or granular cells arranged in tubular (figs. 104–108), papillary (figs. 111–116), solid (figs. 117, 118, 120, 121), and cystic patterns (figs. 109, 111, 119). Rarely, the tumor is focally or completely sarcomatoid resembling fibrosarcoma (figs. 122, 123), or myosarcoma (fig. 124).

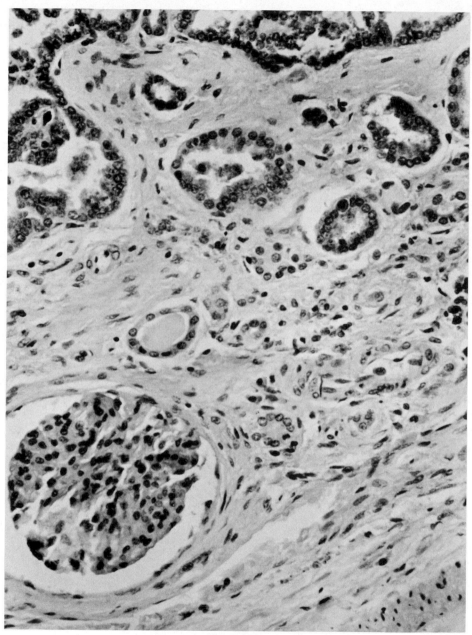

Figure 104
RENAL ADENOCARCINOMA
Malignant tubules are difficult to distinguish from normal proximal convoluted tubules in this well differentiated tubular renal adenocarcinoma. X330.

PLATE II

RENAL ADENOCARCINOMA

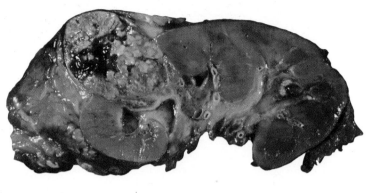

A.   This renal adenocarcinoma is protruding from the cortical surface. The interior is homogeneous yellow-orange with central hemorrhage.

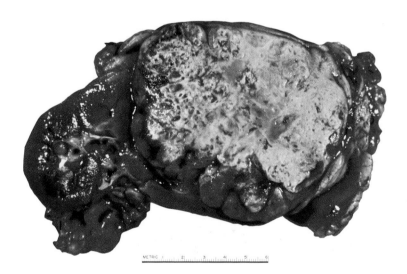

B.   The cut surface of this large renal adenocarcinoma, with irregular bosselated margins, shows focal necrosis and early cystic change.

PLATE III

RENAL ADENOCARCINOMA

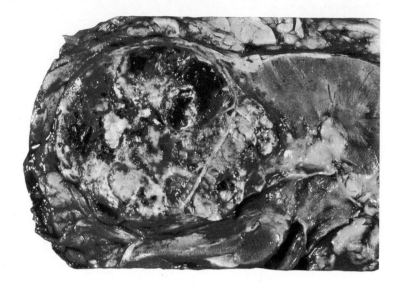

A. A variegated pattern due to old and recent necrosis and extensive subcapsular hemorrhage is seen in this renal adenocarcinoma.

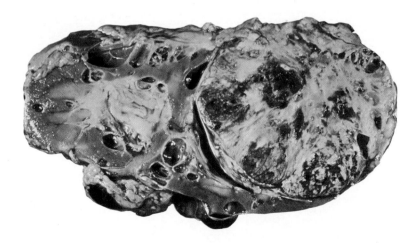

B. Fibrosis, necrosis, cystic change, and hemorrhage are all evident in this renal adenocarcinoma.

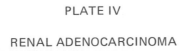

PLATE IV

RENAL ADENOCARCINOMA

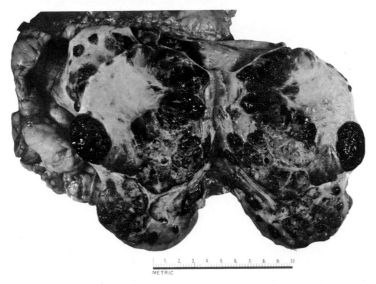

A. There is extensive fibrosis within this renal adenocarcinoma, and hemorrhagic necrosis of a major portion of the remaining parenchyma. (Courtesy of Dr. Seth L. Haber, Santa Clara, Calif.)

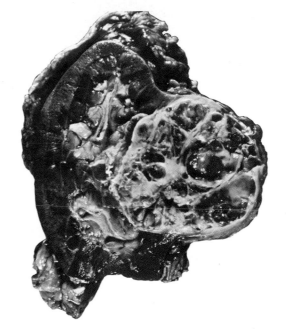

B. Late stages of degenerative change are evident in a renal adenocarcinoma, with extensive cystic change, fibrosis, and no residual gross tumor. (Courtesy of Dr. Seth L. Haber, Santa Clara, Calif.)

B

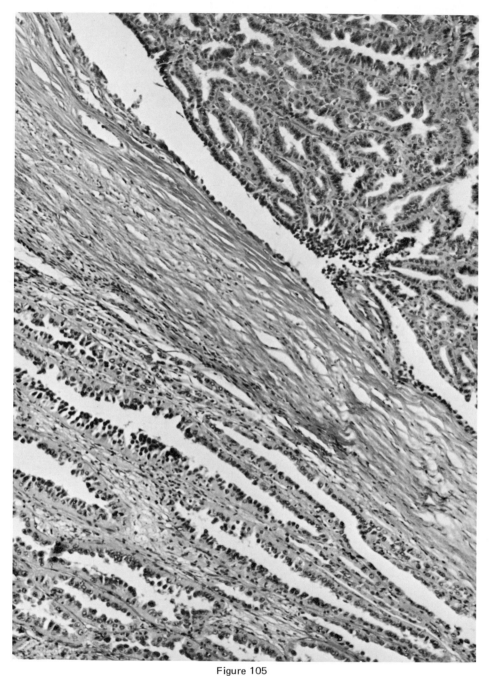

Figure 105
RENAL ADENOCARCINOMA
This illustrates the longitudinal and cross sections of a well differentiated tubular renal adenocarcinoma. X127.

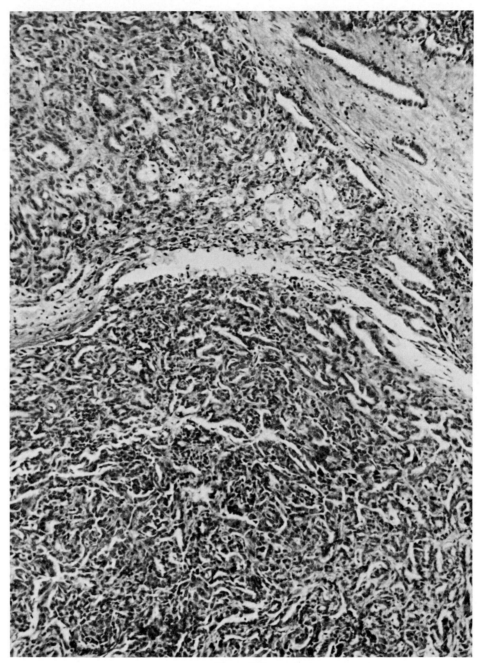

Figure 106
RENAL ADENOCARCINOMA
The upper half of this field is composed of well differentiated tubules separated by stroma and stromal macrophages. The tubules in the lower half of the field are tightly packed and haphazardly arranged. X127.

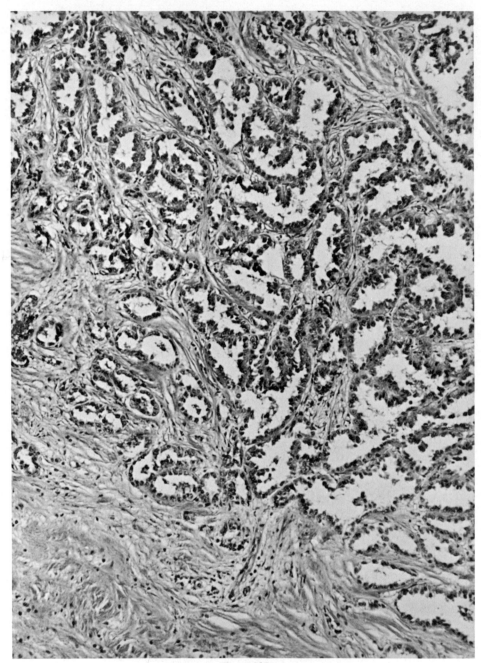

Figure 107
RENAL ADENOCARCINOMA
In this tubular variant of renal adenocarcinoma, tubular cells are moderately pleomorphic and nuclei are prominent. The tubules show considerable variation in size and shape. X127.

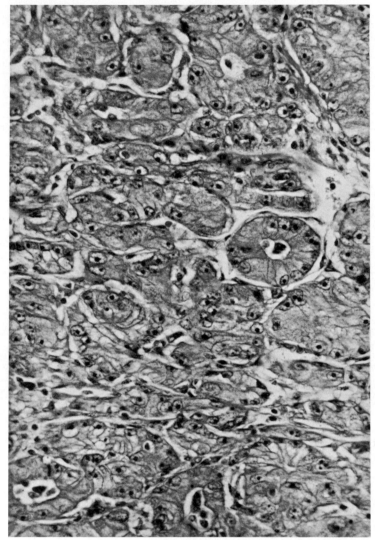

Figure 108
RENAL ADENOCARCINOMA
These tubular structures are composed of large granular cells with little intervening stroma. The tubules are separated by thin-walled vessels. X210.

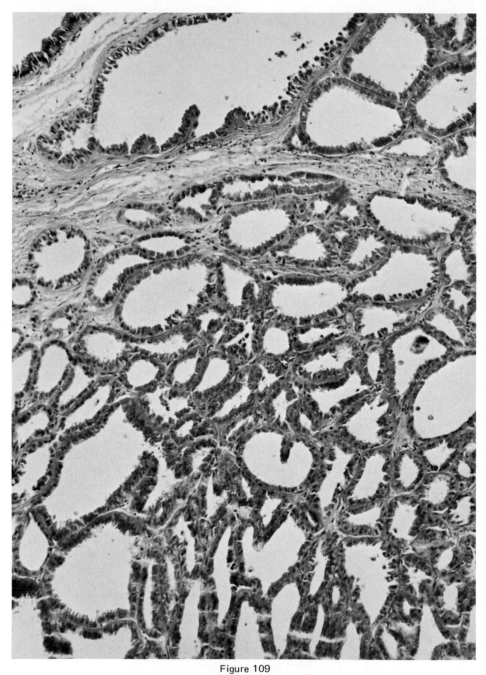

Figure 109
RENAL ADENOCARCINOMA
This renal adenocarcinoma is composed of widely dilated tubules, each lined by a single layer of granular cells. X127.

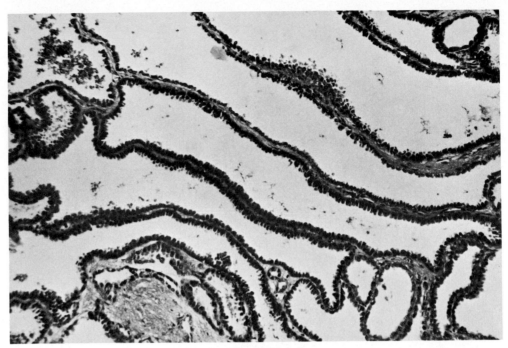

Figure 110
RENAL ADENOCARCINOMA
This tubular renal adenocarcinoma is composed of granular cells with tubules dilated to cystic proportions. Cysts are lined by a single layer of small granular cells. X140.

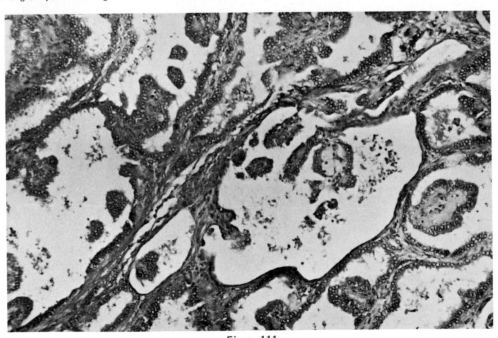

Figure 111
RENAL ADENOCARCINOMA
A papillary pattern in this renal adenocarcinoma is formed by the extensive proliferation of papillary structures into tubular lumens. X140.

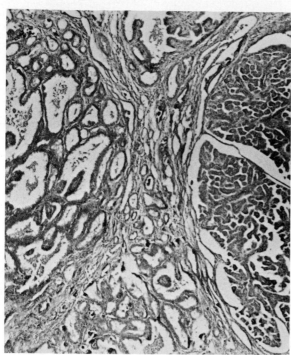

Figure 112

Figure 112
RENAL ADENOCARCINOMA
This mixed tubular and papillary renal adenocarcinoma is composed of small cuboidal granular cells. Papillary structures are complex and compactly arranged. X60.

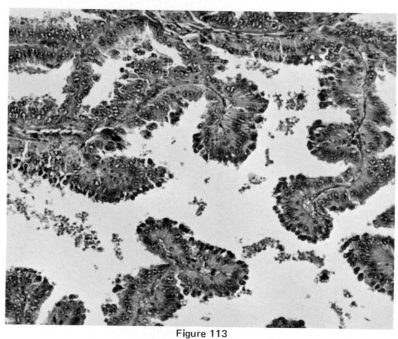

Figure 113
RENAL ADENOCARCINOMA
The intraluminal proliferation of frondlike structures is composed of tall columnar granular cells. The fibrovascular stroma in this renal adenocarcinoma is quite delicate. X127.

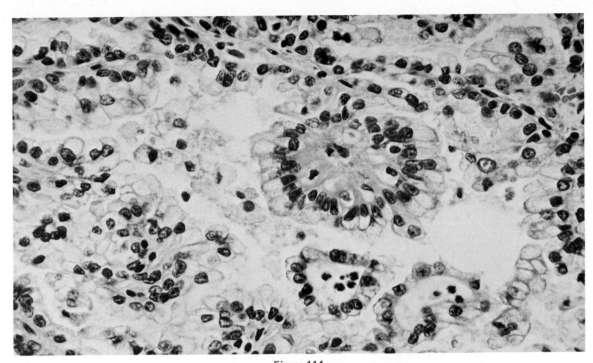

Figure 114
RENAL ADENOCARCINOMA
The formation of branching papillary projections is illustrated in this clear cell renal adenocarcinoma. X280.

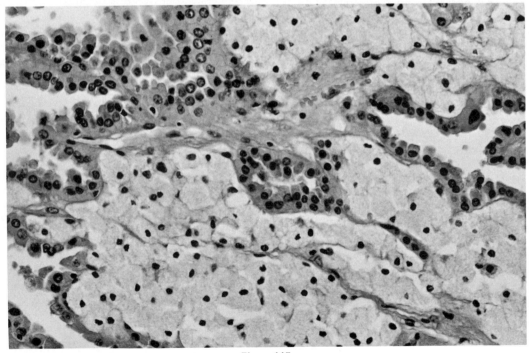

Figure 115
RENAL ADENOCARCINOMA
Broad papillary processes can be seen in this granular cell renal adenocarcinoma. The stroma contains many foamy histiocytes. X240.

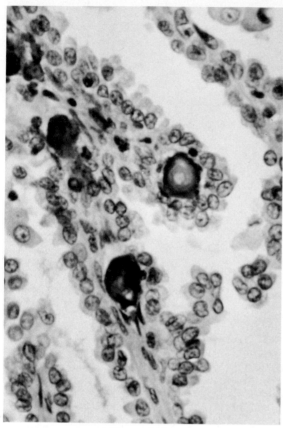

Figure 116

Figure 116
RENAL ADENOCARCINOMA
This papillary granular cell renal adenocarcinoma contains laminated calcified concretions (psammoma bodies) in the stroma of the papillary processes. X530.

Figure 117
RENAL ADENOCARCINOMA
A solid renal adenocarcinoma is composed of small granular cells arranged in islands separated by a myxoid stroma. X127.

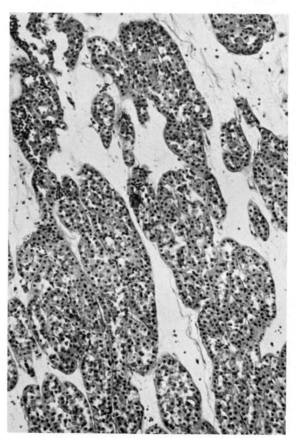

Figure 117

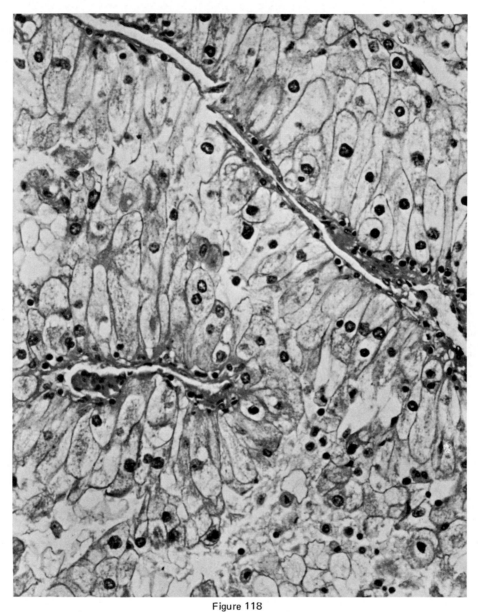

Figure 118
RENAL ADENOCARCINOMA
Sheets of polygonal and oval clear cells form a solid pattern of renal adenocarcinoma interrupted only by occasional thin-walled vessels and fibrous septae. X330.

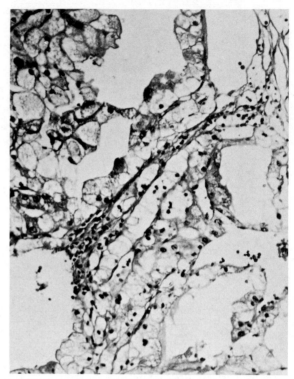

Figure 119
RENAL ADENOCARCINOMA
Focal cystic change and moderate nuclear pleo-morphism are seen in this clear cell renal adenocarcinoma. X185.

Figure 119

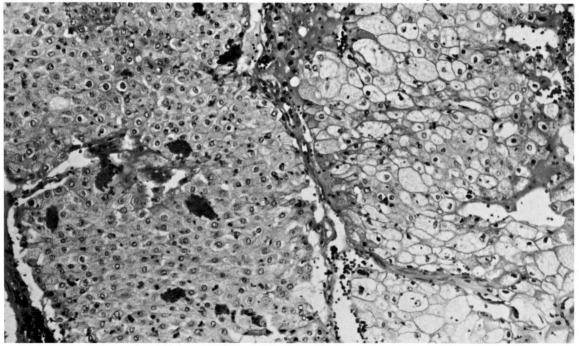

Figure 120
RENAL ADENOCARCINOMA
Clear cells are seen on one side of the field of this renal adenocarcinoma and granular cells on the other, sharply separated by a small vessel. X370.

Figure 121
RENAL ADENOCARCINOMA
A bimorphic renal adenocarcinoma exhibits the typical gross appearance in the area composed of clear cells and a dense gray, fibrous appearance in the sarcomatoid area. (Fig. 2 from Farrow, G. M., Harrison, E. G., Jr., and Utz, D. C. Sarcomas and sarcomatoid and mixed malignant tumors of the kidney in adults—Part III. Cancer 22:556-563, 1968.)

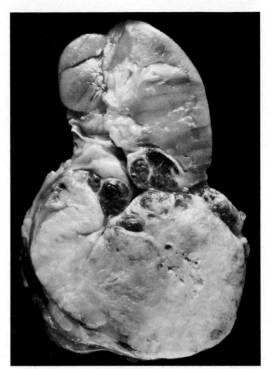

Figure 121

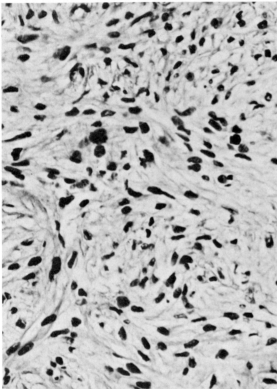

Figure 122
FIBROSARCOMATOID RENAL ADENOCARCINOMA
(Figures 122 and 123 from same case)
This solid fibrosarcomatoid renal adenocarcinoma is composed of spindle cells. The histologic pattern resembles a fibrosarcoma. X245.

Figure 123
FIBROSARCOMATOID RENAL ADENOCARCINOMA
(Figures 122 and 123 from same case)
The fibrosarcomatoid renal adenocarcinoma illustrated in figure 122 metastasized to the liver (upper left). The metastatic focus (lower right) is histologically more typical of a renal adenocarcinoma exhibiting a clear cell tubular pattern. X95.

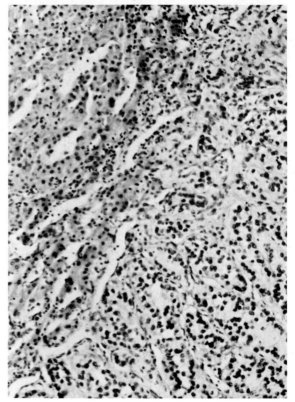

Figure 123

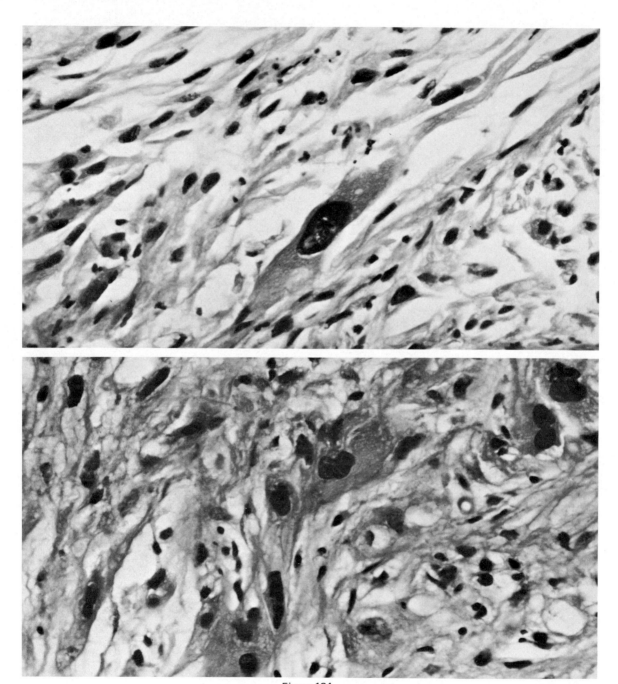

Figure 124
RHABDOMYOSARCOMATOID RENAL ADENOCARCINOMA
Multiple hyperchromatic and giant nuclei are present in this solid rhabdomyosarcomatoid renal adenocarcinoma, particularly in the enlarged straplike cells with a dark fibrillary eosinophilic cytoplasm. Small spindle cells form the background. X464.

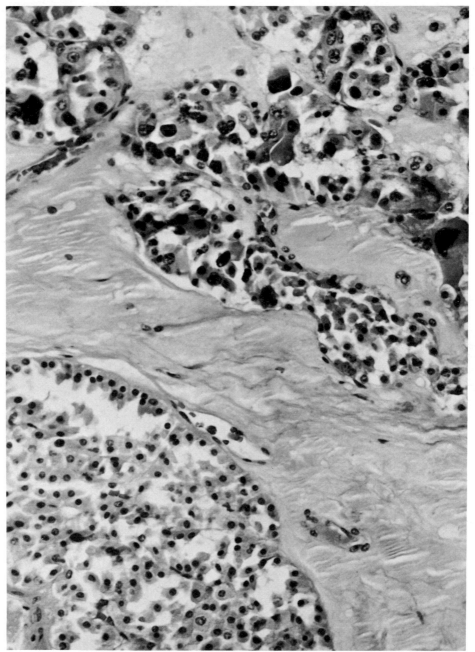

Figure 125
RENAL ADENOCARCINOMA
This renal adenocarcinoma is composed of small granular cells. There is marked fibrosis, and, in areas of entrapment, many of the cells are enlarged and their nuclei pleomorphic and hyperchromatic. X330.

While the overall histologic patterns found in renal adenocarcinomas are quite variable, individual cells are fairly uniform in appearance. Most have a delicate but distinct cytoplasmic membrane and are tightly adherent to neighboring cells. Cells are usually columnar or cuboidal when arranged in papillary or tubular structures and polygonal to ovoid when compressed in solid sheets. Typically, there is little cellular or nuclear pleomorphism and mitotic figures are rare. Pleomorphism appears to be most frequently seen immediately adjacent to areas of fibrosis (fig. 125), possibly representing anoxic effect.

When large amounts of intracellular cholesterol, lipid, and glycogen are present, the cells have a pale, clear cytoplasm examined with the light microscope, since this material is eluted during routine histologic processing. When there are large numbers of cytoplasmic organelles, principally mitochondria, the cytoplasm is brightly eosinophilic and granular (fig. 126).

Within the stroma of renal adenocarcinoma, clusters of foamy histiocytes and foci of calcification are fairly common. Occasionally, one sees scattered psammoma bodies (fig. 116) and cartilaginous or osse-

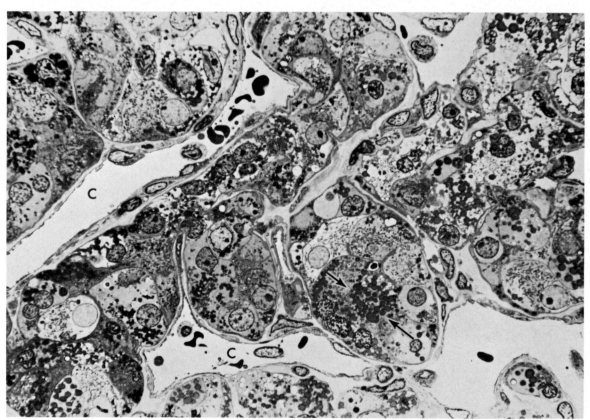

Figure 126
RENAL ADENOCARCINOMA
The presence of small lipid droplets in a granular renal adenocarcinoma is demonstrated by Epon-embedded 1 micron sections stained with toluidine blue. Lipid is indicated by arrows. The finer granularity of the cytoplasm represents mitochondria. Capillaries are identified by C. X742. (Courtesy of Dr. M. D. Lagios, San Francisco, Calif.)

ous metaplasia in the stroma (fig. 127). The accumulation of foamy histiocytes is more frequently seen in papillary rather than solid tumors (fig. 115).

Typically, the accompanying fibrous stroma is inconspicuous, but richly vascular. Stromal vessels are thin-walled, predisposing to the leakage of blood (fig. 128) and accumulation of hemosiderin (fig. 129) in stromal macrophages. Cholesterol clefts and scattered inflammatory cells are seen in areas of necrosis (fig. 130). When hemor-

rhage and necrosis are extensive, there is often a marked reactive fibrosis to the extent that large portions of the tumor may be replaced, leaving only scattered tumor cells entrapped within dense hyalinized collagenous tissue (pl. IV; figs. 125, 131). Spontaneous regression of renal adenocarcinomas, which has been reported many times, may occur by this process, possibly induced by venous invasion and accompanying thrombosis (Everson and Cole).

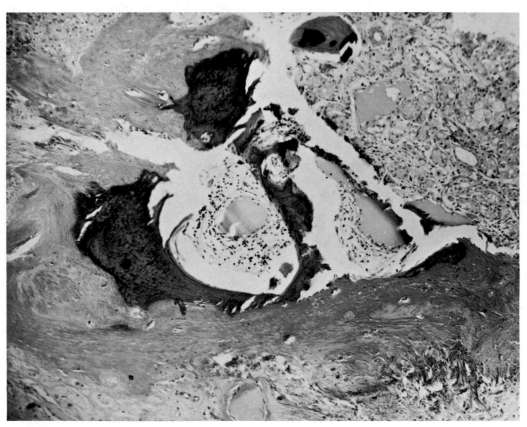

Figure 127
OSSEOUS METAPLASIA IN RENAL ADENOCARCINOMA
Osseous metaplasia is located in the dense fibrous stroma of a renal adenocarcinoma. Marrow elements are present between trabeculae. X87.

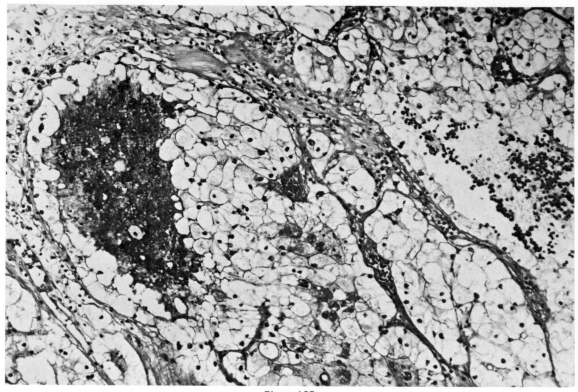

Figure 128
RENAL ADENOCARCINOMA
Fresh hemorrhage is seen in the parenchyma and acinar spaces of a renal adenocarcinoma secondary to leakage from thin-walled tumor vessels. X185.

Histochemical Features. The characteristic histochemical features of renal adenocarcinoma are: (1) Intracytoplasmic glycogen demonstrated by the periodic acid-Schiff reaction (pl. V-A) which is negative with prior diastase digestion (pl. V-B); (2) neutral lipid stainable with oil red O (pl. V-C), Sudan IV, or perchloric acid-naphthoquinone on frozen sections (completely removed by xylene or chloroform with methyl alcohol); and (3) phospholipid stainable with Sudan black (pl. V-D) or luxol fast blue after treatment by xylene or chloroform with methyl alcohol. Cholesterol has been found in renal adenocarcinomas by extraction technics and by electron microscopy, but we have rarely been able to demonstrate cholesterol histochemically in the tumors we have studied.

Mucopolysaccharides are not found in the cytoplasm of renal adenocarcinomas, although they can be demonstrated extracellularly on cell membranes (glycocalix) and may accumulate in the lumens of tumor tubules and acini.

A variety of enzymes have been identified in the cells of renal adenocarcinomas, which are also seen in normal proximal, convoluted tubular cells but are not specific for these tissues and are, therefore, of limited use diagnostically (Braunstein and Adelman).

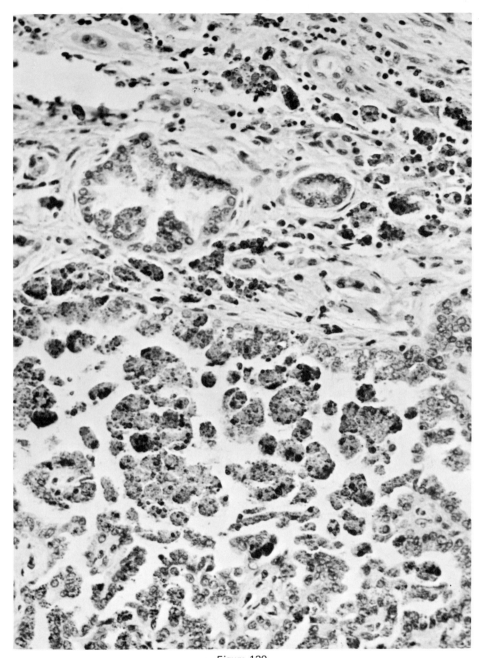

Figure 129
RENAL ADENOCARCINOMA
An accumulation of hemosiderin pigment in macrophages is seen near an area of old hemorrhage in a renal adenocarcinoma. X130.

PLATE V

RENAL ADENOCARCINOMA

The histochemical features of a renal adenocarcinoma are illustrated:

A.   Periodic acid-Schiff (PAS) positive material in the cytoplasm of tumor cells prior to diastase digestion. X64.

B.   Same tumor with PAS positive material (glycogen) removed by prior diastase digestion. X64.

C.   Droplets of oil red 0 positive material within the cytoplasm (neutral lipid). X192.

D.   Droplets and plates of Sudan black positive material (phospholipid) remaining after oil red 0 positive material has been eluted with xylene. X192.

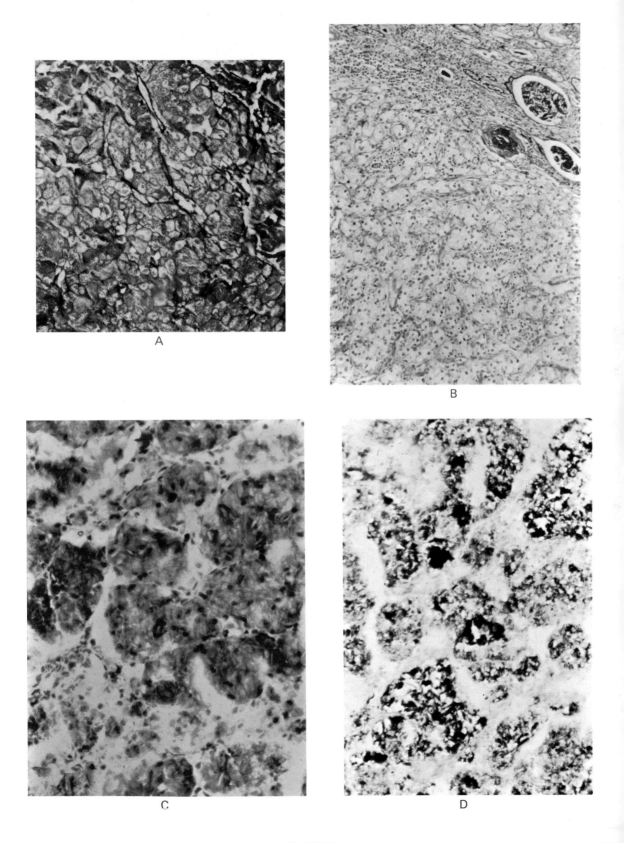

A

B

C

D

PLATE V

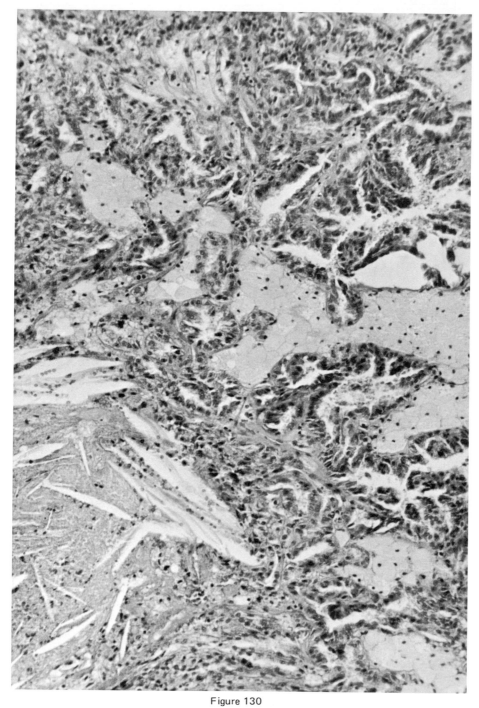

Figure 130
RENAL ADENOCARCINOMA
In this renal adenocarcinoma, areas of focal necrosis are replaced by amorphous debris, scattered inflammatory cells, and cholesterol clefts. X185.

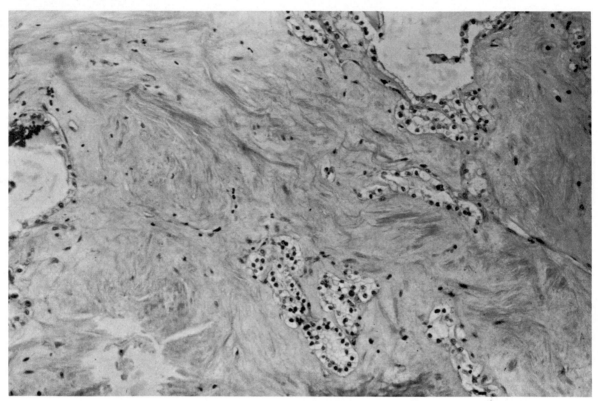

Figure 131
RENAL ADENOCARCINOMA
In this area there is replacement by dense fibrosis in a renal adenocarcinoma which had previously undergone extensive necrosis. Scattered clusters of tumor cells are entrapped in the fibrous stroma. X185.

Electron Microscopic Features. The controversy over the histogenesis of renal adenocarcinoma was laid to rest by electron microscopic studies demonstrating an origin in cells of the proximal convoluted tubule (Oberling et al.). Cells of the renal adenocarcinoma are distinctly unlike those of the adrenal gland or glomerulus (Tannenbaum), loop of Henle, distal convoluted tubule, and collecting tubules, but are essentially identical to the normal epithelial cells of the proximal convoluted tubule (see histogenesis of tumors of the upper urinary tract, p. 93). The electron microscopic features of renal adenocarcinomas and so-called adenomas, whether in humans (adults or children) or lower animals, are essentially indistinguishable (Oberling et al.; Pratt-Thomas et al.; Seljelid; Seljelid and Ericsson; Tannenbaum).

These ultrastructural similarities between normal and neoplastic cells of the proximal convoluted tubule include: (1) A brush border of tightly packed microvilli; (2) membrane-associated vesicles involved in pinocytosis; (3) membrane coatings of extracellular material (glycocalix); (4) infoldings of the plasma membrane; and (5) abundance of tortuous and elongated mitochondria (fig. 132; Oberling et al.; Pratt-Thomas et al.; Seljelid; Seljelid and Ericsson; Tannenbaum).

The mitochondria may be normal, but the majority are atypical with bizarre arrangements, elongation of cristae, and

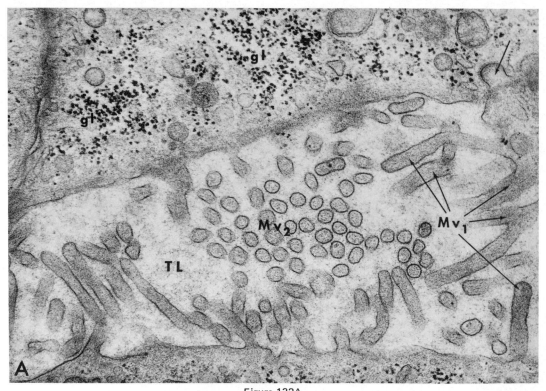

Figure 132A
RENAL ADENOCARCINOMA
A. Parts of two tumor cells are separated by a narrow lumen (TL). The plasma membrane is evaginated to form microvilli (Mv). X32,000.

vacuolation. Numerous branches between elongated cristae are common. Amorphous, electron-dense bodies have been noted in the mitochondrial matrix (fig. 133; Seljelid and Ericsson).

The **clear** and **granular cells** seen in light microscopic preparations are also accounted for by electron microscopic studies (Ericsson et al.). **Clear cells** contain large amounts of particulate glycogen, triglycerides, and phospholipid but little endoplasmic reticulum and Golgi, and relatively few mitochondria and cytosomes. The clear appearance is due to the combination of sparse cytoplasmic organelles and to lipid and glycogen which are eluted during routine histologic processing (fig. 134). **Granular cells** owe their appearance to numerous mitochondria and a more highly developed Golgi and endoplasmic reticulum with more frequent cytosomes. Lipids and glycogen may be present, but usually in small amounts. Electron microscopic evidence points to an origin of the cytosomes directly from vesicles of the Golgi and endoplasmic reticulum. It has not been determined whether or not the observed inverse relationship between the presence of Golgi and smooth endoplasmic reticulum and the accumulation of intracytoplasmic lipids and glycogen are causally related.

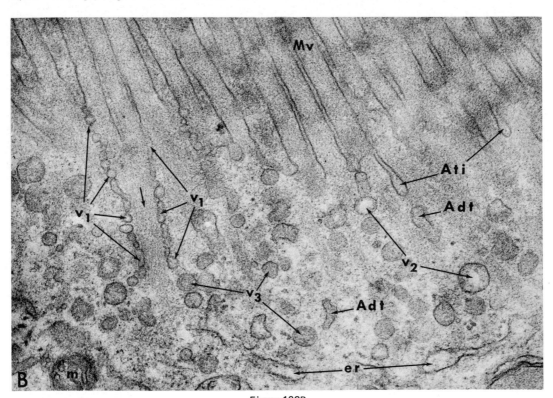

Figure 132B
RENAL ADENOCARCINOMA

B. The higher magnification of microvilli (Mv) and adjacent cytoplasm in a tumor cell are shown. Invaginations of the plasma membrane form apical tubules (Ati). Some elements resemble apical dense tubules (Adt). Small vesicles are present in the cytoplasm (v). Mitochondria (m). Endoplasmic reticulum (er). X40,000. (Figs. 9 and 10 from Seljelid, R., and Ericsson, J. L. E. Electron microscopic observations on specializations of the cell surface in renal clear cell carcinoma. Lab. Invest. 14:435-447, 1965.)

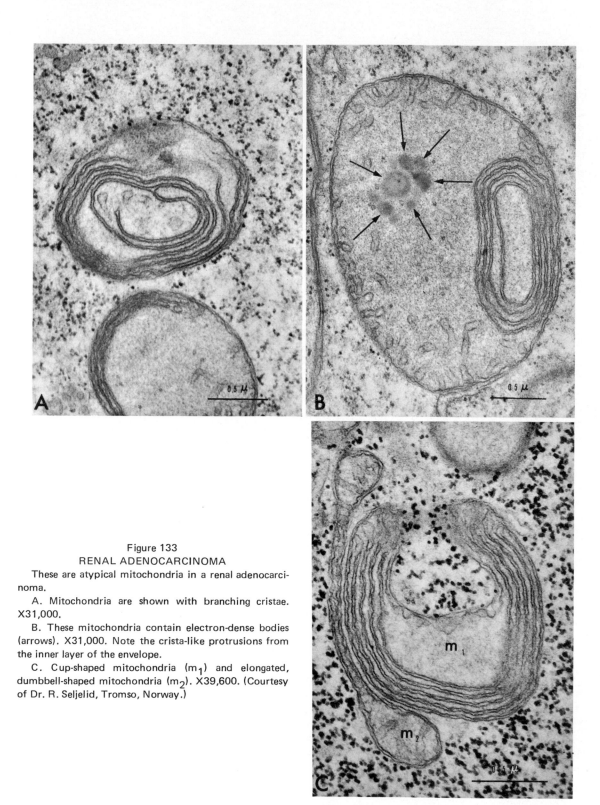

Figure 133
RENAL ADENOCARCINOMA

These are atypical mitochondria in a renal adenocarcinoma.

A. Mitochondria are shown with branching cristae. X31,000.

B. These mitochondria contain electron-dense bodies (arrows). X31,000. Note the crista-like protrusions from the inner layer of the envelope.

C. Cup-shaped mitochondria (m_1) and elongated, dumbbell-shaped mitochondria (m_2). X39,600. (Courtesy of Dr. R. Seljelid, Tromso, Norway.)

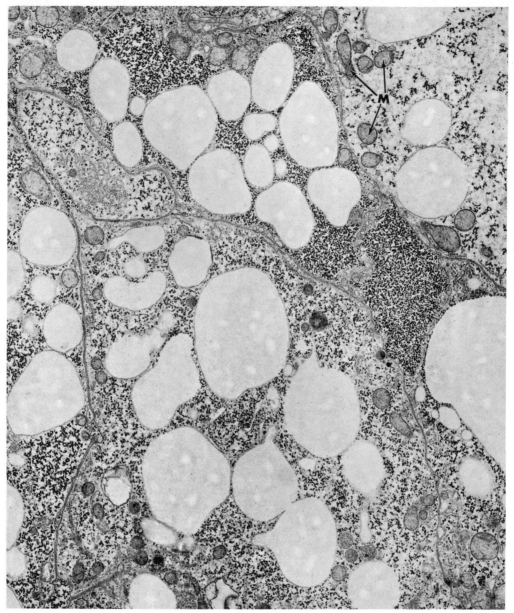

Figure 134
RENAL ADENOCARCINOMA
The electron microscopic appearance of several clear cells shows a content of glycogen and numerous fat vacuoles. Mitochondria (M) and other cytoplasmic organelles are scarce. X9300. (Fig. 11 from Ericsson, J. L. E., Seljelid, R., and Orrenius, S. Comparative light and electron microscopic observations of the cytoplasmic matrix in renal carcinomas. Virchows Arch. (Pathol. Anat.) 341:204-223, 1966.)

DIFFERENTIAL DIAGNOSIS
FROM OTHER PRIMARY TUMORS

Sarcomatoid Tumors. The differential diagnosis of renal adenocarcinoma within the kidney primarily involves distinguishing the poorly differentiated sarcomatoid renal adenocarcinoma from various renal sarcomas, pleomorphic transitional cell carcinomas, and Wilms' tumor, and the clear cell tumors from histiocytic tumors, malakoplakia, and xanthogranulomatous pyelonephritis.

Farrow and associates found 37 sarcomatoid renal adenocarcinomas among 2100 renal adenocarcinomas at the Mayo Clinic (1.8 percent). The most common forms of sarcomatoid renal adenocarcinoma were those mimicking rhabdomyosarcoma (10 cases) and fibrosarcoma (24 cases). The tumors resembling rhabdomyosarcomas are composed of strap cells, giant cells, and multinucleated giant cells intermixed with smaller malignant spindle cells and arranged somewhat haphazardly in sheets and irregular clusters (fig. 124). Special stains fail to reveal myofibrils or cross striations, and frequently intracellular lipids can be demonstrated which assist in the diagnosis.

Those renal adenocarcinomas composed predominantly of spindle cells generally contain many mitotic figures and are accompanied by considerable collagenous tissue, producing a pattern which bears a striking resemblance to fibrosarcoma (figs. 122, 123). Leiomyosarcoma and spindle cell transitional cell carcinoma of the renal pelvis should also be considered.

Tannenbaum has pointed out the difficulty of distinguishing between fibrous tissue and smooth muscle tumors of the kidney even with the aid of histochemical technics and electron microscopy. However, he feels that spindle cell mesenchymal tumors can be distinguished electron microscopically from sarcomatoid renal adenocarcinomas by the presence of: (1) pentalaminar desmosomes; (2) basement membrane formation; and (3) a brush border in cells of sarcomatoid renal adenocarcinomas which establishes an origin from epithelial rather than mesenchymal cells.

The relatively rare liposarcomatoid variant of renal adenocarcinoma is indistinguishable from liposarcoma. Fusiform and anastomosing stellate cells are interspersed with unilocular and multilocular cells containing fat droplets. Multinucleated giant cells, myxomatous changes, and markedly pleomorphic areas are often present. The presence of phospholipid favors the diagnosis of renal adenocarcinoma, while acid mucopolysaccharides (testicular hyaluronidase-labile) support a diagnosis of liposarcoma.

Finally, there are renal adenocarcinomas containing sarcomatoid areas intermixed with components of malignant bone or cartilage. Farrow and associates found three such cases in 37 sarcomatoid renal adenocarcinomas. The malignant mesenchymal components are usually intimately intermingled with sarcomatoid portions of the adenocarcinoma and often multifocal, providing evidence against the diagnosis of collision tumors of diverse types. Whether the sarcomatous portions are derived from the stroma, which is the possibility we favor, or from metaplastic transformation of the cells of the adenocarcinoma as proposed by Farrow and his coworkers has not been established. Whichever is the case, the mesenchymal components are seen in metastases, as well as in the primary tumor, indicating that the inductive or metaplastic forces are also operational outside the kidney.

In many of the sarcomatoid and pleomorphic forms, characteristic patterns of renal adenocarcinoma may be found if enough sections of the tumor are examined (figs. 123, 135). In some cases, the differentiation in distant metastases is better than in the primary tumor. Before making a diagnosis of renal sarcoma, an exhaustive search of the tumor for foci of adenocarcinoma should be made. The majority of tumors classified as renal sarcoma reviewed by us have proved to be sarcomatoid renal adenocarcinomas by histochemical technics and careful examination of multiple sections. If facilities are available, electron microscopy should be carried out, since sarcomatoid renal adenocarcinomas do retain certain features of epithelial cells which help in distinguishing them from sarcomas (Tannenbaum). Wet formalin fixed tissue for electron microscopic examination, although far from ideal, is usually adequate to make the correct diagnosis.

Histiocytic Tumors. Occasionally, tumors included in the spectrum of fibrous histiocytomas are found in the kidney and may simulate clear cell or spindle cell sarcomatoid renal adenocarcinoma. These histiocytic tumors are uncommon as primary lesions of the kidney, but are among the more common primary tumors arising in the retroperitoneum and may extend to involve the kidney. Primary and metastatic histiocytic tumors of the kidney

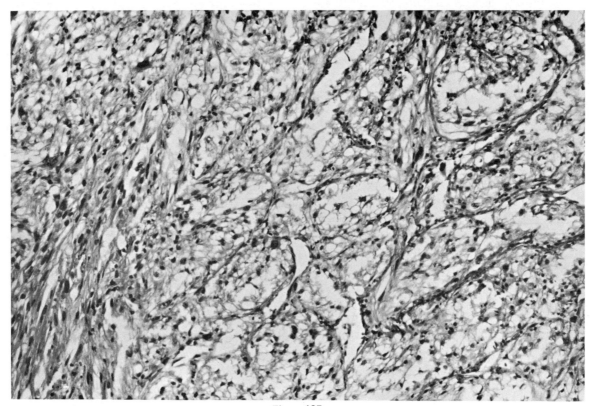

Figure 135
RENAL ADENOCARCINOMA, MIXED PATTERN
A sarcomatoid renal adenocarcinoma is present in the upper right of the field, while the remainder of the field shows the more typical appearance of clear cells in solid sheets and tubular structures. X185.

are discussed on page 234.

Nephroblastoma. Distinguishing a predominantly sarcomatous nephroblastoma from a sarcomatoid renal adenocarcinoma is usually not a problem. Difficulties do arise, however, on the rare occasions when: (1) a nephroblastoma and renal adenocarcinoma occur simultaneously in the same kidney; and (2) when a sarcomatoid renal adenocarcinoma is intermingled with metaplastic malignant mesenchymal components (Farrow et al.).

The diagnosis of nephroblastoma can usually be established by its typical bimorphic histologic pattern, characterized by a background of small spindle cells supported on a fine reticulin network and focal differentiation toward ductlike structures. Histochemical and electron microscopic examination may be necessary in some cases to establish the presence of components of renal adenocarcinoma.

Nonprimary Carcinomas Involving the Renal Parenchyma. In poorly differentiated sarcomatoid or pleomorphic tumors involving both the kidney and renal pelvis, it may be difficult and, occasionally, impossible to determine whether the tumor is primary in the kidney or primary in the renal pelvis, or, in very rare cases, whether it represents collision of two independent tumors (Gillis et al.; Graham and Vynalek; Walker and Jordan). In the last case, it would be most unlikely for both components to present with sarcomatoid or pleomorphic patterns. Usually, a careful search of multiple sections will disclose sufficiently well differentiated tumor to decide its origin. When the tumor is uniformly undifferentiated, histochemical examination for lipids and keratin may help. Unfortunately, transitional cell carcinomas have no distinguishing histochemical features, and those present in renal adenocarcinomas and squamous cell carcinomas are usually lost by the time the tumor is sufficiently undifferentiated, so that it cannot be identified by routine histologic examination. The presence of a sarcomatoid pattern is not a distinguishing feature, since both renal adenocarcinomas and renal pelvic carcinomas may assume this pattern when poorly differentiated, and the tendency for transitional cell carcinomas of the renal pelvis to become sarcomatoid is greater after invasion of the renal parenchyma (Farrow et al.). Electron microscopic examination can help to rule out a sarcoma or sarcomatoid adenocarcinoma (Lichtiger et al.; Tannenbaum). Unfortunately, there have been no reports on ultrastructural features of pleomorphic renal adenocarcinomas or poorly differentiated transitional cell carcinomas, so we have no basis for evaluating the use of the electron microscope in differentiating between these two tumors.

The problem of distinguishing between renal adenocarcinoma and metastatic carcinoma to the kidney in a nephrectomy specimen does not arise often. However, in view of the frequency of metastases to the kidney, this possibility should be kept in mind. Metastases to the kidney have been reported in 4.6 to 7.6 percent of patients with carcinoma examined at autopsy, which is approximately 2 to 3 times as frequent as the incidence of renal adenocarcinoma (Abeshouse and Goldstein; Pine; Willis, 1952). The frequency of bilaterality in metastases (73 to 81 percent; Klinger; Payne) is greater than that of primary bilateral renal adenocarcinoma (0.5 to 1.5 percent; Abeshouse and Weinberg; Moertel et al.), but this is of little help in differential diagnosis, since renal adenocarcinomas frequently metastasize to the opposite kidney (Table V). The sites of the

Table V

FREQUENCY WITH WHICH MALIGNANT TUMORS IN VARIOUS SITES METASTASIZE TO KIDNEY*

Site of Primary Tumor	Percentage Metastasizing to Kidney
Opposite Kidney	27.5
Lung	21.0
Breast	11.0
Stomach	9.6
Ovary	5.5
Intestine	4.5
Uterus	4.4
Pancreas	4.1
Cervix	3.1
Prostate	3.0
Other	0.5

*Modified from Table V-2, p. 80. In: Bennington, J. L., and Kradjian, R. Renal Carcinoma. Philadelphia: W. B. Saunders Co., 1967.

Table VI

PRIMARY SOURCE OF METASTASES IN KIDNEY*

Site of Primary Tumor	Percentage Metastasizing to Kidney
Breast	24.5
Lung	24.0
Intestine	10.5
Opposite Kidney	7.6
Stomach	6.6
Ovary	3.0
Cervix	2.5
Pancreas	2.0
Uterus	1.5
Prostate	1.0
Other	15.8
Total	100.0

*Modified from Table V-1, p. 80. In: Bennington, J. L., and Kradjian, R. Renal Carcinoma. Philadelphia: W. B. Saunders Co., 1967.

primary malignant tumors among 196 patients with carcinoma metastatic to the kidney, listed in order of descending frequency, are given in Table VI. Also for comparison, the frequency with which certain malignant tumors metastasize to the kidney are given in Table V.

Malakoplakia and Xanthogranulomatous Pyelonephritis. Malakoplakia and xanthogranuloma are two inflammatory conditions which are quite rare in adults and even more so in children, but are important because they can occur anywhere in the urinary tract, and in these sites closely mimic carcinoma clinically, radiologically, and morphologically (Lambird and Yardley; Malek et al.; Graivier and Vargas; Rios-Dalenz and Peacock).

In the kidney, either of these inflammatory reactions may replace part, or all of the renal parenchyma and even extend into the perinephric fat. Grossly, they are generally nodular, focally necrotic, or cystic; these lesions are bright yellow to orange due to large amounts of neutral and phospholipid in the cytoplasm of the interstitial macrophages which proliferate to form the tumor (pl. VI; Kerr et al.). The characteristic lesion in the renal pelvis, ureter, and bladder is a plaquelike mass which replaces mucosa, although the entire wall and even the retroperitoneum may be involved. Resolution of the lesions is by fibrosis, which in the ureter can produce stenosis.

Histologically, malakoplakia and xanthogranulomas resemble the clear cell variant of renal adenocarcinoma and may be misdiagnosed as renal adenocarcinoma by the unwary (Graivier and Vargas). They have also been described as a benign cystic adenomatous renal parenchymal tumor, so-called Perlmann's tumor (Dobben). Histologically, both are formed by proliferation of sheets of rounded histiocytes with small,

PLATE VI

MALAKOPLAKIA AND XANTHOGRANULOMATOUS PYELONEPHRITIS OF KIDNEY

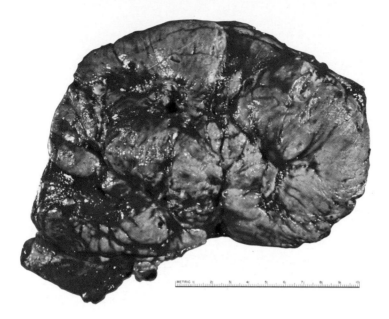

A.   The gross appearance of malakoplakia of the kidney shows complete replacement of the normal renal parenchyma by yellow-orange nodular masses which are focally hemorrhagic and necrotic. (Courtesy of Dr. Vivian Gildenhorn, Los Angeles, Calif.)

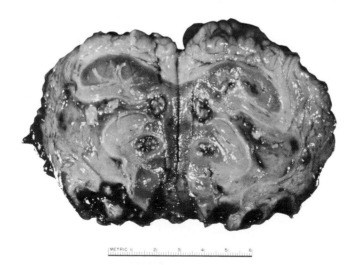

B.   This gross appearance of xanthogranulomatous pyelonephritis shows much of the renal parenchyma being replaced by yellow-gray to tan nodules resembling tumor.

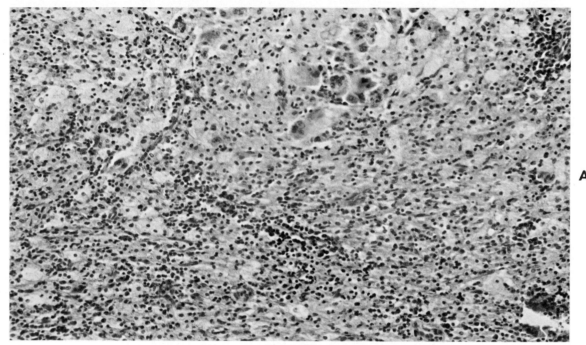

Figure 136
XANTHOGRANULOMATOUS PYELONEPHRITIS

A. This is a low power view of xanthogranulomatous pyelonephritis. There is focal necrosis, infiltration of lympho-cytes, and a background of round to polygonal foamy histiocytes, some of which are multinucleated. Cholesterol clefts are present. X140.

B. This higher magnification demonstrates the foamy cytoplasmic contents, rounded to polygonal cellular configura-tion, distinct cell membranes, and nuclear variability. The stromal and vascular scaffolding typical of renal adenocarcinoma is missing in xanthogranulomatous pyelonephritis. X1300.

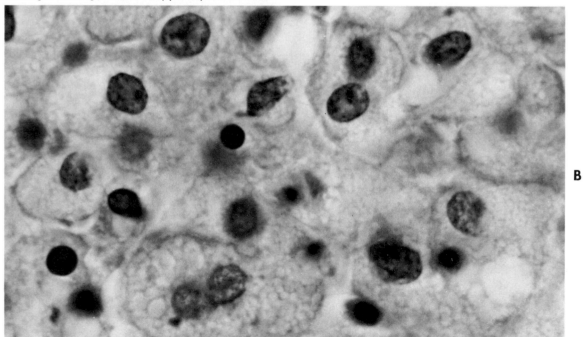

regular, round to oval nuclei, and a granular or foamy clear to brightly eosinophilic cytoplasm. Xanthogranulomatous lesions are said to be characterized by multinucle- ated cells and the presence of cholesterol deposits (fig. 136), while malakoplakia is recognized by the presence of Michaelis-Gutmann bodies (fig. 137).

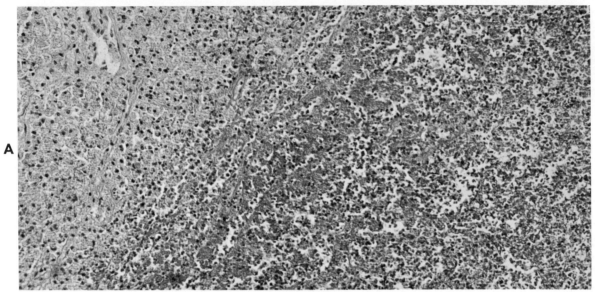

Figure 137
MALAKOPLAKIA

A. This low power view of malakoplakia reveals a similarity to figure 136 of xanthogranulomatous pyelonephritis; there is necrosis, inflammation, and a diffuse infiltrate of histiocytes. Multinucleated giant cells and cholesterol clefts are not seen. X140.

B. This higher magnification shows the cytologic similarity of malakoplakia to xanthogranulomatous pyelonephritis. Characteristic calcospherites (Michaelis-Gutmann bodies) are seen in the cytoplasm (arrows). X1300.

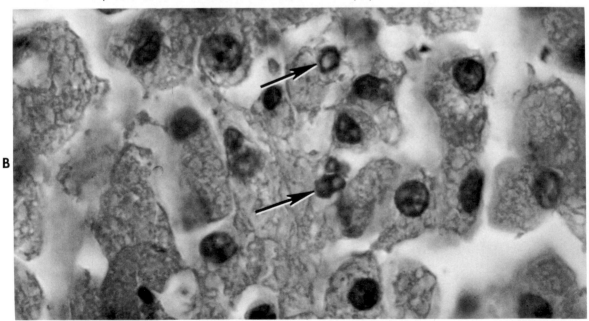

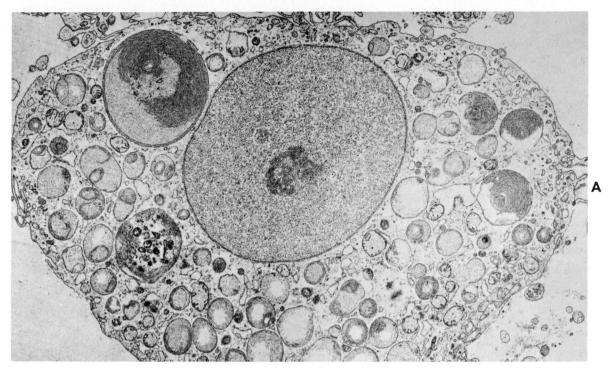

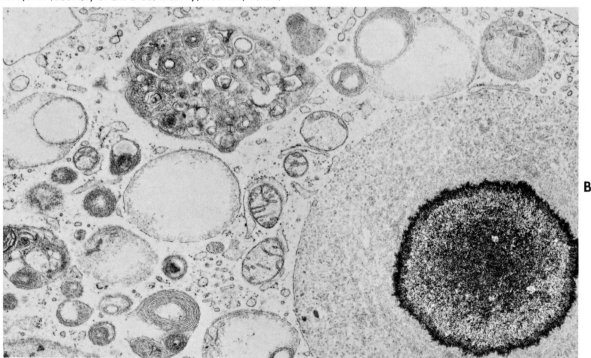

Figure 138
MALAKOPLAKIA

This is the electron microscopic appearance of histiocytes in malakoplakia.

A. In the cytoplasm are numerous vacuoles containing whorled complex parallel membranes and electron dense flocculent material. The structures appear to represent heterophagosomes containing lipid debris. X6500.

B. This higher magnification reveals a portion of a partially calcified heterophagosome (Michaelis-Gutmann body). X17,000. (Courtesy of Dr. Bruce Mackay, Houston, Texas.)

Conventionally, malakoplakia and xanthogranulomatous inflammation are considered as distinct entities; the differentiation is largely based upon the presence of characteristic cytoplasmic calcospherites in the macrophages in malakoplakia. In both conditions, there is prominent increase in the numbers of cytosegresomes (Kerr et al.; Lambird and Yardley). In lesions described as malakoplakia, Michaelis-Gutmann bodies are found (fig. 138) which are thought to arise through phagocytosis of bacterial degradation products by the cytosegresomes, providing a matrix for deposition of needle-like crystals resembling hydroxyapatite. Whether or not the presence of Michaelis-Gutmann bodies is sufficient to warrant designation of two distinct entities is yet to be proved.

Recent evidence suggests that these two conditions may be different expressions of the same or related pathologic changes (Kerr et al.; Lambird and Yardley). Both are frequently associated with urinary tract obstruction, calculi, and urinary tract infection and have been produced experimentally by ureteral ligation and induction of urinary tract infection (Kerr et al.; Lambird and Yardley; Malek et al.; Povysil and Konickova; Tan and Heptinstall). The basic process appears to be bacterial infection most frequently due to *E. coli, Proteus, or Pseudomonas* species.

DISTRIBUTION OF METASTASES FROM RENAL ADENOCARCINOMA

At autopsy, metastases are present in as many as 95 percent of patients with renal adenocarcinoma (Creevy; Harvey; Kozoll and Kirshbaum; Soloway). Statistics relating to the frequency of metastases in various sites of 523 patients with metastatic renal adenocarcinoma are shown in Table VII. The percentage of the total number of metastases to a specific organ or tissue, contributed by renal adenocarcinoma, is shown in Table VIII. Unusual sites for metastases of renal adenocarcinoma have been extensively reviewed by Bennington and Kradjian. At sites in which metastases are relatively common, i.e., brain, lung, and bone, and at sites in which metastases are less common, i.e., ureter, penis, heart, thyroid, skin, vagina, and

Table VII

RENAL ADENOCARCINOMA
SITES AND FREQUENCY OF METASTASES
AT AUTOPSY*

Sites of Metastasis	Percentage of Patients with Metastasis
Lung	55.0
Lymph nodes	34.0
Liver	33.0
Bone	32.0
Adrenal	19.0
Opposite kidney	11.0
Brain	5.7
Heart	5.0
Spleen	4.6
Intestine	3.8
Skin	3.2
Diaphragm	2.3
Pancreas, Thyroid, Ureter, Epididymis, Muscle, Gallbladder	2.0
Mesentery, Corpus cavernosum, Bladder, Dura, Pericardium, Bile duct, Ovary	1.0

*Modified from Table VI-1, p. 157. In: Bennington, J. L., and Kradjian, R. Renal Carcinoma. Philadelphia: W. B. Saunders Co., 1967.

Table VIII

PERCENTAGE OF TOTAL NUMBER
OF METASTASES TO CERTAIN ORGANS
CONTRIBUTED BY RENAL ADENOCARCINOMA*

Site of Metastasis	Percentage of Total Metastases to Site
Ureter	15.0
Penis	11.0
Vagina	9.0
Thyroid	8.6
Heart	8.0
Kidney	7.3
Brain	7.0
Skin	6.8
Intestine	4.9
Lung	4.9
Bone	4.6
Uterus	4.0
Pleura	4.0
Adrenal	2.7
Lymph Node	2.5
Pancreas	2.3
Liver	2.1
Ovary, Peritoneum, Diaphragm, Pericardium	2.0

*Modified from Table VI-4, p. 159. In: Bennington, J. L., and Kradjian, R. Renal Carcinoma. Philadelphia: W. B. Saunders Co., 1967.

intestine, the percentage of metastases contributed by renal adenocarcinoma is greater than would be expected from the frequency of this carcinoma among all carcinomas. This raises several possibilities: (1) Patients with renal adenocarcinoma may live longer than patients with other carcinomas, thus providing a greater opportunity for metastases to develop; (2) cells from renal adenocarcinoma are better able to reach or survive in certain sites than cells from other cancers; (3) one or more routes for dissemination of metastases may be available from renal adenocarcinoma, but not readily available for other carcinomas;

and (4) some combination of these mechanisms, which seems most likely.

Routes of Metastases. The embolic dissemination of malignant cells occurs by three different routes: lymphogenous, lymphohematogenous, and hematogenous. The following are characteristic patterns of spread by these routes in patients with renal adenocarcinoma.

Lymphogenous Spread. This occurs chiefly to the regional lymph nodes. The first to be involved are usually the most proximal nodes among the lymphatics draining the kidney and less frequently to other retroperitoneal, abdominal, and mediastinal lymph nodes, and relatively infrequently to supraclavicular, cervical, axillary, and inguinal nodes.

Lymphohematogenous Spread. Because of the proximity of the lateral aortic nodes to the cisterna chyli, malignant cells carried by the lymphatics may gain access to the thoracic duct, then to the superior vena cava to be carried through the right heart into the pulmonary circulation.

The frequency with which lymphohematogenous spread occurs has not been determined in any large series of patients with renal carcinoma, but has been studied in abdominal and retroperitoneal tumors as a group. In one series of 12 extraperitoneal primary abdominal cancers, one of the carcinomas metastasized via the vena cava, three via the thoracic duct, and five via both vena cava and thoracic duct (Brunner). The overall findings suggest that the thoracic duct was one route of spread for 67 percent of the primary extraperitoneal abdominal carcinomas. Thus, this lymphohematogenous route provides a means for metastases to bypass the liver via the thoracic duct and to reach the lung through the pulmonary arteries (fig. 139).

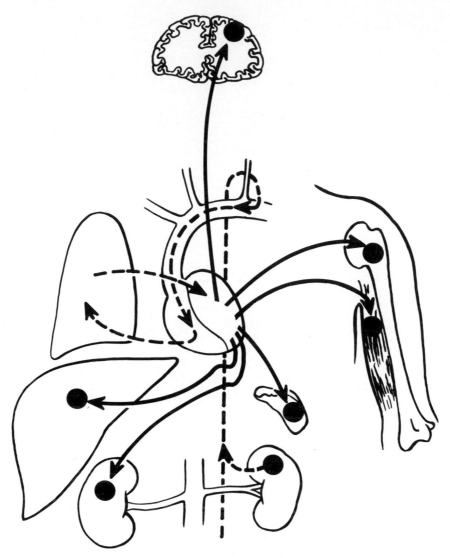

Figure 139
METASTATIC RENAL ADENOCARCINOMA
This illustrates lymphohematogenous dissemination of metastases from a renal adenocarcinoma. Embolic cells gaining access to the thoracic duct are carried cranially, empty into the superior vena cava, and pass to the lungs via the right side of the heart. Cells not filtered out by the pulmonary capillaries enter the systemic circulation and may be carried anyplace in the body.

Occasionally, intraluminal attachment and growth of metastatic renal carcinoma may fill and obstruct the thoracic duct in a manner similar to that seen in the superior vena cava (fig. 140; Schwedenberg; Winkler).

Hematogenous Spread. Spread by this route is probably more important in renal adenocarcinoma than for most other cancers. The venous drainage of the kidney through the caval system and its tributaries helps to explain the frequency and wide distribution of metastases from this tumor (fig. 141). Embolic cells in the renal vein may spread: (1) retrograde to pelvic structures via the left spermatic or ovarian vein;

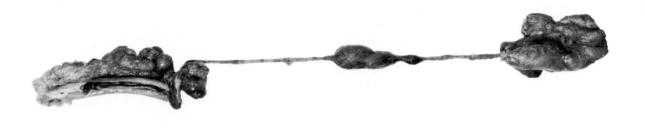

Figure 140
METASTATIC RENAL ADENOCARCINOMA IN THORACIC DUCT
In this specimen from a patient with renal adenocarcinoma, an embolus of metastatic tumor is present midway up the thoracic duct. (Courtesy of Dr. Noel Gowing, London, England.)

(2) along the axial skeleton by way of the paravertebral veins (Batson's plexus); (3) up the vena cava through the right heart to the lungs; and (4) after passing through the pulmonary circulation to multiple sites by the arterial circulation.

Retrograde to Pelvic Structures via Left Spermatic or Ovarian Vein. In 1956, Abeshouse was able to find reports of 50 well documented instances of metastases from renal adenocarcinoma to genito-urinary organs. Because the primary carci-noma was in the left kidney in the great majority of cases—8 of 12 metastases to the ureter; 8 of 8 to the bladder; 3 of 3 to the penis; 2 of 2 to the epididymis; 2 of 3 to the testis; and 20 of 25 to the vagina (not mentioned by him were 2 of 2 metastases to the ovary) (fig. 155), he concluded that connection of the left renal vein with the left testicular (or ovarian) vein provides a means of retrograde venous embolization of metastases to pelvic organs (figs. 141, 142). He discounted lymphatic, arterial, and intraureteral implantation as most unlikely.

Although Abeshouse's arguments against "implantation metastases" are most con-vincing, there are occasional reports of this unlikely phenomenon occurring in the

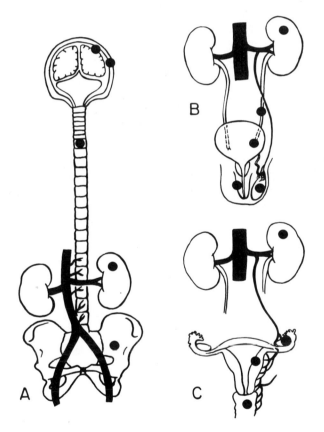

Figure 141
METASTATIC RENAL ADENOCARCINOMA
Hematogenous dissemination of metastases from a renal adenocarcinoma occurs (A) via Batson's plexus to axial structures; (B) by retrograde extension along the left testicular vein to pelvic and genital structures in the male; and (C) by retrograde extension along the left ovarian vein to pelvic and genital structures in the female.

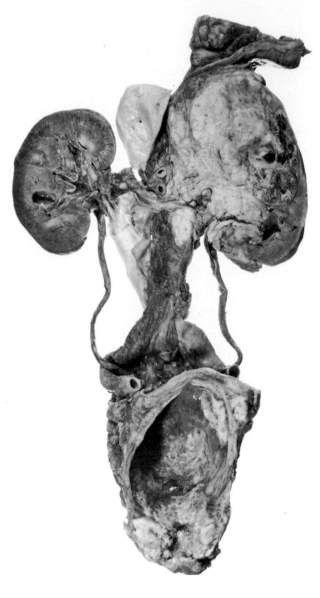

cm

0 1 2 3 4 5

Figure 142
RETROGRADE METASTASIS
OF RENAL ADENOCARCINOMA

A 64 year old man died of renal adenocarcinoma. The tumor which arose in the left kidney had invaded the renal pelvis and renal vein, spread directly to the diaphragm and left adrenal, and metastasized to lymph nodes, lungs, vertebrae, bladder, and prostatic bed. (Courtesy of Dr. Roger Pugh, London, England.)

bladder and the ureter (Suzuki; Heslin et al.; Howell; Macalpine; Sargent). Reports of extension of renal adenocarcinoma in the ureteric vein in conjunction with ureteral metastases indicate what is most likely the actual route of so-called "implantation metastases" (Mitchell).

To Axial Skeleton via Paravertebral Veins. The great frequency of osseous metastases in patients with renal adeno-carcinoma is in large part due to the proximity of the kidney to the paravertebral (Batson's) venous plexus (Batson). Since the paravertebral veins form an extensive system from pelvis to skull, which anastomoses freely with the caval system at each segmental level, it is not surprising that tumor cells entering the vena cava can be shunted into the paravertebral veins (presumably during periods of increased abdominal pressure) where they lodge, producing metastases at various sites along the axial skeleton. This route of metastases not only explains the frequent bony metastases in the pelvis, spine, and skull, but may also account for the relatively high frequency of involvement of the thyroid, which is in close proximity to the paravertebral veins. While our statistics indicate that about 9 percent of metastases to the thyroid are from renal adenocarcinoma, Tuaillon and associates have suggested that as many as 25 percent of metastases to the thyroid are from renal adenocarcinoma, and postulated that they reached the thyroid via the vertebral veins.

Ascending in the Vena Cava. The vena cava undoubtedly provides the channel for the great majority of metastases from renal adenocarcinoma, especially those ultimately reaching the lung. Extension of a column of tumor up the vena cava (fig. 143), and on occasion into the right side of the heart (fig. 144), is one of the more dramatic findings encountered in the post-mortem examination of patients with renal adenocarcinoma. Although a few patients with such findings have lived for many years following nephrectomy, the extension of tumor into the renal veins or vena cava is usually a grave prognostic sign.

Migration Through Pulmonary Circulation to Arterial Circulation. Although the lung is effective in filtering out the major-ity of embolic malignant cells carried to it by blood from the right heart, it apparently does not trap them all. Zeidman and Buss have shown that malignant cells reaching the lung are not necessarily arrested there, but may pass via the pulmonary capillaries as single cells or small emboli into the arterial circulation to produce widespread metastases. Many of the sites of metastasis in renal adenocarcinoma such as the eyes

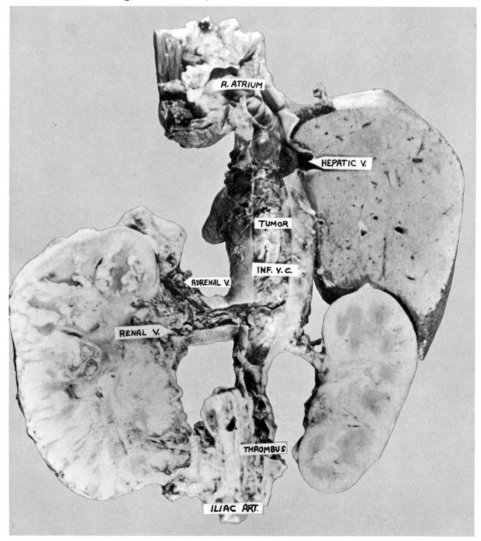

Figure 143
HEMATOGENOUS EXTENSION OF RENAL ADENOCARCINOMA
This shows hematogenous extension of renal adenocarcinoma from the kidney into the renal vein and up the dilated vena cava to the right side of the heart. (Courtesy of Dr. A. Lazar, Leonia, N. J.)

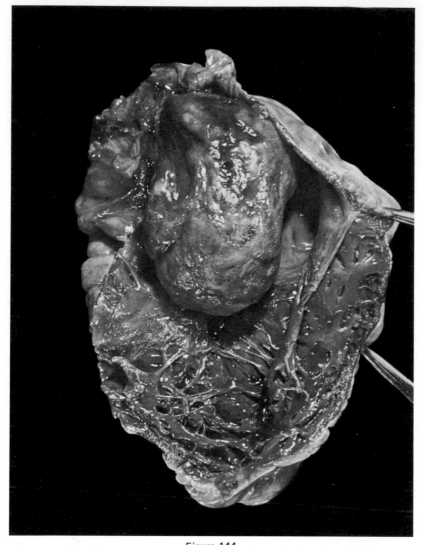

Figure 144
INTRAVENOUS GROWTH OF RENAL ADENOCARCINOMA
This large mass of renal adenocarcinoma had extended up the vena cava into the right atrium and nearly filled it.
(Courtesy of Dr. N. L. Morgenstern, Oakland, Calif.)

(fig. 145), skin (fig. 146), and striated muscles or heart can be accounted for by arterial spread. In experimental animals, introduction of tumor cells into the arterial circulation produces just such a distribution of metastases (fig. 147).

With the reservation that metastases to a particular organ may have reached that site by more than one route, the hematogenous routes usually taken by metastases from renal adenocarcinoma to particular organs and sites are shown in figures 139 and 141.

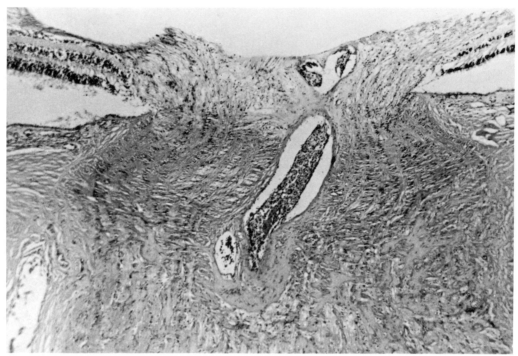

Figure 145
METASTATIC RENAL ADENOCARCINOMA
Metastatic renal adenocarcinoma to the eye resulted from a tumor embolus which lodged in the choroidal artery. X74.
(Courtesy of Dr. Joseph B. Crawford, San Francisco, Calif.)

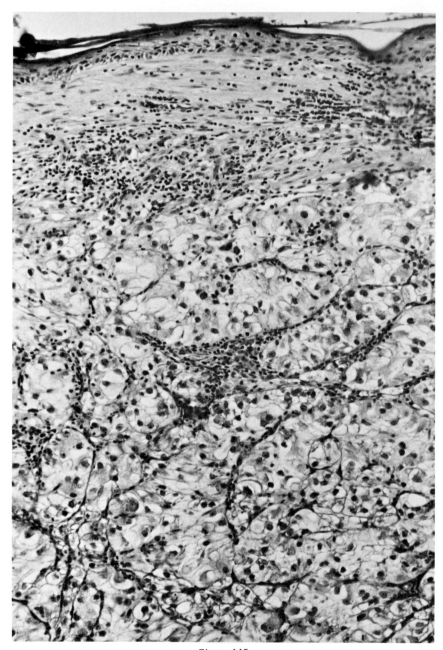

Figure 146
METASTATIC RENAL ADENOCARCINOMA
This renal adenocarcinoma was metastatic to the skin with a trabecular arrangement of clear cells. The fibrovascular stroma is typical of renal adenocarcinoma. X185.

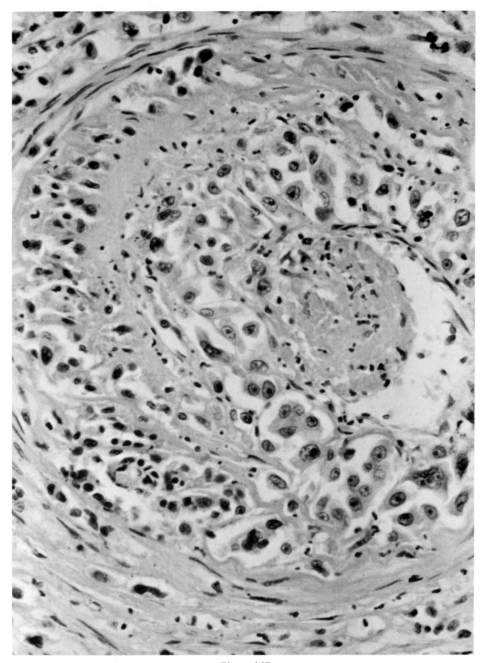

Figure 147
RENAL ADENOCARCINOMA INVOLVING ARTERY
This renal adenocarcinoma infiltrated between the layers of the muscular wall and into the lumen of a small artery. X330.

DIFFERENTIAL DIAGNOSIS OF TUMORS IN OTHER SITES FROM METASTATIC RENAL ADENOCARCINOMA

In general, it is difficult to be certain of the origin of a metastatic carcinoma by histologic examination. Metastatic deposits from renal adenocarcinomas are usually recognized rather easily, especially when composed of large clear cells (fig. 146). Unfortunately, metastases from renal adenocarcinoma are not always of the clear cell type and often may be considerably less well differentiated than the primary tumor. Secondly, the presence of clear cells is not pathognomonic of renal adenocarcinoma and what is thought to be metastatic renal adenocarcinoma may be a primary tumor rather than a metastasis, or a metastasis from a primary tumor of another organ. Tumors that may be confused with metastatic renal adenocarcinoma in various sites are described below.

In the Skin. Since renal adenocarcinomas metastasize to the skin relatively frequently and make up a disproportionately large number of skin metastases, it is important to distinguish these metastases from primary skin tumors to prevent a diagnosis of carcinomatosis and subjecting the patient to an exhaustive and unnecessary search for a primary renal adenocarcinoma.

Several skin tumors may be confused with metastatic renal adenocarcinoma. The two most important are sebaceous carcinoma and nodular hidradenoma, and occasionally "balloon cell melanoma" (Ranchod). In general, the solitary appendage tumors are found in older individuals as asymptomatic growths of long duration in an otherwise healthy patient, whereas metastatic renal adenocarcinoma usually grows more rapidly. Even though it may be a presenting nodule in a patient who is relatively well, careful examination or history may reveal systemic complaints referable to the primary neoplasm.

Sebaceous carcinoma is rare and is generally found on the eyelids or scalp, but may occur anyplace on the skin, usually as an ulcerating nodule. Rulon and Helwig accepted only 6 of 38 lesions cross indexed as sebaceous carcinoma in the Armed Forces Institute of Pathology Registry. Two of the 32 excluded cases represented metastatic renal adenocarcinoma. Characteristically, sebaceous carcinoma is lobulated and the nests of tumor cells, while irregular in size and shape, tend to mimic the maturation of normal sebaceous lobules. Cells at the margin of individual lobules are usually poorly differentiated, while those nearer the center resemble sebaceous cells, but with pronounced nuclear pleomorphism and hyperchromasia. Occasionally, foci of keratinization are present (fig. 148).

Both renal adenocarcinoma and sebaceous carcinoma contain intracellular glycogen, neutral and phospholipids, and cholesterol; both may be composed of clear and eosinophilic granular cells. Histologic differentiation between these two tumors is based largely upon the characteristic lobulation, resemblance to sebaceous cells, foci of keratinization, and nuclear pleomorphism seen in the sebaceous carcinoma.

The nodular hidradenoma also presents as a solitary skin nodule and may be found anyplace on the body. Typically, it is multilobular and composed of sheets of clear cells interspersed with ductal structures. Individual cells have distinct cell membranes and small, oval to pyknotic nuclei with infrequent mitoses. Histochemically, most of the cells contain glycogen, but none contain lipid. Muco-

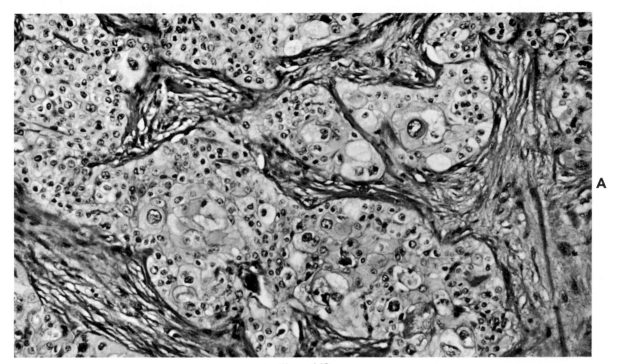

A

Figure 148
SEBACEOUS CARCINOMA OF SKIN

A. This sebaceous carcinoma is composed of large nests of clear cells. Centrally, the cells and nuclei are large with clear cytoplasm and pleomorphic nuclei. Peripherally, the cells and nuclei are small and regular in size and shape. X185.

B. This higher magnification demonstrates a coarse, amorphous, collagenous stroma surrounding the nests of tumor cells which is unusual for renal adenocarcinoma. Cells in the center of tumor cell nests are large with pleomorphic nuclei compared to the cells at the margins of the nests. X465.

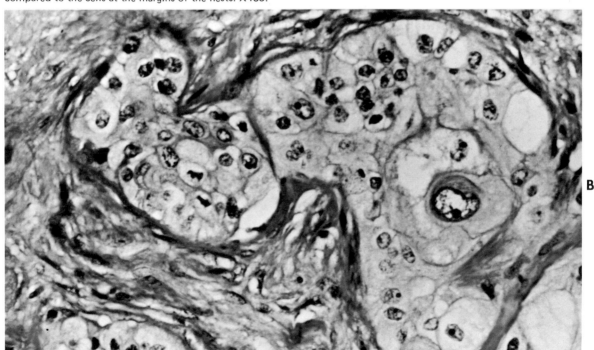

B

polysaccharides are present within duct lumens, but not within individual cells. This tumor can be distinguished from metastatic renal adenocarcinoma by its characteristic multilobular pattern which is usually not seen in metastatic renal adenocarcinoma, and by its lack of any papillary organization and absence of intracellular lipid, which are usually present in renal adenocarcinoma. Glycogen and intraluminal mucopolysaccharides are seen in both tumors and are of no help in differential diagnosis (fig. 149).

It is unlikely that a primary balloon cell melanoma would be confused with a metastatic renal adenocarcinoma, since melanomas usually can be traced to an epithelial origin while metastases involve the dermis and subcutaneous tissue. If there is any doubt, the presence of melanin pigment and the absence of lipids help to confirm the diagnosis of melanoma.

In the Region of the Salivary Glands. While metastases to the salivary glands are rare, metastases to the soft tissue of the neck occur frequently from renal adenocarcinoma and may metastatically invade the salivary glands, making it necessary to distinguish metastatic disease from an invasive primary salivary gland carcinoma.

The two salivary gland tumors most likely to be confused with metastatic renal adenocarcinoma are the mucoepidermoid carcinoma (fig. 150) and variants of the acinic cell tumor (fig. 151). The mucoepidermoid carcinoma is usually not a problem unless the tumor is predominantly formed of clear cells, and even then a diligent search will generally reveal the characteristic mucosecretory and focally keratinizing cells. Histochemically, intracellular PAS-diastase resistant material will be noted (Evans and Cruickshank).

The acinic cell tumor, either in the salivary gland or in metastatic sites, may closely simulate metastatic renal adenocarcinoma by showing a trabecular or tubular arrangement of clear cells supported by a delicate vascular stroma. Since both tumors may contain intracellular glycogen and lipid, the most useful distinguishing feature is the presence of PAS-positive, diastase-resistant intracellular material in acinic cell tumors, which is not found in renal adenocarcinomas, although such material may be present in duct lumens in both tumors (Evans and Cruickshank).

In the Lung. The benign clear cell (sugar) tumor of the lung was first described by Liebow and Castleman in 1963, but is apparently not a well known entity. It is important to distinguish this tumor (fig. 152) from renal adenocarcinoma, since it is benign; obviously, the prognostic and therapeutic implications are quite different for the two tumors. The clear cell tumor of the lung closely resembles renal adenocarcinoma histologically, and both may contain large amounts of glycogen, which has led to the many confusing reports of renal adenocarcinoma metastatic to the lung, with a mysteriously disappearing primary tumor.

The important histologic features that set these tumors apart are the scanty or absent lipid in the clear cell tumor and the presence of PAS-positive, diastase-resistant intracellular material. At the electron microscopic level, characteristic neurosecretory-type granules are seen in the cytoplasm which are not seen in renal adenocarcinoma, thereby justifying the extra expense and effort of electron microscopy (Becker and Soifer). At times, bronchiolo-alveolar adenocarcinoma of the lung may be composed of clear cells and mimic metastatic renal adenocarcinoma

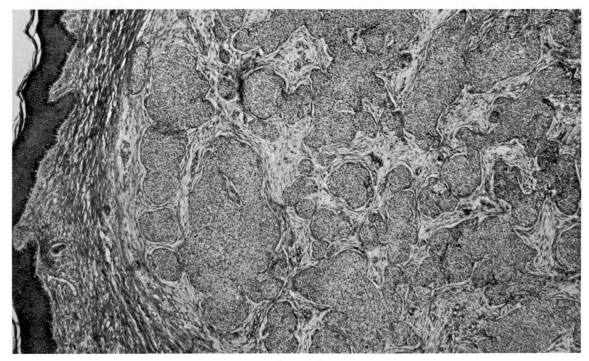

Figure 149
NODULAR HIDRADENOMA OF SKIN

A. At low magnification this nodular hidradenoma shows nests of small clear cells and pyknotic nuclei. The loose connective tissue stroma between nests of cells is a characteristic feature of this neoplasm. X72.

B. At higher magnification an amorphous membrane-like structure, similar to that seen in sebaceous carcinoma, is evident around nests of tumor cells. Cells are haphazardly arranged with little stroma within the nests. Nuclei are small, folded, and angulated. X465.

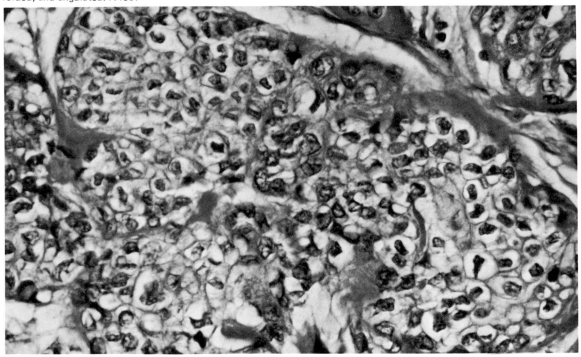

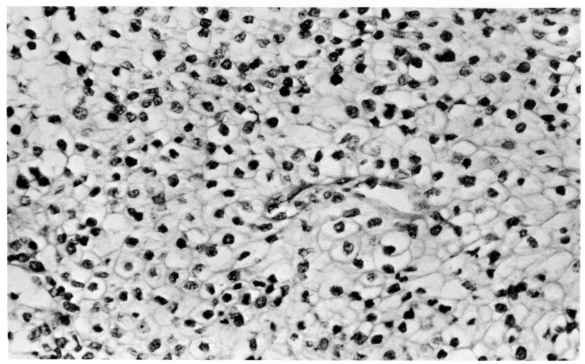

Figure 150
MUCOEPIDERMOID CARCINOMA OF SALIVARY GLAND
In this clear cell variant of mucoepidermoid carcinoma of the salivary gland, the cell membranes are distinct, revealing round to polygonal cell contours. Nuclei are small, dark, and somewhat irregular. The pattern is difficult to distinguish from a renal adenocarcinoma. X280.

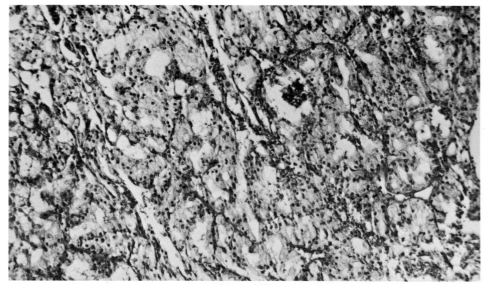

Figure 151
ACINIC CELL CARCINOMA OF SALIVARY GLAND
The tubular and trabecular structures, supported by a delicate fibrovascular stroma, closely mimic the pattern of renal adenocarcinoma. The cytoplasm in the large cells ranges from clear to granular and is typically basophilic rather than eosinophilic, as seen in renal adenocarcinoma. X95.

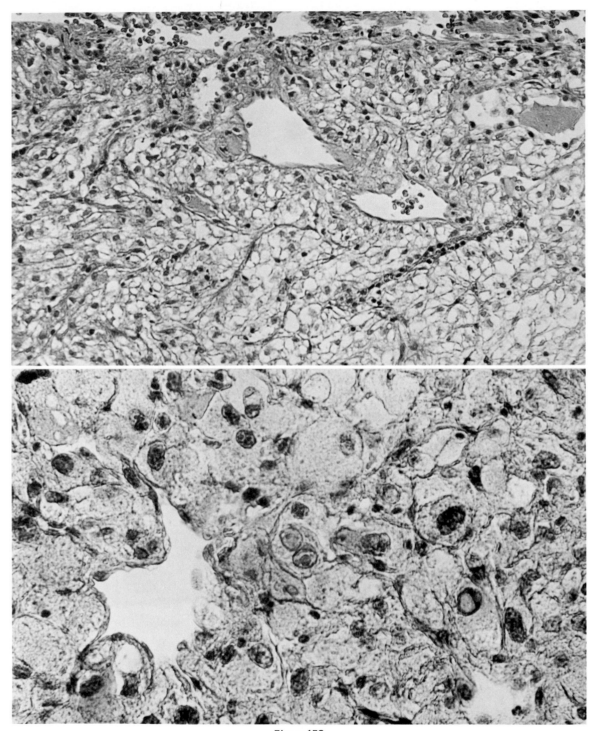

Figure 152
BENIGN CLEAR CELL TUMOR OF LUNG
This tumor is composed of large clear cells with distinct cellular membranes and small hyperchromatic nuclei. The cells are arranged in a trabecular pattern around thin-walled blood vessels. Upper, X280; lower, X800. (Courtesy of Dr. Averill A. Liebow, San Diego, Calif.)

(fig. 153). Special stains for mucins and lipids are of help, since mucins but not lipids are found in the bronchiolo-alveolar carcinoma while the opposite is true of renal adenocarcinoma.

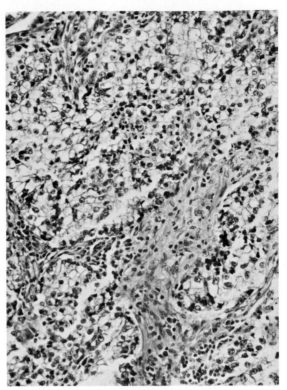

Figure 153

Figure 153
BRONCHIOLO-ALVEOLAR ADENOCARCINOMA
The clear cell variant of bronchiolo-alveolar adenocarcinoma reveals alveoli lined by slender cylindrical cells which frequently form papillary proliferations. Individual cells are clear with small vesicular nuclei. X185.

In the Central Nervous System. While metastases to the brain from carcinomas of a wide variety of primary sites can provide diagnostic problems, one of the more difficult histologic problems is the differentiation of the primary hemangioblastoma of the brain from metastatic renal adenocarcinoma. This is particularly confusing because of the histologic similarities between these two tumors, the propensity for renal adenocarcinoma to metastasize to the brain, and the well known association of hemangioblastoma, usually in the cerebellum, and renal adenocarcinoma in patients with **von Hippel-Lindau syndrome** (see p. 107).

The microscopic features of hemangioblastoma include numerous thin-walled vessels of capillary size and a stroma containing many round to polygonal clear cells with a foamy cytoplasm and small, round to oval nuclei (fig. 154; Kawamura et al.).

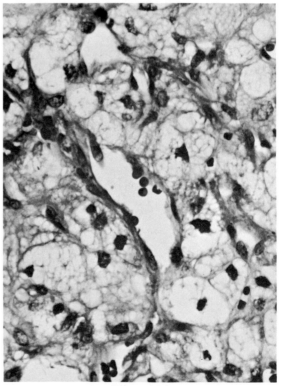

Figure 154

Figure 154
CEREBELLAR HEMANGIOBLASTOMA
This cerebellar hemangioblastoma is composed of haphazardly arranged foamy to granular histiocytes. The stroma is richly vascular and a prominent feature of the tumor. The variation in cellular size, indistinct cellular membranes, and disorganized pattern help to distinguish this tumor from a metastatic renal adenocarcinoma. X464.

The clear cells contain glycogen and lipids and are of histiocytic origin. Considering the difficulty of distinguishing xanthogranulomatous pyelonephritis from renal adenocarcinoma, and the still debated issue whether stromal foam cells in papillary renal adenocarcinomas are of epithelial or histiocytic origin, it is not surprising that it is difficult to distinguish renal adenocarcinoma metastatic to the brain from hemangioblastoma.

Because both tumors contain intracellular glycogen and lipid in the clear cells, histochemical stains are of limited use, although demonstration of the prominent endothelial proliferation in hemangioblastoma with a reticulin stain may be helpful. More important is the absence in hemangioblastomas of papillary, tubular, or trabecular patterns which are usually found in renal adenocarcinoma.

In the Ovary. A host of primary neoplasms of the ovary, including the spectrum of lipoid cell tumors and clear cell (mesonephric) carcinoma, may enter into the differential diagnosis of primary ovarian tumor versus metastatic renal adenocarcinoma (fig. 155). It is beyond the scope of this fascicle to review all these entities, which are adequately covered, together with important distinguishing features, in the reports of Scully and of Taylor and Norris.

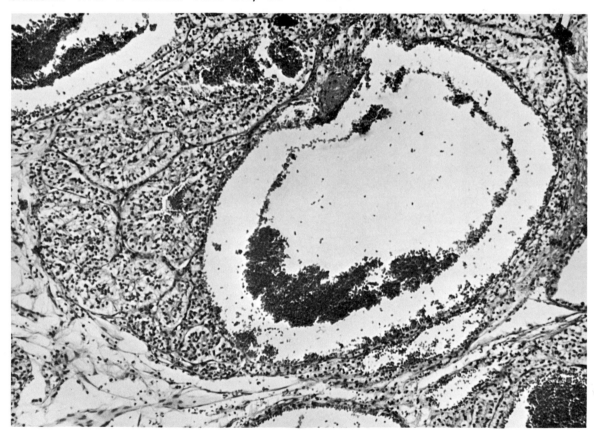

Figure 155
METASTATIC RENAL ADENOCARCINOMA
Metastasis of this renal adenocarcinoma to the right ovary had an identical histologic appearance to that of the primary tumor. X130.

In the Adrenal Gland. The problem of differentiating a primary adrenal cortical carcinoma from metastatic renal adenocarcinoma is probably academic, except in the unlikely circumstance when an endocrinologically inactive adrenal cortical tumor is discovered and a primary renal adenocarcinoma is missed at the time of surgery.

Distinction between these two possibilities would be difficult histologically, since both tumors contain intracytoplasmic fat and glycogen and neither contains intracellular mucins. Characteristically, the adrenal cortical carcinomas are usually histologically much more bizarre than renal adenocarcinomas with marked pleomorphism, frequent mitoses, numerous giant cells, and prominent nuclear hyperchromasia and, at times, they may be sarcomatoid (fig. 156). While this is not the usual pattern, renal adenocarcinomas may also be poorly differentiated and even sarcomatoid, so these features cannot be relied upon to distinguish one from the other. If differentiation is important, electron microscopic examination may be required (Tannenbaum).

PROGNOSIS

In general, the prognoses for patients with renal adenocarcinoma are poor. In most series, the overall survival rate is 18 to 27 percent 10 years after nephrectomy (Kaufman). Since there is considerable evidence that this tumor grows slowly, the unfavorable outcome is not attributable solely to aggressiveness, but in part to: (1) Silent growth until the tumor reaches a relatively large size, frequently with metastases responsible for the presenting symptoms; and (2) the patient's delay to seek medical aid after these symptoms appear.

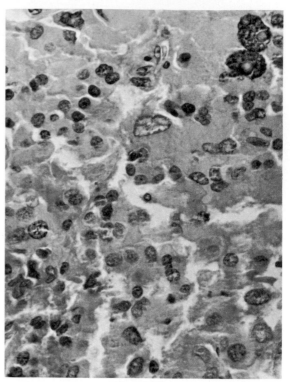

Figure 156
ADRENAL CORTICAL ADENOCARCINOMA
This adrenal cortical adenocarcinoma is composed of rounded cells showing poor cohesion, indistinct cell membranes, and considerable variation in size and shape. Nuclei show marked pleomorphism and focal hyperchromasia. The cytoplasm, which is typically eosinophilic, is smudgy rather than granular, but the stroma is scanty. X464.

Occult Growth and Metastases. At nephrectomy, the average size of renal adenocarcinomas has been reported between 5 to 7.5 cm. (Riches et al., 1951; Strauss and Welt). At that time, about 40 percent have grown through the renal capsule (pl. IV-B), 36 percent have invaded the renal vein (fig. 157), and 40 percent will have produced distant metastases unsuspected prior to surgery (Riches et al., 1951; Mostofi). In spite of the extensive local growth, vascular infiltration and invasion symptoms are late features of the disease and may be referable to metastases rather than the primary tumor.

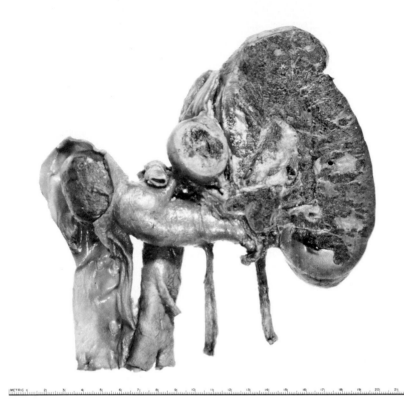

Figure 157
RENAL ADENOCARCINOMA INVADING VEINS
Extension of a column of renal adenocarcinoma fills a renal vein and extends into the vena cava. (Courtesy of Dr. Noel Gowing, London, England.)

Delay in Seeking Medical Attention. For a number of reasons, the patient with symptoms related to renal adenocarcinoma usually does not seek medical attention immediately. Graham estimated the average delay from onset of symptoms to treatment to be 1.8 years. Carcinoma of almost any other organ would be far advanced at this stage and a patient would be considered inoperable with a history of symptoms for nearly two years, a primary tumor 5 to 7.5 cm. in diameter, with vascular invasion and extension to adjacent structures. Yet, nephrectomy for renal adenocarcinoma is performed in such circumstances, and, in spite of the high rate of occult metastases at the time of surgery,

the overall 10-year survival rates are 18 to 27 percent. In the context of experience with carcinomas of other organs, these survival rates are remarkable; they provide considerable impetus for discovering technics which will allow earlier diagnosis of renal adenocarcinoma in a more curable stage.

The following are among the many features suggested that relate to the prognosis for patients with renal adenocarcinoma: (1) Age and sex; (2) gross features of the tumor, including location, number, size, local extension, renal vein invasion, regional lymph node metastasis, and distant metastasis; and (3) microscopic features, including cell type and histologic grade.

Age and Sex. There is little evidence to suggest that age and sex influence the prognosis for patients with renal adenocarcinoma. A better prognosis for younger individuals has been suggested by several investigators (Fetter and Snyder; Mostofi), although Hand and Broders observed a greater frequency of poorly differentiated tumors in patients under 40 years of age, and Griffiths could find no difference in survival rates according to age.

Mostofi reported in his series that while 5-year survival rates were nearly identical for men (48 percent) and women (50 percent), the 10-year survival rates were significantly better for women (42 percent) than for men (32 percent). However, other authors have found no significant differences in survival between men and women in either localized or locally invasive renal adenocarcinomas at 5 or 10 years (Flocks; Griffiths).

Gross Features

Number and Location of Tumors. Petkovic and Mostofi have both demonstrated poorer survival rates for patients with multiple rather than solitary tumors in the same kidney. Mostofi reported a 40 percent 10-year survival for patients with multiple tumors in contrast to 50 percent for patients with solitary tumors. With respect to location, Hand and Broders found a better prognosis for patients with tumors of the upper pole, while Mostofi found a more favorable prognosis for patients with tumors located in the midportion of the kidney. The differences are not great and at this time the findings with respect to location appear inconclusive.

Presence of Calcification. Gross and microscopic calcification is found in approximately 15 to 20 percent of renal adenocarcinomas. It may be present anyplace in the stroma or the capsule of the tumor, and occasionally in foci of metaplastic ossification. While a number of authors have attempted to relate the presence of calcification with prognosis, there is no agreement whether such presence makes the prognosis better or worse. Most likely, calcification has little or no prognostic significance (Griffiths).

Size. There are now many reports demonstrating that the larger the renal adenocarcinoma, the poorer the prognosis. This has been shown in relation to estimates of tumor size, actual measurements of maximum diameter, and determinations of tumor weight (Hand and Broders; Arner et al.; Böttiger; Kay; Bixler et al.; Priestley). However, the inverse relationship between increasing tumor size and survival is a rule to which there are notable exceptions. As Riches and associates (1951) have observed, tumor size alone is not indicative of its degree of malignancy. Bell, for example, although demonstrating a direct correlation between increasing tumor size and increasing frequency of metastases, also found that of tumors greater than 10 cm. in diameter, nearly 20 percent had not yet metastasized. In general, however, the larger the tumor, the greater the likelihood of local extension and vascular invasion and metastasis (Graph V).

Local Extension. There is general agreement that the extension of tumor beyond the renal capsule has an adverse effect on the patient's chances for survival. This has been demonstrated by significantly longer periods of survival and more survivors at 5 and 10 years for those patients without invasion. Hand and Broders found the average survival in the absence of perinephric invasion was 72 months and with invasion, 39 months. Kaufman reported a

GRAPH V

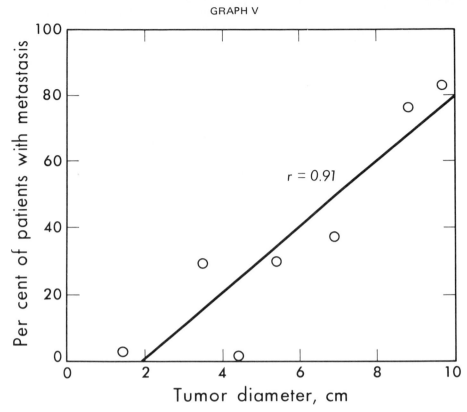

This graph shows the relation of the frequency of metastasis to the diameter of renal adenocarcinomas with a fitted regression line computed by the method of the least number of squares. (Prepared from data in: Bell, E. T. Renal Diseases, 2d ed., p. 435. Philadelphia: Lea & Febiger, 1950.)

56 percent 10-year survival in the absence of perirenal invasion against 14 percent with invasion.

If the tumor is well circumscribed, prognosis is more favorable for patients with renal adenocarcinoma confined to the kidney. Prognosis is poorer when the tumor is grossly or microscopically infiltrating the surrounding renal parenchyma.

Renal Vein Invasion. Some authors feel that renal vein involvement is a more important prognostic feature than perinephric invasion (Bell), but most contend that it is significant, but less important than perirenal invasion (Arner et al.; Flocks; Griffiths; Hand and Broders; Kaufman). There are still others who feel that renal vein involvement has no prognostic significance (Skinner et al.). How-

ever, most investigators have found that patients with renal vein involvement have a significantly poorer prognosis than those with tumors confined to the kidney. Graph VI shows the effects of renal vein invasion and perinephric invasion on 10-year survival rates for patients with renal adenocarcinoma.

Regional Lymph Node Metastases. Regional lymph node metastases offer about the same prognostic significance as renal vein invasion. Because regional lymph node metastases may be unsuspected and an appreciable number of patients with such metastases survive 10 years, Robson and associates have recommended extensive lymphadenectomy at the time of nephrectomy for renal adenocarcinoma.

Distant Metastases. If distant metastases

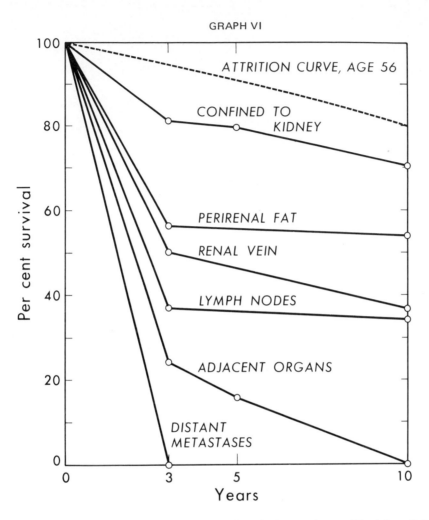

GRAPH VI

The survival of patients is shown in relation to the stage of renal adenocarcinoma. (Fig. 1 from Robson, C. J., Churchill, B. M., and Anderson, W. The results of radical nephrectomy for renal cell carcinoma. J. Urol. 101:297-301, 1969.)

are found at the time of nephrectomy, the chances of cure are almost nonexistent. Flocks and Kadesky reported 3.5 percent and 1.3 percent, and Kaufman and Mims reported 5 percent and 0 percent survival at 5 and 10 years for their patients with distant metastases. The rare exception may be the fortunate patient with a surgically resectable solitary metastasis (Riches, 1964; Straus and Scanlon).

Staging. The important gross features relating to prognosis have been incorporated into various staging systems which are closely related and differ primarily in the relative importance placed on renal vein and perinephric fat invasion. The most comprehensive staging system is that of Robson and associates (fig. 158). In their experience, invasion of perinephric fat is less important than renal vein involvement, and this is reflected in their system which follows:

STAGING OF RENAL CELL CARCINOMA

STAGE I

TUMOR WITHIN CAPSULE

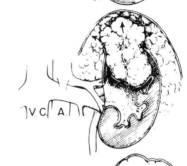

STAGE II

TUMOR INVASION OF PERINEPHRIC FAT (CONFINED TO GEROTA'S FASCIA)

STAGE III

TUMOR INVOLVEMENT OF REGIONAL LYMPH NODES AND/OR RENAL VEIN AND CAVA

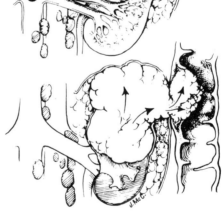

STAGE IV

ADJACENT ORGANS OR DISTANT METASTASES

Figure 158
CLINICAL STAGES OF RENAL ADENOCARCINOMA
This is a diagrammatic presentation of the clinical stages of renal adenocarcinoma. (Fig. 3 from Holland, J. M. Cancer of the kidney—natural history and staging. Cancer 32:1030-1042, 1973.)

Stage 1.   Confined to kidney.
Stage 2.   Invasion of perinephric fat, but confined to Gerota's fascia.
Stage 3.
    A.   Invasion of renal vein or vena cava.
    B.   Metastases to regional lymph nodes.
    C.   Invasion of renal vein or vena cava and metastases to regional lymph nodes.
Stage 4.
    A.   Invasion of adjacent organs other than adrenal gland.
    B.   Distant metastases.

Survival figures from 87 patients with renal adenocarcinoma in Robson and associates' series based on their staging system are shown in Graph VI. The progressively diminishing survival rates with each succeeding stage follows naturally from the usual biologic behavior of malignant tumors.

Microscopic Features

Compared with most other carcinomas, renal adenocarcinoma is usually remarkably well differentiated with relatively little pleomorphism and only infrequent mitoses.

Riches (1964), in grading 110 renal adenocarcinomas, found that 45 percent were very well differentiated, 36 percent were of intermediate differentiation, and only 18 percent were pleomorphic.

Because of the varied and distinctive histologic features of renal adenocarcinoma, many authors have attempted to classify this neoplasm on the basis of cell type and histologic configurations. This subject has been covered in many papers and with conflicting results (Melicow and Uson; Riches, 1964). Classifications based on the presence of cystic, solid, tubular,

GRAPH VII

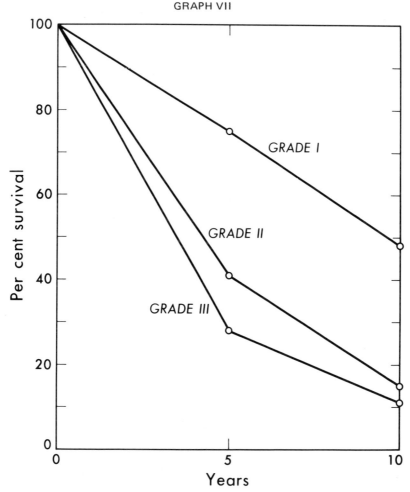

Crude survival rates for patients with renal adenocarcinoma are correlated with histologic grade. (Modified from Griffiths, I. H. In: Monographs on Neoplastic Disease at Various Sites. Vol. V, Tumours of the Kidney and Ureter. (Ed.) Riches, E. W. Baltimore: Williams & Wilkins Co.; Edinburgh: E. & S. Livingstone, Ltd., 1964.)

and papillary patterns have shown no correlation with survival. Furthermore, Böttiger has shown that there is no prognostic significance attributable to a tumor composed predominantly of clear or granular cells.

It is our opinion that neither the presence of clear or granular cells nor the patterns of organization (papillary, tubular, cystic) have any prognostic significance, and while histologic grading can be used to assess prognosis (Graph VII), it carries no greater accuracy than staging; to be reliable, it requires considerable experience and extensive sampling of every tumor. The subject of histologic grading has been exhaustively reviewed by Mostofi, who stated that, in his experience, grading was both difficult and of very little value so he simply classified renal adenocarcinomas as "well differentiated" and "not well differentiated."

Nevertheless, there does appear to be a close correlation between histologic grading and survival rates (Arner et al.; Böttiger; Riches, 1964). But because of the relative infrequency with which this tumor is encountered in the average laboratory, and the lack of a well established, uniform method of grading, the technic is not widely used. Assessing prognosis on the basis of staging, i.e., tumor size, extent of local invasion, vascular involvement, and metastases, requires less experience, is less time consuming, and correlates better with survival (Flocks and Kadesky; Petkovic). It is likely that eventually a computer-based system for analyzing the multiple variables of gross and histologic features of the tumor, as well as clinical and biochemical data, will provide even greater accuracy in estimating prognosis (Newman and Schulman).

References

Abeshouse, B. S. Metastasis to ureters and urinary bladder from renal carcinoma. Report of 2 cases. J. Int. Coll. Surg. 25:117-126, 1956.

............, and Goldstein, A. E. Metastatic malignant tumors of the kidney: a review of the literature and report of 23 cases. Urol. Cutan. Rev. 45:163-186, 1941.

............, and Weinberg, T. Malignant renal neoplasms. A clinical and pathologic study. Arch. Surg. 50:46-55, 1945.

Abrams, H. L., Spiro, R., and Goldstein, N. Metastases in carcinoma: Analysis of 1000 autopsied cases. Cancer 3:74-85, 1950.

Ali, M. Y., and Muir, C. S. Malignant renal neoplasms in Singapore: survey of incidence, mortality, and pathological features. Br. J. Urol. 36:465-481, 1964.

Alken, C. E., Roucayrol, J. C., Oberhausen, E., Taupitz, A., and Ueberberg, H. On the problem of carcinogenesis following thorotrast pyelography. Urol. Int. 10:137-156, 1960.

Amador, E., Zimmerman, T. S., and Wacker, W. E. C. Urinary alkaline phosphatase activity. I. Elevated urinary LDH and alkaline phosphatase activities for the diagnosis of renal adenocarcinomas. J.A.M.A. 185:769-775, 1963.

Apitz, K. Die Geschwülste und Gewebsmissbildungen der Nierenrinde. I. Die intrarenalen Nebenniereninseln. Virchows Arch. (Pathol. Anat.) 311:285-431, 1944.

Arison, R. N., and Feudale, E. L. Induction of renal tumour by streptozotocin in rats. Nature 214:1254-1255, 1967.

Arner, O., Blanck, C., and Schreeb, T. von. Renal adenocarcinoma; morphology—grading of malignancy—prognosis. A study of 197 cases. Acta Chir. Scand. (Suppl.) 346:1-51, 1965.

Azzopardi, J. G. Systemic Effects of Neoplasia, pp. 98-184. In: Recent Advances in Pathology, by Various Authors. (Ed.) Harrison, C. V. Boston: Little, Brown and Company, 1966.

Barch, S. H., Shaver, J. R., and Wilson, G. B. Some aspects of the ultrastructure of cells of the Lucke renal adenocarcinoma. Ann. N. Y. Acad. Sci. 126:188-203, 1965.

Batson, O. V. The role of the vertebral veins in metastatic processes. Ann. Intern. Med. 16:38-45, 1942.

Becker, N. H., and Soifer, I. Benign clear cell tumor ("Sugar Tumor") of the lung. Cancer 27:712-719, 1971.

Bell, E. T. Renal Diseases, 2d ed., p. 435. Philadelphia: Lea & Febiger, 1950.

Bengtsson, U., Angervall, L., Ekman, H., and Lehmann, L. Transitional cell tumors of the renal pelvis in analgesic abusers. Scand. J. Urol. Nephrol. 2:145-150, 1968.

Bennington, J. L., and Kradjian, R. M. Renal Carcinoma, pp. 38-42; 180-196. Philadelphia: W. B. Saunders Co., 1967.

............, and Laubscher, F. A. Epidemiologic studies on carcinoma of the kidney. I. Association of renal adenocarcinoma with smoking. Cancer 21:1069-1071, 1968.

............, Ferguson, B. R., and Campbell, P. B. Epidemiologic studies of carcinoma of the kidney. II. Association of renal adenoma with smoking. Cancer 22:821-832, 1968.

Berdjis, C. C. Kidney tumors and irradiation pathogenesis of kidney tumors in irradiated rats. Oncologia 16:312-324, 1963.

Berger, L., and Sinkoff, M. W. Systemic manifestations of hypernephroma. A review of 273 cases. Am. J. Med. 22:791-796, 1957.

Bernstein, J. Developmental abnormalities of the renal parenchyma: renal hypoplasia and dysplasia. Pathol. Annu. 3:213-247, 1968.

Bixler, L. C., Stenstrom, K. W., and Creevy, C. D. Malignant tumors of the kidney: review of 117 cases. Radiology 42:329-345, 1944.

Bjelke, E. Malignant neoplasms of the kidney in children. Cancer 17:318-321, 1964.

Bjornberg, O. Hypernephroma in old age. Nord Med. 64:1005-1007, 1960.

Blackard, C. E., and Mellinger, G. T. Cancer in a horseshoe kidney. A report of two cases. Arch. Surg. 97:616-627, 1968.

Blanchard, L., and Montpellier, J. M. Contribution à l'etude des tumeurs epitheliales du rein chez le cheval. Bull. Cancer 18:173-183, 1929.

Bloom, H. J. G. Medroxyprogesterone acetate (provera) in the treatment of metastatic renal cancer. Br. J. Cancer 25:250-265, 1971.

Bogaert, R., De Loecker, W., and Tverdy, G. Amyloidosis secondary to renal carcinoma. Clinical study of 3 cases. Acta Clin. Belg. 15:81-95, 1960.

Borski, A. A., and Kimbrough, J. C. Bilateral carcinoma in polycystic renal disease—an unique case. J. Urol. 71:677-681, 1954.

Böttiger, L. E. Prognosis in renal carcinoma. Cancer 26:780-787, 1970.

............, and Ivemark, B. I. The structure of renal carcinoma correlated to its clinical behavior. J. Urol. 81:512-514, 1959.

............, Blanck, C., and Schreeb, T. von. Renal carcinoma. An attempt to correlate symptoms and findings with the histopathologic picture. Acta Med. Scand. 180:329-338, 1966.

Bowman, H. S., and Martinez, E. J. Fever, anemia, and hyperhaptoglobinemia. An extrarenal triad of hypernephroma. Ann. Intern. Med. 68:613-620, 1968.

Boyland, E., Dukes, C. E., Grover, P. L., and Mitchley, B. C. V. The induction of renal tumours by feeding lead acetate to rats. Br. J. Cancer 16:283-288, 1962.

Brandt, P. W., Dacie, J. V., Steiner, R. E., and Szur, L. Incidence of renal lesions in polycythaemia. A survey of 91 patients. Br. Med. J. 2:468-472, 1963.

Brannan, W., Miller, W., and Crisler, M. Coexistence of renal neoplasms and renal cyst. South. Med. J. 55:749-752, 1962.

Braunstein, H., and Adelman, J. U. Histochemical study of the enzymatic activity of human neoplasms. II. Histogenesis of renal cell carcinoma. Cancer 19:935-938, 1966.

Brenner, B. M., and Gilbert, V. E. Elevated levels of lactic dehydrogenase, glutamic-oxalacetic transaminase, and catalase in infected urine. Am. J. Med. Sci. 245:31-42, 1963.

Breslow, L., and Milmore, B. K. Cancer Registration and Survival in California. California Tumor Registry, State of California, Department of Public Health, 1963.

Brinton, L. F. Hypernephroma-familial occurrence in one family. J.A.M.A. 173:888-890, 1960.

Brunner, U. The role of the thoracic duct as a pathway of metastasis of abdominal tumors. Schweiz. Med. Wochenschr. 90:554-561, 1960.

Buch, H., Häuser, H., Pfleger, K., and Rüdiger, W. Bestimmung von Phenacetin und N-Acetyl-p-aminophenol über Stoffwechselprodukte im Harn. Z. Klin. Chem. Klin. Biochem. 4:288-290, 1966.

Butler, W. H., and Barnes, J. M. Carcinogenic action of groundnut meal containing aflatoxin in rats. Food Cosmet. Toxicol. 6:135-141, 1968.

Case, R. A. M. Monographs on Neoplastic Disease at Various Sites, Vol. V. Tumours of the Kidney and Ureter, p. 8. (Ed.) Riches, E. W. Baltimore: Williams & Wilkins Co.; Edinburgh: E. & S. Livingstone, Ltd., 1964.

Claude, A. Adénocarcinome rénal endémique chez une souche pure de souris. Rev. Fr. Etud. Clin. Biol. 3:261-262, 1958.

Clarke, B. G., and Goade, W. J., Jr. Fever and anemia in renal cancer. N. Engl. J. Med. 254:107-110, 1956.

Cohnheim, J. Lectures on General Pathology. Handbook for Practitioners and Students. Translated from 2d German ed. by McKee, A. B. London: New Sydenham Society, 1889.

Cole, P. Coffee-drinking and cancer of the lower urinary tract. Lancet 1:1335-1337, 1971.

Cooray, G. H. Observations on malignant disease in Ceylon based on a study of 2,295 biopsies of malignant tumors. Indian J. Med. Res. 32:71-91, 1944.

Creevy, C. D. Confusing clinical manifestations of malignant renal neoplasms. Arch. Intern. Med. 55:895-916, 1935.

Cresson, S. L., and Pilling, G. P. Renal tumors. Pediatr. Clin. North Am. 6:473-490, 1959.

Cristol, D. S., McDonald, J. R., and Emmett, J. L. Renal adenomas in hypernephromatous kidneys: A study of their incidence, nature and relationship. J. Urol. 55:18-27, 1946.

Dalgaard, O. Z. Polycystic Disease of the Kidneys, pp. 907-937. In: Diseases of the Kidney. (Eds.) Strauss, M. B., and Welt, L. G. Boston: Little, Brown & Company, 1963.

Damon, A., Holub, D. A., Melicow, M. M., and Uson, A. C. Polycythemia and renal carcinoma. Report of ten new cases, two with long hematologic remission following nephrectomy. Am. J. Med. 25:182-197, 1958.

Dehner, L. P., Leestma, J. E., and Price, E. B., Jr. Renal cell carcinoma in in children: A clinicopathologic study of 15 cases and review of the literature. J. Pediatr. 76:358-368, 1970.

deVeer, J. A., and Hamm, F. C. Tumors of the kidney. I. Adenomas and carcinomas derived from renal parenchyma. Brooklyn Hosp. J. 8:53-84, 1950.

Dingwall-Fordyce, I., and Lane, R. E. A follow-up study of lead workers. Br. J. Ind. Med. 20:313-315, 1963.

Dobben, G. D. Benign adenomatous polycystic kidney tumor (Perlmann's tumor). Radiology 76:100-103, 1961.

Dorfman, L. E., Amador, E., and Wacker, W. E. Urinary lactic dehydrogenase activity. II. Elevated activities for the diagnosis of carcinomas of the kidney and bladder. Biochem. Clin. 2:41-55, 1963.

Druckrey, H., Preussmann, R., and Ivankovic, S. N-nitroso compounds in organotropic and transplacental carcinogenesis. Ann. N. Y. Acad. Sci. 163:676-696, 1969.

Eker, R. Familial renal adenomas in Wistar rats. A preliminary report. Acta Pathol. Microbiol. Scand. 34:554-562, 1954.

............, and Mossige, J. A dominant gene for renal adenomas in the rat. Nature 189:858-859, 1961.

Ellner, H. J., Bergman, H., and Alfonso, G. Two cases of solitary giant tubular adenoma of the kidney simulating carcinoma of the renal parenchyma. J. Urol. 84:706-709, 1960.

Emmett, J. L., Levine, S. R., and Woolner, L. B. Coexistence of renal cyst and tumour: incidence in 1,007 cases. Br. J. Urol. 35:403-410, 1963.

Epstein, S. M., Bartus, B., and Farber, E. Renal epithelial neoplasms induced in male Wistar rats by oral Aflatoxin B1. Cancer Res. 29:1045-1050, 1969.

Ericsson, J. L. E., Seljelid, R., and Orrenius, S. Comparative light and electron microscopic observations of the cytoplasmic matrix in renal carcinomas. Virchows Arch. (Pathol. Anat.) 341:204-223, 1966.

Evans, J. A., Halpern, M., and Finby, N. Diagnosis of kidney cancer. An analysis of 100 consecutive cases. J.A.M.A. 175:201-203, 1961.

Evans, R. W. Histologic Appearances of Tumors, with a Consideration of their Histogenesis and Certain Aspects of their Clinical Features and Behaviour, 2d ed. Baltimore: Williams & Wilkins Co., 1967; Edinburgh and London: E. & S. Livingstone, Ltd., 1966.

............, and Cruickshank, A. H. Epithelial Tumours of the Salivary Glands, pp. 98-141. In: Major Problems in Pathology, Vol. 1. Philadelphia: W. B. Saunders Co., 1970.

Everson, T. C., and Cole, W. H. Spontaneous Regression of Cancer; a Study and Abstract of Reports in the World Medical Literature and of Personal Communications Concerning Spontaneous Regression of Malignant Disease, pp. 11-87. Philadelphia: W. B. Saunders Co., 1966.

Farrow, G. M., Harrison, E. G., Jr., and Utz, D. C. Sarcomas and sarcomatoid and mixed malignant tumors of the kidney in adults—Part III. Cancer 22:556-563, 1968.

Ferber, B., Handy, V. H., Gerhardt, P. R., and Solomon, M. Cancer in New York State, Exclusive of New York City, 1941-60. Bureau of Cancer Control, New York State Department of Health, 1962.

Fetter, T. R., and Snyder, A. I. Survival study in renal cell carcinoma. Surg. Gynecol. Obstet. 117:7-9, 1963.

Fisher, E. R., and Horvat, B. Comparative ultrastructural study of so-called renal adenoma and carcinoma. J. Urol. 108:382-386, 1972.

Fite, G. L. Classifications of tumors of the kidney. Arch. Pathol. 39:37-41, 1945.

Flocks, R. H. Renal tumors. Proc. Natl. Cancer Conf. 6:247-256, 1970.

............, and Kadesky, M. C. Malignant neoplasms of the kidney: an analysis of 353 patients followed five years or more. J. Urol. 79:196-201, 1958.

Folin, J. Angiography in renal tumours. Its value in diagnosis and differential diagnosis as a complement to conventional methods. Acta Radiol. (Diag.) Suppl. 267:7-96, 1967.

Foot, N. C., Papanicolaou, G. N., Holmquist, N. D., and Seybolt, J. F. Exfoliative cytology of urinary sediments. A review of 2,829 cases. Cancer 11:127-137, 1958.

Frey, W. G., III. Polycythemia and hypernephroma. Review and report of a case with apparent surgical cure. N. Engl. J. Med. 258:842-844, 1958.

Geschickter, C. F., and Widenhorn, H. Nephrogenic tumors. Am. J. Cancer 22:620-658, 1934.

Gillis, D. J., Finnerty, P., and Maxted, W. C. Simultaneous occurrence of hypernephroma and transitional cell carcinoma with development of transitional cell carcinoma in the opposite kidney: case report. J. Urol. 106:646-647, 1971.

Goldberg, M. F., Tashjian, A. H., Jr., Order, S. E., and Dammin, G. J. Renal adenocarcinoma containing a parathyroid hormone-like substance and associated with marked hypercalcemia. Am. J. Med. 36:805-814, 1964.

Gordon, D. A. The extrarenal manifestations of hypernephroma. Can. Med. Assoc. J. 88:61-67, 1963.

Grabstald, H., Whitmore, W. F., and Melamed, M. R. Renal pelvic tumors. J.A.M.A. 218:845-854, 1971.

Graham, A. P. Malignancy of the kidney, survey of 195 cases. J. Urol. 58:10-21, 1947.

Graham, J. B., and Vynalek, W. J. Renal cell and transitional cell carcinomas in the same kidney. J. Urol. 76:137-141, 1956.

Graivier, L., and Vargas, M. A. Xanthogranulomatous pyelonephritis in childhood. Am. J. Dis. Child. 123:156-158, 1972.

Grawitz, P. A. Die sogenannten Lipome der Niere. Virchows Arch. (Pathol. Anat.) 93:39-63, 1883.

Greene, L. F., and Rosenthal, M. H. Multiple hypernephromas of the kidney in association with Lindau's disease. N. Engl. J. Med. 244:633-634, 1951.

Greene, R. H., and Brooks, H. Tumors of the Kidney, pp. 243-251. In: Diseases of the Genitourinary Organs and the Kidney, 2d ed. Philadelphia: W. B. Saunders Co., 1908.

Griffiths, I. H. Factors in Prognosis of Renal Adenocarcinoma as Indicated by Published Reports, p. 347. In: Monographs on Neoplastic Disease at Various Sites, Vol. V. Tumours of the Kidney and Ureter. (Ed.) Riches, E. W. Baltimore: Williams & Wilkins Co.; Edinborough: E. & S. Livingstone, Ltd., 1964.

............, and Thackray, A. C. Parenchymal carcinoma of the kidney. Br. J. Urol. 21:128-151, 1949.

Guérin, M., Chouroulinkov, I., and Rivière, M. R. Experimental Kidney Tumors, pp. 199-268. In: The Kidney: Morphology, Biochemistry, Physiology, Vol. II. (Eds.) Rouiller, C., and Muller, A. F. New York and London: Academic Press, 1969.

Hajdu, S. I., and Thomas, A. G. Renal cell carcinoma at autopsy. J. Urol. 97:978-982, 1967.

Halpern, M. Renal cell carcinoma. N. Engl. J. Med. 270:108-109, 1964.

Hand, J. R., and Broders, A. C. Carcinoma of the kidney: the degree of malignancy in relation to factors bearing on prognosis. J. Urol. 28:199-216, 1932.

Hard, G. C., and Butler, W. H. Ultrastructural aspects of renal adenocarcinoma induced in the rat by dimethylnitrosamine. Cancer Res. 31:366-372, 1971.

Harvey, N. A. Kidney tumors. A clinical and pathological study, with special reference to the "hypernephroid" tumor. J. Urol. 57:669-692, 1947.

Heslin, J. E., Milner, W. A., and Garlick, W. B. Lower urinary tract implants or metastases from clear cell carcinoma of the kidney. J. Urol. 73:39-46, 1955.

Hewlett, J. S., Hoffman, G. C., Senhauser, D. A., and Battle, J. D., Jr. Hypernephroma with erythrocythemia. Report of a case and assay of the tumor for an erythropoietic-stimulating substance. N. Engl. J. Med. 262:1058-1062, 1960.

Hicks, W. K. Benign tubular adenoma with malignant transformation. J. Urol. 71:162-165, 1954.

Higgins, C. C. Adenoma of the kidney. Report of six cases. Am. J. Surg. 65:3-14, 1944.

Howell, R. D. Ureteral implantation of renal adenocarcinoma. J. Urol. 66:561-564, 1951.

Jabara, A. G. Three cases of primary malignant neoplasms arising in the canine urinary system. J. Comp. Pathol. 78:335-339, 1968.

Johnson, D. E., Millar, J. D., and Rhoades, J. W. Nitrosamines in tobacco smoke. Natl. Cancer Inst. Monogr. 28:181-189, 1968.

Johnson, W. F. Carcinoma in a polycystic kidney. J. Urol. 69:10-12, 1953.

Jones, N. F., Payne, R. W., Hyde, R. D., and Price, T. M. L. Renal polycythaemia. Lancet 1:299-303, 1960.

Judd, E. S., and Hand, J. R. Hypernephroma. J. Urol. 22:10-21, 1929.

Kahn, P. C., Wise, H. M., Jr., and Robbins, A. H. Complete angiographic evaluation of renal cancer. J.A.M.A. 204:753-757, 1968.

Kaufman, J. J. Reasons for nephrectomy. Palliative and curative. J.A.M.A. 204:607-608, 1968.

............, and Mims, M. M. Current Problems in Surgery. Tumors of the Kidney. Chicago: Year Book Medical Publishers, Inc., 1966.

Kawamura, J., Garcia, J. H., and Kamijyo, Y. Cerebellar hemangioblastoma: Histogenesis of stroma cells. Cancer 31:1528-1540, 1973.

Kay, S. Renal carcinoma. A 10-year study. Am. J. Clin. Pathol. 50:428-432, 1968.

Kent, S. P. Spontaneous and induced malignant neoplasms in monkeys. Ann. N. Y. Acad. Sci. 85:819-827, 1960.

Kernohan, J. W., Woltman, H. W., and Adson, A. W. Intramedullary tumors of the spinal cord: a review of fifty-one cases, with an attempt at histologic classification. Arch. Neurol. Psychiatr. 25:679-701, 1931.

Kerr, J. F. R., Gaffney, T. J., McGeary, H. M., Duhig, R. E. T., and Nicolaides, N. J. Malakoplakia: an electron-microscope and chemical study. J. Pathol. 107:289-294, 1972.

Kirkman, H. Estrogen-induced tumors of the kidney in the Syrian hamster. Natl. Cancer Inst. Monogr. 1:1-139, 1959.

Klinger, M. E. Renal-cell carcinoma in siblings: A case report. J. Am. Geriatr. Soc. 16:1047-1052, 1968.

König, G. Pracktische Abhandlung über die Krankheiten der Nieren, durch Krankheitsfalle erlautert, pp. 246-248. Leipzig: Knobloch, 1826.

Korst, D. R., Whalley, B. E., and Bethell, F. H. Erythropoietic activity of plasma in polycythemia. J. Lab. Clin. Med. 54:916, 1959.

Kozoll, D. D., and Kirshbaum, J. D. Relationship of benign and malignant hypernephroid tumors of kidney. Clinical and pathological study of 77 cases in 12,885 necropsies. J. Urol. 44:435-449, 1940.

Kristensen, J. K., Gammelgaard, P. A., Holm, H. H., and Rasmussen, S. N. Ultrasound in the demonstration of renal masses. Br. J. Urol. 44:517-527, 1972.

Krueckemeyer, K., Lessmann, H. D., and Pudwitz, K. R. Carcinoma of the kidney as thorotrast injury. Fortschr. Roentgenstr. 93:313-321, 1960.

Lambird, P. A., and Yardley, J. H. Urinary tract malakoplakia: report of a fatal case with ultrastructural observations of Michaelis-Gutmann bodies. Johns Hopkins Med. J. 126:1-14, 1970.

Lang, E. K. The differential diagnosis of renal cysts and tumors. Cyst puncture, aspiration, and analysis of cyst content for fat as diagnostic criteria for renal cysts. Radiology 87:883-888, 1966.

Lee, L. W., and Davis, E., Jr. Gross urinary hemorrhage: a symptom, not a disease. J.A.M.A. 153:782-784, 1953.

Lehman, C. J., Erslev, A. J., and Myerson, R. M. Erythrocytosis associated with hepatocellular carcinoma. Am. J. Med. 35:439-442, 1963.

Lichtiger, B., Mackay, B., and Tessmer, C. F. Spindle-cell variant of squamous carcinoma. A light and electron microscopic study of 13 cases. Cancer 26:1311-1320, 1970.

Liebow, A. A., and Castleman, B. Benign "clear cell tumors" of the lung. Am. J. Pathol. (Abstr.) 43: 13a-14a, 1963.

Lindau, A. Studien uber Kleinhirncysten, Bau, Pathogenese und Bezienhungen zur Angiomatosis Retinae. Acta Pathol. Microbiol. Scand. (Suppl.) 1:1-128, 1926.

Long, R. J., Utz, D. C., and Dockerty, M. B. Malignant transformation of a renal adenoma: Report of a case. Can. J. Surg. 9:266-268, 1966.

Love, L., Neumann, H. A., Szanto, P. B., and Novak, G. M. Malignant renal tumors in adolescence. Radiology 92:855-860, 1969.

Lucke, B. Kidney carcinoma in the leopard frog: a virus tumor. Ann. N. Y. Acad. Sci. 54:1093-1109, 1952.

............, and Schlumberger, H. G. Tumors of the Kidney, Renal Pelvis and Ureter. Fascicle 30, Atlas of Tumor Pathology. Washington: Armed Forces Institute of Pathology, 1957.

Lytton, B., Rosof, B., and Evans, J. S. Parathyroid hormone-like activity in a renal carcinoma producing hypercalcemia. J. Urol. 93:127-131, 1965.

Macalpine, J. B. Papillomatous disease of the renal pelvis. Br. J. Surg. 35:113-132, 1947.

Magee, P. N. In vivo reactions of nitroso compounds. Ann. N. Y. Acad. Sci. 163:717-729, 1969.

Malament, M. The diagnosis of renal cyst versus renal carcinoma. Surg. Clin. North Am. 45:1377-1392, 1965.

Malek, R. S., Greene, L. F., DeWeerd, J. H., and Farrow, G. M. Xanthogranulomatous pyelonephritis. Br. J. Urol. 44:296-308, 1972.

Mao, P., and Molnar, J. J. The fine structure and histochemistry of lead-induced renal tumors in rats. Am. J. Pathol. 50:571-603, 1967.

McDonald, J. R., and Priestley, J. T. Malignant tumors of the kidney; surgical and prognostic significance of tumor thrombosis of the renal vein. Surg. Gynecol. Obstet. 77:295-306, 1943.

Melicow, M. M., and Becker, J. A. Radiographic simulation of certain solid tumors of the renal corpus to renal cyst. J. Urol. 97:592-610, 1967.

............, and Uson, A. C. Nonurologic symptoms in patients with renal cancer. J.A.M.A. 172:146-151, 1960.

Melmon, K. L., and Rosen, S. W. Lindau's disease. Review of the literature and study of a large kindred. Am. J. Med. 36:595-617, 1964.

Miller, E. C., and Miller, J. A. Studies on the mechanism of activation of aromatic amine and amide carcinogens to ultimate carcinogenic electrophilic reactants. Ann. N. Y. Acad. Sci. 163:731-750, 1969.

Mitchell, J. E. Ureteric secondaries from a hypernephroma. Br. J. Surg. 45:392-394, 1958.

Moertel, C. G., Dockerty, M. B., and Baggenstoss, A. H. Multiple primary malignant neoplasms. III. Tumors of multicentric origin. Cancer 14:238-248, 1961.

Monlux, A. W., Anderson, W. A., and Davis, C. L. A survey of tumors occurring in cattle, sheep, and swine. Am. J. Vet. Res. 17:646-677, 1956.

Morbidity from Cancer in the United States, pp. 151-154. Public Health Monograph No. 56, United States Department of Health, Education, and Welfare, 1947.

Morlock, C. G., and Horton, B. T. Variations in systolic blood pressure in renal tumor: a study of 491 cases. Am. J. Med. Sci. 191:647-658, 1936.

Morris, J. G., Coorey, G. J., Dick, R., Evans, W. A., Smitananda, N., Pearson, B. S., Loewenthal, J. I., Blackburn, C. R. B., and McRae, J. The diagnosis of renal tumors by radioisotope scanning. J. Urol. 97:40-54, 1967.

Mostofi, F. K. Pathology and Spread of Renal Cell Carcinoma, pp. 41-85. In: Renal Neoplasia. (Ed.) King, J. S., Jr. Boston: Little Brown and Company, Inc., 1967.

Mugera, G. M., and Nderito, P. Tumours of the liver, kidney and lungs in rats fed Encephalartos hildebrandtii. Br. J. Cancer 22:563-568, 1968.

Murphy, F. J., Mau, W., and Zelman, S. Nephrogenic polycythemia. J. Urol. 91:474-477, 1964.

Newcomb, W. D. The search for truth, with special reference to the frequency of gastric ulcer-cancer and the origin of Grawitz tumours of the kidney. Proc. R. Soc. Med. 30:113-136, 1936.

Newman, H. R., and Schulman, M. L. Renal cortical tumors: a 40-year statistical study. Urol. Survey 19:2-12, 1969.

Nicholson, G. W. Kidney tumors. Guys Hosp. Rep. 63:331-363, 1909.

Nixon, R. K., O'Rourke, W., Rupe, C. E., and Korst, D. R. Nephrogenic polycythemia. Arch. Intern. Med. 106:797-802, 1960.

Oberling, C., Riviere, M., and Haguenau, F. Ultrastructure of the clear cells in renal carcinomas and its importance for the demonstration of their renal origin. Nature (London) 186:402-403, 1960.

Ochsner, M. G. Renal cell carcinoma: five year followup study of 70 cases. J. Urol. 93:361-363, 1965.

O'Grady, A. S., Morse, L. J., and Lee, J. B. Parathyroid hormone-secreting renal carcinoma associated with hypercalcemia and metabolic alkalosis. Ann. Intern. Med. 63:858-868, 1965.

Olovson, T. Die Senkungsreaktion beim Hypernephrom. Erfahrungen von 109 operierten Fällen. Acta Chir. Scand. 93:503-512, 1946.

Omland, G. Polycythemia in renal carcinoma. Acta Med. Scand. 164:451-454, 1959.

Osborn, S. H., Griswold, M. H., Wilder, C. S., Cutler, S. J., and Pollack, E. S. Cancer in Connecticut 1935—1951, pp. 28-38. Connecticut State Department of Health, 1955.

Ostrum, H. W., and Fetter, J. S. Silent nephroma. J. Urol. 43:39-51, 1940.

Palma, L. D., Kenny, G. M., and Murphy, G. P. Childhood renal carcinoma. Cancer 26:1321-1324, 1970.

Payne, R. A. Metastatic renal tumours. Br. J. Surg. 48:310-315, 1960.

Penman, H. G., and Thomson, K. J. Amyloidosis and renal adenocarcinoma. A post-mortem study. J. Pathol. 107:45-47, 1972.

Petkovic, S. D. An anatomical classification of renal tumors in the adult as a basis for prognosis. J. Urol. 81:618-623, 1959.

Pinals, R. S., and Krane, S. M. Medical aspects of renal carcinoma. Postgrad. Med. J. 38:507-519, 1962.

Pine, L. F. Metastatic renal malignancy. Journal Lancet 70:301-302, 1950.

Plaine, L. I., and Hinman, F., Jr. Malignancy in asymptomatic renal masses. J. Urol. 94:342-347, 1965.

Povysil, C., and Konickova, L. Experimental xanthogranulomatous pyelonephritis. Invest. Urol. 9:313-318, 1972.

Pratt-Thomas, H. R., Spicer, S. S., Upshur, J. K., and Greene, W. B. Carcinoma of the kidney in a 15-year-old boy. Unusual histologic features with formation of microvilli. Cancer 31:719-725, 1973.

Priestley, J. T. Survival following removal of malignant renal neoplasms. J.A.M.A. 113:902-906, 1939.

Quinland, W. S., and Cuff, J. R. Primary carcinoma in the Negro. Anatomic distribution of three hundred cases. Arch. Pathol. 30:393-402, 1940.

Radosevic, Z., Saric, M., Beritic, T., and Knezevic, J. The kidney in lead poisoning. Br. J. Ind. Med. 18:222-230, 1961.

Ranchod, M. Metastatic melanoma with balloon cell changes. Cancer 30:1006-1013, 1972.

Ratcliffe, H. L. Familial occurrence of renal carcinoma in Rhesus monkeys (Macaca mulatta). Am. J. Pathol. 16:619-624, 1940.

Reidbord, H. E. Metaplasia of the parietal layer of Bowman's capsule. Am. J. Clin. Pathol. 50:240-242, 1968.

Reiss, O. Leukemoid reaction due to hypernephroma. J.A.M.A. 180:1126-1127, 1962.

Riches, E. On carcinoma of the kidney. Ann. R. Coll. Surg. Engl. 32:201-208, 1963.

Riches, E. W. Monographs on Neoplastic Disease at Various Sites, Vol. V. Tumours of the Kidney and Ureter. Baltimore: Williams & Wilkins Co.; Edinburgh: E. & S. Livingstone, Ltd., 1964.

............, Griffiths, I. H., and Thackray, A. C. New growths of the kidney and ureter. Br. J. Urol. 23:297-356, 1951.

Rios-Dalenz, J. L., and Peacock, R. C. Xanthogranulomatous pyelonephritis. Cancer 19:289-296, 1966.

Robson, C. J., Churchill, B. M., and Anderson, W. The results of radical nephrectomy for renal cell carcinoma. J. Urol. 101:297-301, 1969.

Rothman, D., and Rennard, M. Myoma-erythrocytosis syndrome. Report of a case. Obstet. Gynecol. 21:102-105, 1963.

Rulon, D. B., and Helwig, E. B. Cutaneous sebaceous neoplasms. Cancer 33:82-102, 1974.

Rusche, C. Silent adenocarcinoma of the kidney with solitary metastases occurring in brothers. J. Urol. 70:146-151, 1953.

Sandison, A. T., and Anderson, L. J. Tumors of the kidney in cattle, sheep and pigs. Cancer 21:727-742, 1968.

Sargent, J. W. Ureteral metastasis from renal adenocarcinoma presenting a bizarre urogram. J. Urol. 83:97-99, 1960.

Schreck, W. R., and Holmes, J. H. Ultrasound as a diagnostic aid for renal neoplasms and cysts. J. Urol. 103:281-285, 1970.

Schwedenberg, T. J. Ueber die Carcinose des Ductus thoracicus. Virchows Arch. (Pathol. Anat.) 181:295-338, 1905.

Scotti, D. W. Malignancies in infancy and childhood; clinical and pathological survey of 64 consecutive cases. N. Y. State J. Med. 39:1188-1208, 1939.

Scully, R. E. Recent progress in ovarian cancer. Hum. Pathol. 1:73-98, 1970.

Seljelid, R. An electron microscopic study of the formation of cytosomes in a rat kidney adenoma. J. Ultrastruct. Res. 16:569-583, 1966.

............, and Ericsson, J. L. E. An electron microscopic study of mitochondria in renal clear cell carcinoma. J. Microscopie 4:759-770, 1965.

............, and Ericsson, J. L. E. Electron microscopic observations on specializations of the cell surface in renal clear cell carcinoma. Lab. Invest. 14:435-447, 1965.

Sempronj, A., and Morelli, E. Carcinoma of the kidney in rats treated with beta-anthraquinoline. Am. J. Cancer 35:534-537, 1939.

Serfontein, W. J., and Hurter, P. Nitrosamines as environmental carcinogens. II. Evidence for the presence of nitrosamines in tobacco smoke condensate. Cancer Res. 26:575-579, 1966.

Skinner, D. G., Colvin, R. B., Vermillion, C. D., Pfister, R. C., and Leadbetter, W. F. Diagnosis and management of renal cell carcinoma. A clinical and pathologic study of 309 cases. Cancer 28:1165-1177, 1971.

Smith, E., and Young, A. Kidney tumours: an analysis of series of 118 cases. Can. Med. Assoc. J. 44:149-152, 1941.

Soloway, H. M. Renal tumors. A review of one hundred thirty cases. J. Urol. 40:477-490, 1938.

Spatz, M. Toxic and carcinogenic alkylating agents from cycads. Ann. N. Y. Acad. Sci. 163:848-859, 1969.

Stauffer, M. H. Nephrogenic hepatosplenomegaly. Gastroenterology 40:694, 1961.

Steiner, P. E. Sources, Materials, Racial Composition, Age, Sex, Methods, Comments, and Comparisons with Sedentes, pp. 9-23; Carcinoma of the Kidney, pp. 255-264. In: Cancer: Race and Geography. Baltimore: Williams & Wilkins Co., 1954.

Sternberg, S. S., Philips, F. S., and Cronin, A. P. Renal tumors and other lesions in rats following a single intravenous injection of Daunomycin. Cancer Res. 32:1029-1036, 1972.

Stoerk, O. Zur Histogenese der Grawitzschen Nierengeschwülste. Beitr. Pathol. 43:393-437, 1908.

Straus, F. H., and Scanlon, E. F. Five-year survival after hepatic lobectomy for metastatic hypernephroma. Arch. Surg. 72:328-331, 1956.

Strauss, M. B., and Welt, L. G. Diseases of the Kidney, p. 990. Boston: Little, Brown and Company, 1963.

Sudeck, P. Zwei Fälle von Adenosarcom der Niere. Virchows Arch. (Pathol. Anat.) 133:558-562, 1893.

Suzuki, S. Implantationscarcinom in der Harnblasenschleimhaut. Berl. klin. Wchnschr. 46:294-297, 1909.

Swann, P. F., and Magee, P. N. Induction of rat kidney tumours by ethyl methanesulphonate and nervous tissue tumours by methyl methanesulphonate and ethyl methanesulphonate. Nature 223:947-949, 1969.

Tan, H. K., and Heptinstall, R. H. Experimental pyelonephritis. A light and electron microscopic study of the periodic acid-Schiff positive interstitial cell. Lab. Invest. 20:62-69, 1969.

Tannenbaum, M. Ultrastructural pathology of human renal cell tumors. Pathol. Annu. 6:249-277, 1971.

Taylor, H. B., and Norris, H. J. Lipid cell tumors of the ovary. Cancer 20:1953-1962, 1967.

Terracini, B., Palestro, G., Gigliardi, M. R., and Montesano, R. Carcinogenicity of dimethylnitrosamine in Swiss mice. Br. J. Cancer 20:871-876, 1966.

Thomson, W. H., and Karat, A. B. Hypercalcaemia associated with adenocarcinoma of the kidney without demonstrable bone lesions. Br. Med. J. 2:745-746, 1966.

Thorling, E. B., and Ersbak, J. Erythrocytosis and hypernephroma. Scand. J. Haematol. 1:38-46, 1964.

Tonning, H. O., Warren, R. F., and Barrie, H. J. Familial haemangiomata of the cerebellum. Report of three cases in a family of four. J. Neurosurg. 9:124-132, 1952.

Tuaillon, M. M., Colson, P., and Plauchu, M. Les metastases intrathyroidiennes des tumeurs à cellules claires du rein. Lyon Med. 91:939-966, 1959.

Umiker, W. Accuracy of cytologic diagnosis of cancer of the urinary tract. Acta Cytol. 8:186-193, 1964.

Utz, D. C., Warren, M. M., Gregg, J. A., Ludwig, J. A., and Kelalis, P. P. Reversible hepatic dysfunction associated with hypernephroma. Mayo Clin. Proc. 45:161-169, 1970.

Van Duuren, B. L. Carcinogenic epoxides, lactones, and halo-ethers and their mode of action. Ann. N. Y. Acad. Sci. 163:633-651, 1969.

Vesselinovitch, S. D., and Mihailovich, N. The development of neurogenic neoplasms, embryonal kidney tumors, harderian gland adenomas, Anitschkow cell sarcomas of the heart, and other neoplasms in urethan-treated newborn rats. Cancer Res. 28:888-897, 1968.

Wacker, W. E. C., Dorfman, L. E., and Amador, E. Urinary lactic dehydrogenase activity. IV. Screening test for detection of renal disease dissociated and in association with arterial hypertension. J.A.M.A. 188:671-676, 1964.

Waldmann, T. A., Levin, E. H., and Baldwin, M. The association of polycythemia with a cerebellar hemangioblastoma. The production of an erythropoiesis stimulating factor by the tumor. Am. J. Med. 31:318-324, 1961.

Walker, D., and Jordan, W. P., Jr. Renal carcinoma and transitional cell carcinoma in the same kidney. South. Med. J. 61:829-832, 1968.

Wallace, A. C., and Nairn, R. C. Renal tubular antigens in kidney tumors. Cancer 29:977-981, 1972.

Walsh, P. N., and Kissane, J. M. Nonmetastatic hypernephroma with reversible hepatic dysfunction. Arch. Intern. Med. 122:214-222, 1968.

Ward, A. M. Tubular metaplasia in Bowman's capsule. J. Clin. Pathol. 23:472-474, 1970.

Weitzner, S. Clear cell carcinoma of the free wall of a simple renal cyst. J. Urol. 106:515-517, 1971.

West, M., Schwartz, M. A., Cohen, J., and Zimmerman, H. J. Serum enzymes in disease. XV. Glycolytic and oxidative enzymes and transaminases in patients with carcinoma of the kidney, prostate and urinary bladder. Cancer 17:432-437, 1964.

Willis, R. A. Pathology of Tumours, 4th ed., pp. 456-485. New York: Appleton-Century-Crofts, 1968.

............, The Spread of Tumours in the Human Body, p. 196. London: Butterworth and Co., Ltd., 1952.

Winkler, K. Ueber die Betheiligung des Lymphgefässsystems an der Verschleppung bösartiger Geschwülste. Virchows Arch. (Pathol. Anat.) (Suppl.) 195-271, 1898.

Wynder, E. L., Kiyohiko, M., and Whitmore, W. F., Jr. Epidemiology of adenocarcinoma of the kidney. J. Natl. Cancer Inst. 53:1619-1634, 1974.

Xipell, J. M. The incidence of benign renal nodules (a clinicopathologic study). J. Urol. 106:503-506, 1971.

Zeidman, I., and Buss, J. M. Transpulmonary passage of tumor cell emboli. Cancer Res. 12:731-733, 1952.

MESENCHYMAL TUMORS OF THE KIDNEY

INTRODUCTION

The relative frequencies of benign and malignant mesenchymal neoplasms of the kidney are difficult to estimate from reports in the literature. Benign neoplasms are almost invariably incidental findings at autopsy, while their malignant counterparts usually are diagnosed during the lifetime of the patient. While this makes direct comparison of incidences impossible, an indirect comparison can be attempted. Approximately 1.9 to 3.4 percent of necropsies are for malignant tumors of the kidney and, in most series, it is reported that sarcomas comprise 2 to 3 percent of malignant renal tumors (Abrams et al.; Lucké and Schlumberger; Steiner; Willis;

Riches et al.). Therefore, no more than 0.1 percent of necropsies should be for renal sarcoma. Since benign mesenchymal tumors are found in the kidneys of 8 to 11 percent of patients at autopsy, it would appear that benign mesenchymal tumors are about 100 times as frequent as sarcomas of the kidney (Reese and Winstanley; Xipell).

Because benign mesenchymal tumors are usually small, asymptomatic, and not detected in life, they are of little practical importance. They are of interest chiefly because their study may shed some light on the origin of sarcomas of the kidney.

TUMORS OF MUSCLE AND ADIPOSE TISSUE

LEIOMYOMA AND LIPOMA

Benign tumors of fat and smooth muscle represent the most common mesenchymal tumors of the kidney. They are found frequently in kidneys examined at autopsy, almost always in patients over the age of 40 years. Those tumors found at autopsy are usually clinically silent and average less than 5 mm. in diameter. Larger benign tumors of fat and smooth muscle do occur, but appear to be relatively uncommon since less than 50 leiomyomas and lipomas large enough to produce clinical symptoms have been reported in patients without

tuberous sclerosis (Beadles and Urich; Clinton-Thomas; Gordon et al.; Robertson and Hand). Among these patients, the majority are middle-aged or older women.

Whether small and discovered incidentally at autopsy or large enough to produce symptoms, benign mesenchymal tumors are much more common in women than men. In the series reported by Reese and Winstanley, small renal cortical nodules of fat and/or smooth muscle were six times as frequent in women as men (Table I, p.21). The distinction between leiomyoma and mesoblastic nephroma is aided by the finding that leiomyomas are sharply circumscribed, do not contain entrapped tubular and glomeruloid structures, and usually occur in adults, while mesoblastic nephroma tends to infiltrate the adjacent renal parenchyma, frequently contains tubular structures, and usually occurs in children.

Because pure leiomyomas and pure lipomas may be found in the same kidney and because a large number of renal cortical mesenchymal tumors contain both fat and smooth muscle, it seems that any proposed origin for such tumors should account for both the presence of fat and smooth muscle (Reese and Winstanley; Xipell). The alternatives worth considering are that these nodules represent (1) choristomas, (2) benign neoplasms arising from retained metanephric blastema, as is postulated for the mesoblastic nephroma (p. 231), or (3) benign neoplasms arising from indifferent mesenchyme in the renal cortex or renal capsule.

In view of the fact that the mesoblastic nephroma is found almost exclusively during the first few months of life and is more frequent in boys than girls, while the clinically silent as well as symptomatic leiomyomas, lipomas, and myolipomas are found after middle age and are more fre-

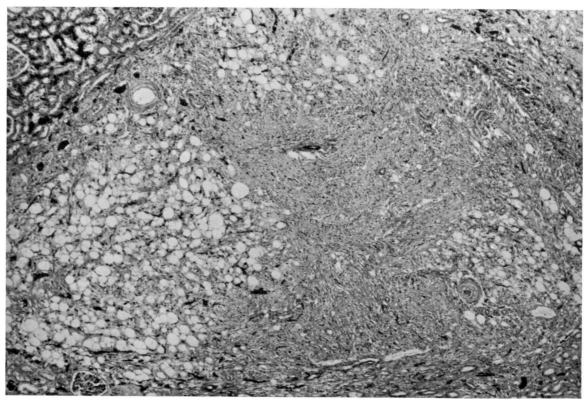

Figure 159
RENAL CORTICAL NODULE
(Figures 159 and 160 from same case)
This small renal cortical nodule is composed of adipose tissue admixed with sheets of smooth muscle. Although not a prominent feature, several thick-walled eccentric sclerotic vessels are present in the tumor. The histologic appearance is indistinguishable from the symptomatic angiomyolipoma associated with tuberous sclerosis. X42.

quent in women than men, it seems unlikely that the tumors of smooth muscle and fat are analogous to mesoblastic nephroma. On the other hand, these tumors do appear closely related to angiomyolipomas and other mesenchymal tumors associated with the tuberous sclerosis complex (Critchley and Earl; Fischer; Klapproth et al.; Price and Mostofi). The possibility that some arise directly from multipotential mesenchymal cells of the renal cortex or renal capsule has not been ruled out.

A large proportion of the benign mixed mesenchymal tumors of the kidney in patients without tuberous sclerosis are myolipomas (pl. VII-A), and nearly one-half have a prominent angiomatous component of poorly formed vessels (pl. VII-C; figs. 159, 160; Klapproth et al.; Reese and Winstanley; Xipell). This pattern makes

them histologically indistinguishable from angiomyolipomas seen in patients with the tuberous sclerosis complex (figs. 163–167). In addition, pure leiomyomas (pl. VIII-A) and lipomas, as well as typical angiomyolipomas, are found in patients with tuberous sclerosis, which indicates that the same spectrum of tumors containing fat and smooth muscle may be found in patients with or without tuberous sclerosis (Lucké and Schlumberger). For this reason, we favor the possibility that the majority of tumors of smooth muscle and fat, whether small or symptomatic, and whether associated with tuberous sclerosis or not, are **choristomas.** On the other hand, for reasons that will be discussed, we believe that most sarcomas of the kidney arise *de novo* from indifferent mesenchyme in the kidney or its capsule.

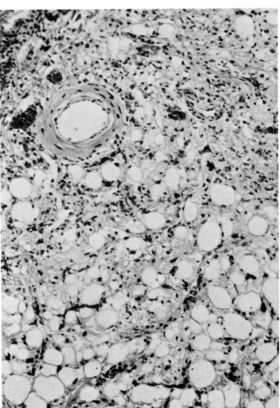

Figure 160
RENAL CORTICAL NODULE
(Figures 159 and 160 from same case)
This higher magnification of the same field shown in figure 159 reveals a poorly formed thick-walled vessel. An integral part of the nodule is surrounded by smooth muscle cells which are continuous with those interspersed throughout the adipose tissue. X95.

Figure 160

ANGIOMYOLIPOMA

Angiomyolipoma is one of the more interesting and controversial tumors found in the kidney. It is formed of heterotopic tissue and as such is probably most appropriately regarded as a choristoma rather than as a neoplasm (see p. 203). The term angiomyolipoma was first used by Morgan and associates in 1951; however, this tumor was initially described in 1911 by Fischer, who also documented its frequent association with the triad of mental retardation, epilepsy, and adenoma sebaceum (tuberous sclerosis complex).

Since the first report of the association of angiomyolipoma with tuberous sclerosis, it has become apparent that the two conditions do not invariably coexist. While as many as 80 percent of patients with tuberous sclerosis may have angiomyolipomas, less than 40 percent of patients with angiomyolipomas have one or more features of the tuberous sclerosis complex, i.e., cutaneous lesions, retinal phacomas, and visceral or cerebral angiomas and cerebral neoplasms (Critchley and Earl; Farrow et al.). However, if small (less than I cm.) angiomyolipomas are included, the number of patients with tuberous sclerosis may be even less (Hajdu and Foote).

Among surgically excised renal tumors, angiomyolipomas are relatively uncommon. Farrow and associates reported 23 cases among 2409 renal tumors found at surgical exploration of the kidney over a 50-year period at the Mayo Clinic. The mean age for patients was 41 years, with a range of 26 to 72 years; the female to male ratio was 2.6 to 1.

Angiomyolipomas are usually unilateral and solitary. While it is frequently stated that the tumor is large and clinically symptomatic in patients with tuberous sclerosis, the converse is often true. In patients without tuberous sclerosis, size of the tumor and clinical symptoms are also quite varied.

Frequently, angiomyolipomas are not recognized as benign tumors, most likely due to their propensity for capsular extension and the presence of atypical histologic features. They have been misdiagnosed as malignant tumors under such headings as fibrosarcoma, liposarcoma, leiomyosarcoma, rhabdomyosarcoma, and malignant mesenchymoma (Hajdu and Foote; Price and Mostofi). Liposarcomas have been misdiagnosed as angiomyolipomas in many reports from the older literature. Unfortunately, this confusion has left the persisting impression that liposarcomas are relatively frequent among sarcomas of the kidney.

CLINICAL FEATURES. Among patients who are symptomatic, the presenting symptom is usually flank or abdominal pain, which may be sudden and severe or less intense and sporadic over a number of years (Farrow et al.; Hajdu and Foote). The pain is apparently due to intrarenal and perirenal hemorrhage or to extrarenal extension. Occasionally, hematuria or hypertension may be the initial symptom which directs attention to the presence of the renal tumor (Farrow et al.; Hajdu and Foote).

GROSS FEATURES. In a series of 30 patients with symptomatic angiomyolipomas, Price and Mostofi found a range in size from 3 cm. to 20 cm. in greatest diameter, with a mean of 9.4 cm. Tumors arose within the medulla as well as in the cortex (fig. 161) without special predilection for upper, lower, or middle portions of the kidney, and occurred in both kidneys with equal frequency.

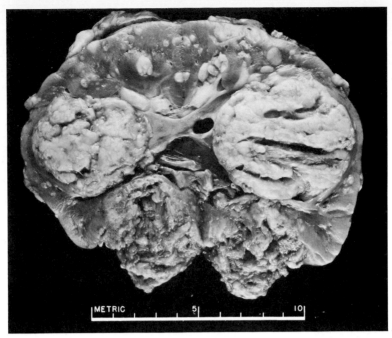

Figure 161
ANGIOMYOLIPOMAS
These two examples of symptomatic angiomyolipoma demonstrate a medullary origin in one and an eccentric cortical origin in the other. (Figs. 2A and B from Farrow, G. M., Harrison, E. G., Jr., Utz, D. C., and Jones, D. R. Renal angiomyolipoma. A clinicopathologic study of 32 cases. Cancer 22:564-570, 1968.)

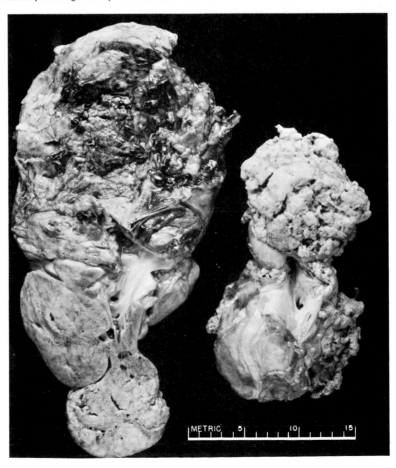

PLATE VII

ANGIOMYOLIPOMA ASSOCIATED WITH TUBEROUS SCLEROSIS

A. This small, incidentally discovered angiomyolipoma of the renal cortex was found in a patient with no obvious stigmata of tuberous sclerosis.

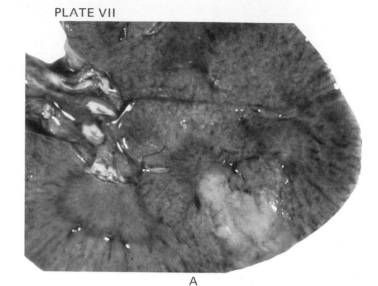

A

ANGIOMYOLIPOMA

B. The external surface of this large symptomatic angiomyolipoma is lobulated, and a portion extends through the renal capsule into the retroperitoneum. The interior is variegated yellow to gray with focal hemorrhage and cystic change. (Courtesy of Dr. Seth L. Haber, Santa Clara, Calif.)

B

ANGIOMYOLIPOMA

C. This angiomyolipoma demonstrates the characteristic features of prominent, irregular, thick-walled blood vessels surrounded by collarettes of smooth muscle, and a background of mature adipose tissue. Trichrome stain. X40.

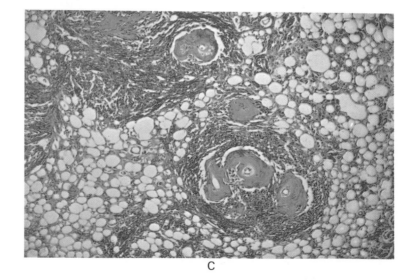

C

PLATE VIII

LEIOMYOMA

A. This subcapsular well circumscribed gray-white leiomyoma contains abundant
areas of fibrosis.

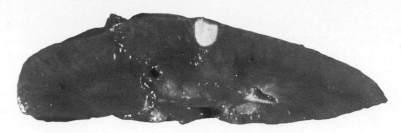

A

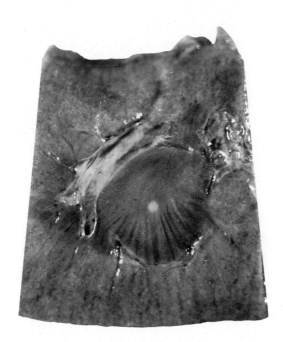

B

RENOMEDULLARY
INTERSTITIAL CELL TUMOR
(MEDULLARY FIBROMA)

B. This illustrates the gross appearance of a
renomedullary interstitial cell tumor
(medullary fibroma) which was located in
the usual position in the midportion of the
renal medulla.

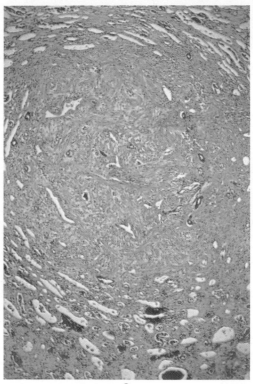

C

RENOMEDULLARY
INTERSTITIAL CELL TUMOR
(MEDULLARY FIBROMA)

C. The histologic appearance of this renomedullary
interstitial cell tumor (medullary fibroma) reveals
well demarcated margins and an interior formed predominantly of collagenous tissue intermixed with
scattered spindle-shaped fibroblasts. Occasional
renal tubules are entrapped within the nodule. Trichrome stain. X100.

The frequency with which angiomyolipomas are multiple or bilateral is not well established. In the same series, it was found that 13 percent of the tumors were multiple in the same kidney but none were bilateral. In a study of 23 patients with symptomatic angiomyolipomas, Farrow and associates found that 30 percent of the tumors were multiple and, of these, one-half (15 percent) were bilateral (fig. 162). This difference may be related to the fact that none of the patients in Price and Mostofi's series had tuberous sclerosis, while over one-third of the patients that Farrow and coworkers studied had tuberous sclerosis. Also, among these patients, the frequency of multiple and bilateral tumors was disproportionately high, although the numbers were not large enough to be statistically significant.

The gross features of this tumor are fairly characteristic. Generally, they are round to oval and elevate the renal capsule, producing a bulging, smooth, or bosselated mass. The cut surface is yellow to gray, depending upon the proportion of fat and smooth muscle in the tumor, and, frequently, masses of pure lobulated fat can be recognized in the predominantly yellow areas (pl. VII-B; fig. 161). A large percentage of surgically removed symptomatic tumors have focal hemorrhage within the tumor, particularly around the margin beneath the capsule (pl. VII-B), and some will have evidence of old hemorrhage with variable amounts of necrosis, cystic change, and calcification.

Growth is usually expansile, although it can be locally invasive. In the series reported by Price and Mostofi, there was extension to the perirenal structures in 23 percent of the cases, but no invasion of the renal calices or pelvis. Among those reported by Farrow and associates, 6 percent

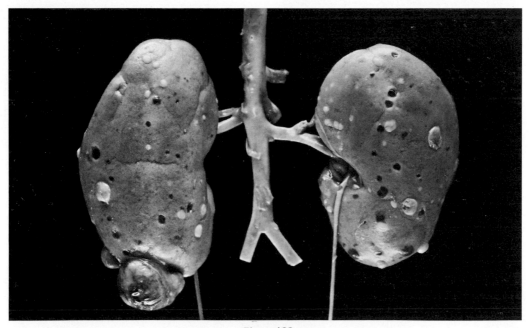

Figure 162
ANGIOMYOLIPOMAS
This illustrates multiple bilateral angiomyolipomas. (Fig. 2C from Farrow, G. M., Harrison, E. G., Jr., Utz, D. C., and Jones, D. R. Renal angiomyolipoma. A clinicopathologic study of 32 cases. Cancer 22:564-570, 1968.)

invaded the pelvis, 25 percent extended beyond the capsule, and 6 percent were adherent to the perirenal structures. In neither series was there any evidence of vascular invasion or metastasis. Documented malignant angiomyolipomas are rare, and those instances reported have been based on extensive destruction of the kidney and invasion of adjacent structures rather than on distant metastases (Berg; Bulkley and Drinker; Hartveit and Hallerbraker).

MICROSCOPIC FEATURES. The microscopic appearance of angiomyolipomas is remarkably constant from patient to patient and does not appear to be affected by tumor size or the degree of tumor extension. The overall pattern is characterized by a variable admixture of mature adipose tissue, tangles of tortuous thick-walled blood vessels, and collarettes and sheets of smooth muscle (pl. VII-C; figs. 163—165). The organization of the components may vary considerably in different parts of the tumor and from patient to patient. Some tumors are composed predominantly of adipose tissue (fig. 166); others are largely formed of muscle (fig. 167), and in still others all gradations of intermixture are found. If sufficient sections are examined, usually all three components can be identified.

Adipose tissue is of the adult type, characterized by large central lipoid vacuole and eccentric pyknotic nucleus. Occasional lipoblasts are seen with vacuolated cytoplasm and an eccentrically placed prominent nucleus. The spaces between fat cells may be filled with small amounts of reticulum and smooth muscle. The smooth muscle component is much more variable. There is considerable variation in size and shape of the smooth muscle cells; however, they are usually arranged in typical interlacing fascicles, and longitudinal myofibrils

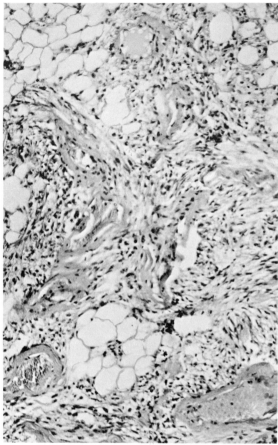

Figure 163
ANGIOMYOLIPOMA
The histologic appearance of this angiomyolipoma contains numerous small, poorly formed sclerotic vessels, each surrounded by haphazardly arranged sheets of smooth muscle. X95.

are recognizable within the cytoplasm. The nuclei are frequently hyperchromatic, moderately pleomorphic, and often worrisome because of the presence of frequent mitotic figures, and both mononuclear and multinuclear giant cells may be present. Smooth muscle may be distributed throughout the tumor, not only between the fat cells but as mantles around tortuous vessels (figs. 164, 165) and in large solid sheets of loosely arranged, whorled, and interlacing fascicles (fig. 167). The vascular

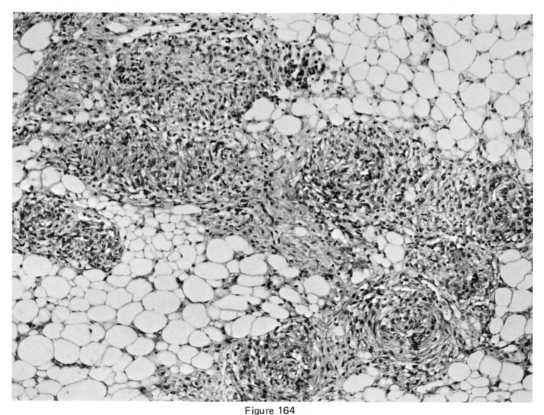

Figure 164
ANGIOMYOLIPOMA
(Figures 164 and 165 from same case)
This angiomyolipoma is composed of whorled collarettes of smooth muscle which surround small muscular vessels with inconspicuous lumens. X112.

component consists of large thick-walled muscular vessels resembling arteries which are extremely tortuous. Many of the vessels are imperfect with walls of varying thickness, eccentrically placed lumens, subintimal fibrosis, hyalinization of media, and lack of normal elastic membranes (fig. 163).

The incorrect diagnosis of malignancy of these tumors is usually based on one or more of the following features: (1) The tumors may be multiple or bilateral, or both; (2) the smooth muscle cells exhibit variation in size and shape, nuclear hyperchromatism, mitoses, and bizarre giant cells; and (3) the tumors exhibit what is interpreted as venous invasion.

TREATMENT AND PROGNOSIS. The usual method of treatment is complete nephrectomy, although complete surgical removal may not be possible due to extrarenal extension (fig. 168). There is not sufficient evidence to indicate whether postoperative radiation is useful in these cases. However, examination of the opposite kidney should be made to determine whether the patient has bilateral angiomyolipomas and, if so, whether there is adequate renal reserve.

When the tumor can be completely excised, the response to therapy is excellent, with nearly a hundred percent cure rate (Farrow et al.; Hajdu and Foote; Price and Mostofi).

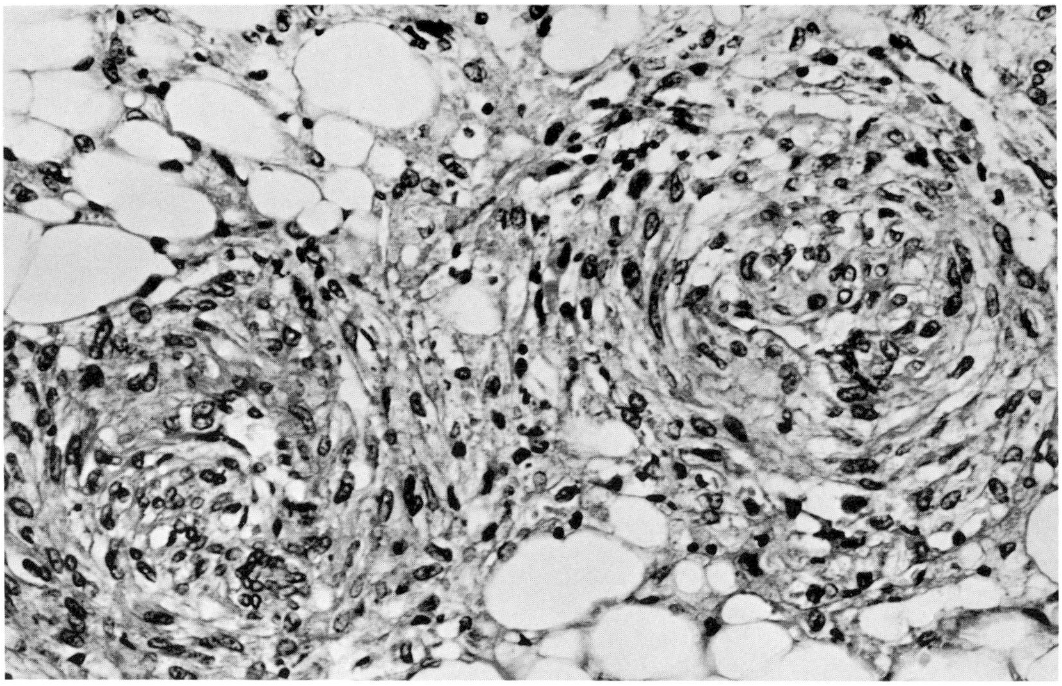

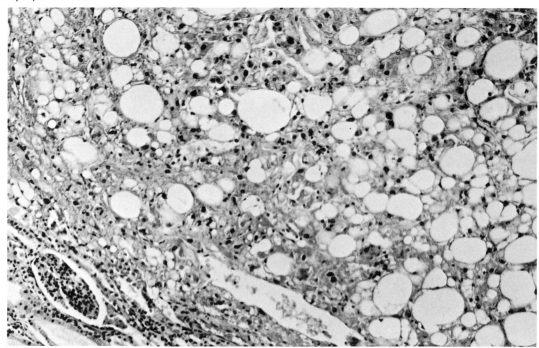

Figure 165
ANGIOMYOLIPOMA
(Figures 164 and 165 from same case)
This higher magnification of figure 164 demonstrates the typical perivascular mantle of smooth muscle cells seen in angiomyolipomas. X330.

Figure 166
ANGIOMYOLIPOMA
This angiomyolipoma is composed predominantly of adipose tissue. Moderate nuclear pleomorphism and hyperchromasia are evident. X210.

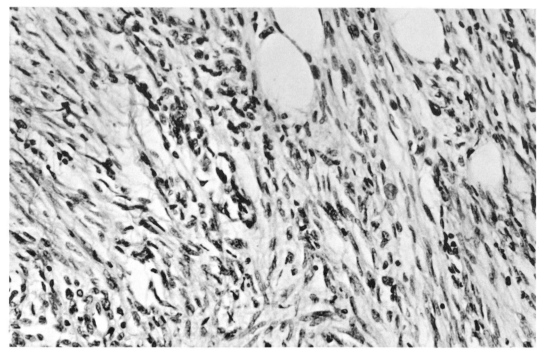

Figure 167
ANGIOMYOLIPOMA

This angiomyolipoma is formed almost entirely of smooth muscle with only occasional small aggregates of adipose tissue. X330.

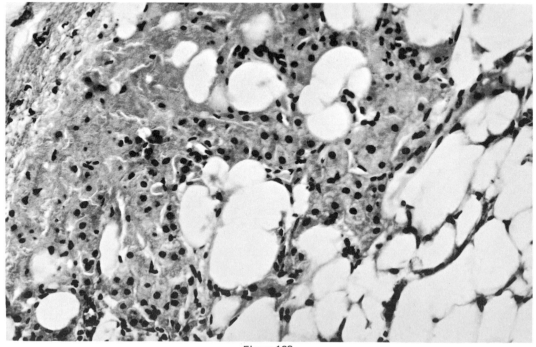

Figure 168
ANGIOMYOLIPOMA
Extrarenal extension of an angiomyolipoma invaded along the retroperitoneum and infiltrated the liver. X330.

LEIOMYOSARCOMA

The first leiomyosarcoma of the kidney was reported by Berry in 1919. A total of 43 of these tumors had been reported by 1972 (Bazaz-Malik and Gupta; Gupta and Dube; Jenkins et al.; Loomis). However, the frequency is undoubtedly higher than indicated by these figures. Early reports made no mention of leiomyosarcoma; renal sarcomas were invariably diagnosed as fibrosarcoma (Mintz). With improved histochemical technics, the diagnosis of fibrosarcoma has disappeared. In a careful study of all renal sarcomas seen at the Mayo Clinic over a 60-year period, Farrow and associates (Part I) found that 15 of 26 sarcomas were leiomyosarcomas. Based on these figures, it would appear that leiomyosarcoma is the most common sarcoma of the kidney.

This tumor has not been observed in children, and only one instance has been reported in an individual under the age of 20 years. After the second decade, leiomyosarcoma increases in frequency with advancing age. The majority have been reported in women. The female to male ratio of reported cases is 1.4 to 1 (Bazaz-Malik and Gupta; Gupta and Dube; Jenkins et al.; Loomis).

CLINICAL FEATURES. Leiomyosarcoma of the kidney is rarely detected while still small and confined to the kidney. The three most common clinical signs, i.e., flank pain, abdominal mass, and hematuria, are all indicative of a large and usually invasive tumor. Patients may present with any combination of these signs, but most frequently with the entire triad. The pain may be dull and aching, developing gradually due to slow enlargement of the tumor; it may be sudden and intense secondary to hemorrhage and necrosis within the tumor, or acute and colicky, due to the passage of blood clots into the renal pelvis and ureter. Nonurologic symptoms include weight loss and fever. The reported duration of clinical signs before seeking medical attention ranges from one week to five years, but is generally less than one year.

Renal leiomyosarcomas frequently extend into the caliceal system and pelvis, producing filling defects demonstrated by excretory urography. Calcification may be present, but has no characteristic pattern or distribution. Roentgenographically, it may be impossible to distinguish this tumor from a renal adenocarcinoma.

GROSS FEATURES. Leiomyosarcomas are found with equal frequency in the right and left kidneys and may arise anyplace within the renal parenchyma, but, like leiomyomas of the kidney, they are usually found near the cortical surface, often in continuity with the renal capsule. When there is invasion into perirenal structures, it may be difficult or impossible to distinguish a primary renal leiomyosarcoma from a leiomyosarcoma arising in the retroperitoneum and extending or metastasizing to the kidney (fig. 169). Renal leiomyosarcomas located mainly in the hilum probably arise in the renal pelvis rather than in the renal parenchyma.

The typical gross appearance is that of an eccentric, firm, bosselated mass protruding from the cortical surface of the kidney, elevating or invading through the capsule. Cut surfaces are glistening tan to light gray, whorled, and lobulated. Areas of hemorrhage, cystic change, fibrosis, and calcification may be present.

MICROSCOPIC FEATURES. The microscopic appearance of a leiomyosarcoma in the kidney is the same as that of a leiomyosarcoma in other sites. Well differentiated tumors are composed of plump,

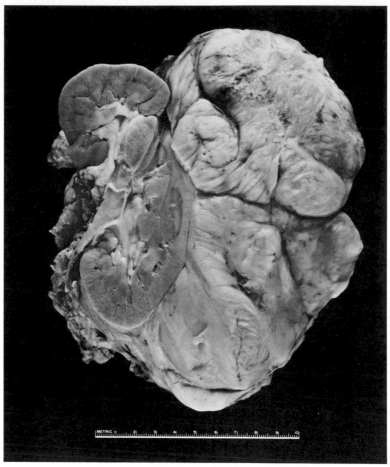

Figure 169
LEIOMYOSARCOMA
This large extrarenal ovoid mass compresses, distorts, and displaces the kidney, but does not appear to invade it. The tumor is surrounded by a pseudocapsule, and on cut section is coarsely lobulated with bulging parenchyma and central scarring with focal hemorrhage in the lobulations. (Fig. 1 from Farrow, G. M., Harrison, E. G., Jr., Utz, D. C., and ReMine, W. H. Sarcomas and sarcomatoid and mixed malignant tumors of the kidney in adults—Part 1. Cancer 22:545-550, 1968.)

spindle-shaped cells containing rod-shaped or elongated oval nuclei (fig. 170). The cytoplasm is eosinophilic, fibrillary, and usually ample, but may be scanty in very cellular tumors. The structure and presence of longitudinal myofibrils are best demonstrated by PTAH and trichrome stains. Poorly differentiated variants are composed of larger cells with rounded or irregular contours. Their nuclei are usually large, hyperchromatic, and may be single or multiple. Electron microscopically, renal leiomyosarcomas have been shown to contain glycogen, numerous mitochondria, and 60 angstrom myofilaments. Typically, basement membranes are scanty or absent and there is little intercellular collagen (Tannenbaum). Differential diagnosis must be made from sarcomatoid renal adenocarcinoma, malignant fibroxanthosarcoma, nephroblastoma, and sarcomas invading the kidney from the retroperitoneum.

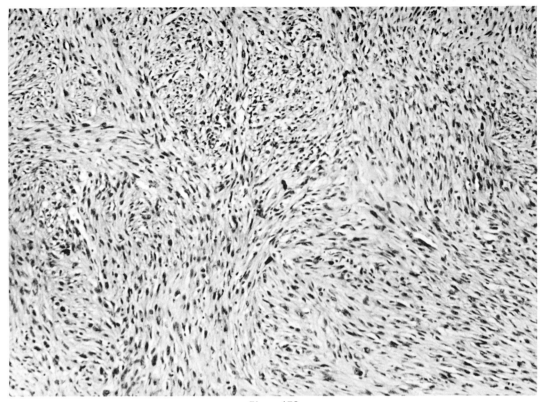

Figure 170
LEIOMYOSARCOMA
Leiomyosarcoma of the kidney is characterized by interlacing fascicles of spindle cells resembling smooth muscle cells. There is moderate nuclear pleomorphism and mitotic figures are present. X112.

TREATMENT AND PROGNOSIS. Of 15 patients with renal leiomyosarcoma at the Mayo Clinic, treated by nephrectomy, 14 died of their tumor in 4 months to 5½ years; one patient was alive and free of tumor at six years (Farrow et al., Part I). Although the results are not good, nephrectomy is presently the treatment of choice since radiation and chemotherapy have nothing to offer.

The number of cases is quite small in which survival figures can be correlated with gross and microscopic features of the tumor. However, it appears that factors which correlate well with survival in leiomyosarcomas of the uterus also apply to those of the kidney. In general, the degree of differentiation of the tumor, as measured by the presence or absence of cellular atypia and nuclear pleomorphism, is not a good indicator of prognosis. The number of mitotic figures seen is probably the best histologic criterion of malignancy. Grossly, those tumors which invade adjacent structures offer a poorer prognosis than those confined to the kidney; the smaller the tumor and the more completely it is circumscribed or encapsulated, the better the prognosis.

At the time of autopsy, local recurrence or metastases have occurred in a large percentage of patients. The most frequent site of metastases is the lung, but metastases to the liver, regional lymph nodes, peritoneum, and mesentery have also been found.

RHABDOMYOSARCOMA

Malignant striated muscle is found as a component in about one-half of all nephroblastomas. However, we are aware of only seven reports of rhabdomyosarcoma of the kidney (Farrow et al., Part I; Herzog; Messinger and Jarman; Seabury). The relative frequency of rhabdomyosarcoma among renal sarcomas is not known. Farrow and associates (Part I) found one rhabdomyosarcoma in a series of 26 renal sarcomas (figs. 171, 172). However, in view of the very few renal rhabdomyosarcomas reported to date, the frequency may be considerably lower than that found by Farrow and associates.

Because rhabdomyoblasts are frequently found as a component of nephroblastoma, many authors feel that the apparently pure rhabdomyosarcomas of the kidney are actually nephroblastomas in which there is an overgrowth of malignant striated muscle. This theory is an attractive one, but there is no evidence to support it. While there is no intrinsic striated muscle in the kidney, rhabdomyosarcomas have been reported in other sites, including the ureter, bronchus, middle ear, extrahepatic biliary tree, liver, and pelvic connective tissue, which are also normally devoid of striated muscle (Evans). To our way of thinking, the most likely explanation of the histogenesis of renal rhabdomyosarcomas is that they arise from indifferent mesenchymal cells which possess the capacity to differentiate into a variety of malignant mesenchymal tissues, including striated muscle.

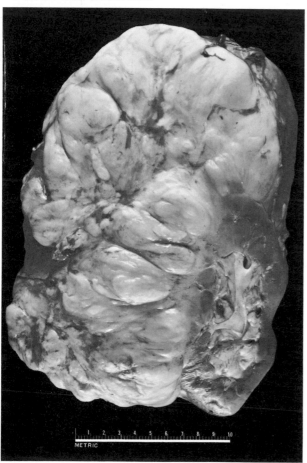

Figure 171

Figure 171
RHABDOMYOSARCOMA
(Figures 171 and 172 from same case)
This primary rhabdomyosarcoma of the kidney weighed 4385 Gm. The multinodular gray-pink tumor invades the renal capsule and the outer cortex along the convex surface of the kidney. (Fig. 8 from Farrow, G. M., Harrison, E. G., Jr., Utz, D. C., and ReMine, W. H. Sarcomas and sarcomatoid and mixed malignant tumors of the kidney in adults—Part I. Cancer 22:545-550, 1968.)

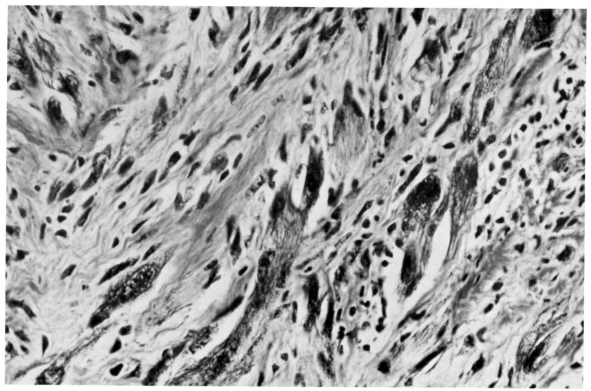

Figure 172
RHABDOMYOSARCOMA
(Figures 171 and 172 from same case)
The histologic appearance of the rhabdomyosarcoma seen in figure 171 shows large tapering cells with an eosinophilic fibrillary cytoplasm and abundant giant hyperchromatic nuclei. Cross striations in the cytoplasm are evident in occasional cells. Small spindle-shaped cells with hyperchromatic nuclei form the background of the tumor. X450.

LIPOSARCOMA

The frequency of liposarcoma of the kidney is greatly overestimated in the older literature due to confusion in distinguishing between retroperitoneal liposarcoma and those tumors primary in the kidney; confusion also results because many angiomyolipomas of the kidney are mistakenly reported as liposarcomas (Farrow et al.). As late as 1958, Williams and Savage accepted 29 cases as examples of renal liposarcoma; however, one-third of these patients had tuberous sclerosis, which suggests that some, or all these tumors were angiomyolipomas. Of these patients, none had any evidence of recurrence or metastases from their renal tumor.

Because the number of well documented cases is small, there is little reliable data on the epidemiology of renal liposarcoma. Among the cases reviewed by Williams and Savage in which there was no stigmata of tuberous sclerosis, 6 patients were male and 14 were female. The majority of tumors occurred between the ages of 40 and 60, with only one patient under 20 years and one over 70 years. In Farrow and associates' (Part I) series, renal liposarcoma ranked with hemangiopericytoma after leiomyosarcoma in relative frequency among renal sarcomas.

The origin of these tumors has not been determined. It is tempting to postulate an origin in preexisting lipomas or mixed mesenchymal tumors containing fat, which are frequently found in the kidney. This may indeed occur on occasion, but the frequency of malignant change in angiomyolipomas is known to be extremely rare. Lipomas in general rarely undergo malignant change. The tendency for liposarcomas to arise in areas generally devoid of fat, i.e., intermuscular planes and deep perivascular tissue, favors the concept that liposarcomas arise from nondifferentiated perivascular adventitial mesenchymal cells. This could explain the origin of liposarcomas in the renal parenchyma or renal capsule without the need to postulate an origin in retained metanephric blastema, residual fat in the renal capsule, or preexisting lipomas. Because liposarcomas, the most common retroperitoneal sarcoma (Ackerman), are frequent in the retroperitoneum and often invade adjacent structures, some liposarcomas of the kidney with extrarenal involvement may be extrarenal in origin.

GROSS FEATURES. Renal liposarcomas usually are localized in the periphery of the cortex or between the renal capsule and kidney (fig. 173). They are typically large and bulky, usually larger than the other forms of renal sarcoma, and often extend into the perirenal fat. They are characteristically multilobular with a variegated appearance. The tumor may be uniform in color or multicolored with areas which are bright yellow, gray or white, and pink to red. Cut surfaces are often mucoid or slimy and frequently show areas of cystic change, hemorrhage, and necrosis. The tumor may appear well circumscribed, but the extent of invasion is difficult to determine grossly.

MICROSCOPIC FEATURES. Microscopically, renal liposarcomas exhibit any

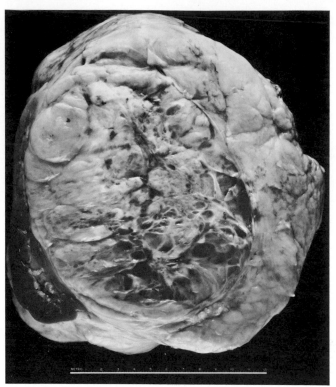

Figure 173
LIPOSARCOMA

This liposarcoma was located peripherally and encircled the kidney beneath the renal capsule. There was no invasion of the renal parenchyma or the perirenal tissues. (Fig. 7 from Farrow, G. M., Harrison, E. G., Jr., Utz, D. C., and ReMine, W. H. Sarcomas and sarcomatoid and mixed malignant tumors of the kidney in adults—Part I. Cancer 22:545-550, 1968.)

of the histologic patterns seen in liposarcomas elsewhere in the body (fig. 174). Histologically, they may be confused with retroperitoneal xanthogranuloma, xanthogranulomatous pyelonephritis, or poorly differentiated renal adenocarcinoma.

TREATMENT AND PROGNOSIS. Nephrectomy appears to offer the best chance for cure, but there is little information on survival figures for this tumor. In the series reported by Farrow and associates (Part I), 3 of 5 patients with renal liposarcoma died of their tumor within periods of 1 month, 1½ years, and 13 years. Two patients were apparently free of tumor 9 months and 2½ years after nephrectomy.

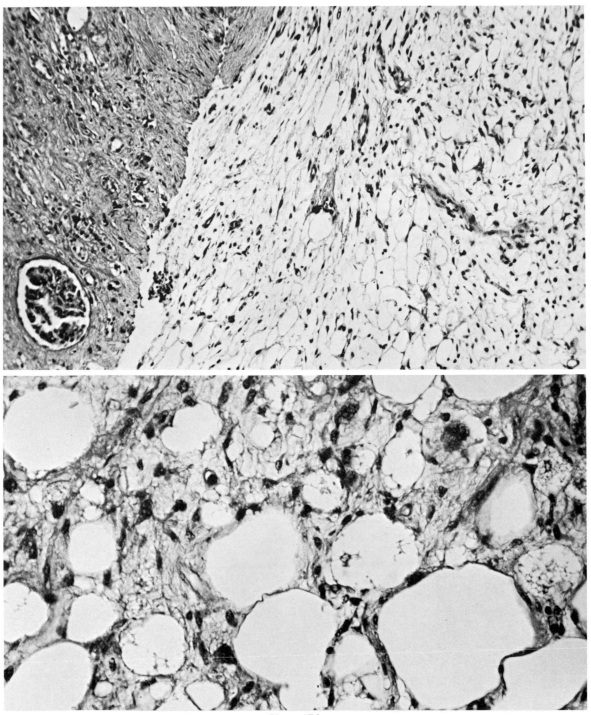

Figure 174
LIPOSARCOMA
This well differentiated liposarcoma was removed from the right kidney of an 80 year old woman. The tumor is composed of cells resembling normal adult fat cells intermixed with immature spindle-shaped and signet ring fat cells. Upper, X60; lower, X185.

TUMORS OF VASCULAR TISSUE

HEMANGIOMA

Hemangiomas of the kidney are relatively uncommon. McCrea found a total of 72 renal hemangiomas reported up to 1951, and added one case of his own. Because these lesions are usually 3 to 4 mm. in greatest diameter and rarely over one centimeter, they are easily missed grossly. This probably accounts for their low incidence in most autopsy series. The right and left kidneys are involved with equal frequency; rarely, hemangiomas are bilateral. Males and females are affected equally. The majority of tumors are detected during the third and fourth decades. The presenting symptom in 95 percent of cases is hematuria. Approximately 40 percent of patients have colicky pain due to the passage of blood clots (Friedman and Solis-Cohen). Since the lesions are small, they are easily missed on excretory urograms, although even small hemangiomas can produce demonstrable filling defects in the renal pelvis (Friedman and Solis-Cohen). These changes are frequently interpreted as carcinoma or tuberculosis (McCrea). Angiomas as well as hemangiopericytomas may be demonstrated by arteriography because of their rich vascularity.

GROSS FEATURES. Hemangiomas may be single or multiple and are occasionally bilateral. They may occur anyplace in the renal parenchyma, but usually are located at the apex of the pyramids (fig.

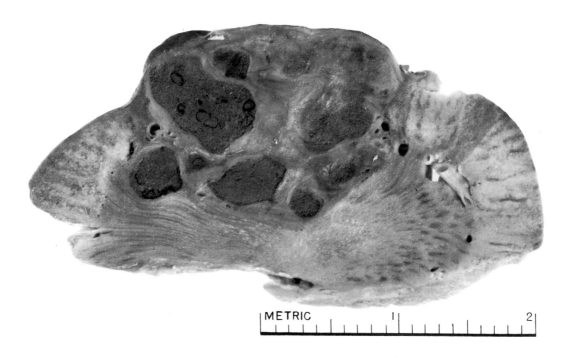

METRIC

Figure 175
CAVERNOUS HEMANGIOMA
A cavernous hemangioma was found incidentally in the renal cortex of the right kidney of a 66 year old man. (Fig. 115 from Lucké, B., and Schlumberger, H. G. Tumors of the Kidney, Renal Pelvis and Ureter. Fascicle 30, Atlas of Tumor Pathology, First Series. Washington: Armed Forces Institute of Pathology, 1957.)

175; Swan and Balme). Occasionally, they present as a small berry-like projection on the caliceal mucosa.

MICROSCOPIC FEATURES. Most renal hemangiomas are of the capillary type, composed of haphazardly arranged capillary size vessels interspersed among more compact clusters of endothelial cells in which there are incomplete or inconspicuous vascular lumens (fig. 176). When the vessels are widely dilated, the tumor is referred to as a cavernous hemangioma. The stroma in older lesions is often fibrous, causing contraction of the tumor.

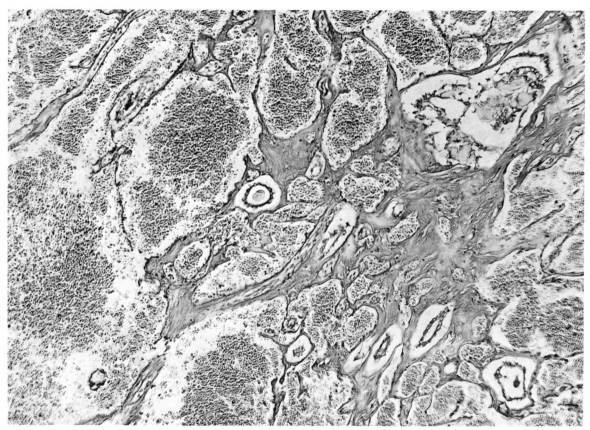

Figure 176
CAPILLARY HEMANGIOMA
This is the histologic appearance of a capillary hemangioma found in the kidney of a 29 year old man. The vascular channels are dilated and lined by a single layer of endothelial cells. The supporting stroma is largely hyalinized. X100. (Fig. 116 from Lucké, B., and Schlumberger, H. G. Tumors of the Kidney, Renal Pelvis and Ureter. Fascicle 30, Atlas of Tumor Pathology, First Series. Washington: Armed Forces Institute of Pathology, 1957.)

ANGIOSARCOMA

SYNONYMS AND RELATED TERMS: **Malignant hemangioendothelioma.**

This is apparently a very rare tumor of the kidney. While there are many references in the older literature to "endothelioma" and "angiosarcoma" of the kidney, such cases have proved to be richly vascular renal adenocarcinomas or angiomyolipomas. We are aware of only one report which may represent renal hemangiosarcoma (Prince).

HEMANGIOPERICYTOMA*

The hemangiopericytoma is an uncommon, richly vascular tumor, first described by Stout and Murray in 1942, which may arise anyplace in the body. There have been only nine reports of this tumor in the kidney, although the incidence may be greater than indicated by these figures (Berk et al.; Black and Heinemann; Farrow et al., Part II; Lee and Kay; Simon and Greene). Nearly 20 percent of the "renal sarcomas" found in the files at the Mayo Clinic were hemangiopericytomas (Farrow et al., Part I).

Farrow and associates (Part I) made no mention of age or sex of the five patients with hemangiopericytoma in their series of renal sarcomas. Among the other four patients, three were women (two aged 41 years; one, 29 years) and one was an 18 year old man. Of the nine patients, two had hypoglycemia relieved by removal of the tumor (Farrow et al.; Simon and Greene). In one of these two patients, hypoglycemia returned with recurrence of the tumor (Farrow et al., Part I).

GROSS FEATURES. The majority of renal hemangiopericytomas reported to date have been firmly attached to the external surface of the kidney, apparently arising from the renal capsule, but not invading the renal parenchyma (fig. 177). Most have been multinodular, firm, and encapsulated, with variable coloration of cut surfaces including pale gray-pink, reddish brown, and yellow areas. Only two have been described as unencapsulated and invading the renal parenchyma (Farrow et al., Part I). Because of the extrarenal location of the hemangiopericytoma, it is difficult to be certain whether they arise from the kidney or its capsule or are primarily retroperitoneal, extending to the kidney. While hemangiopericytoma of the retroperitoneum is relatively uncommon among retroperitoneal sarcomas, an appreciable proportion of all hemangiopericytomas are retroperitoneal. Stout and Murray found 5 of 25 cases and Lee and Kay, 4 of 23 cases of hemangiopericytoma which were primary in the retroperitoneum.

MICROSCOPIC FEATURES. Hemangiopericytoma contains many vascular channels lined by endothelial cells and separated by solid aggregates of rounded to fusiform cells with pale cytoplasm, indistinct cellular membranes, and prominent, round to oval, vesicular nuclei. The tumor cells, thought to be pericytes, are usually oriented around the tumor vessels as whorls or collarettes—a pattern which is best demonstrated by a reticulin stain. Silver staining not only accentuates the outlines of individual vessels, but also demonstrates that the tumor cells are perivascular, and that the vessels are lined by a single layer of endothelial cells. This pattern differentiates this tumor from hemangiosarcoma in which tumor cell proliferation is within the lumens of the vessels.

TREATMENT AND PROGNOSIS. In the cases reported, nephrectomy has been the only form of initial treatment. Four

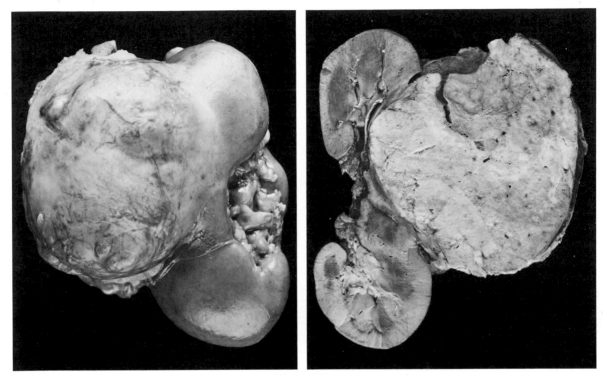

Figure 177
HEMANGIOPERICYTOMA

This hemangiopericytoma is a firm, nodular, circumscribed, eccentric mass which compressed, but did not invade the renal parenchyma. (Fig. 4 from Farrow, G. M., Harrison, E. G., Jr., Utz, D. C., and ReMine, W. H. Sarcomas and sarcomatoid and mixed malignant tumors of the kidney in adults—Part I. Cancer 22:545-550, 1968.)

patients died as a result of the tumor, at 5 months, 10 months, 2½ years, and 10 years postoperatively. One patient was alive with known metastases at 7 months, and three patients were alive with no evidence of tumor at 1, 2, and 10 years following nephrectomy.

As with hemangiopericytomas elsewhere in the body, the outcome is difficult to predict. The histologic picture is a poor indicator of the aggressiveness of the tumor. Generally, the differentiation is good; mitotic figures are scarce in tumors that do not recur and those that subsequently metastasize.

It has been suggested that lymph node dissection has little to offer, since metastases are more frequently hematogenous than lymphogenous in hemangiopericytoma. However, no actual experience has been reported using lymph node dissection in patients with renal hemangiopericytoma.

JUXTAGLOMERULAR TUMOR

SYNONYMS AND RELATED TERMS: Tumor of granular epithelioid cell; cortical juxtaglomerular tumor.

Recognition of neoplasms of juxtaglomerular (granular epithelioid) cell origin was made in 1967 by Robertson and associates, who described a tumor of the kidney resembling hemangiopericytoma which contained large amounts of extractable renin. The tumor was found in a young man with severe diastolic hypertension and hypokalemia. Since the initial report, five additional case reports have helped to establish the clinical presentation and histologic characteristics of this tumor (Schambelan et al.).

Juxtaglomerular cell tumors occur in a much younger age group than the usual renal adenocarcinoma. The mean age of patients in the six reported cases is 19

years, with a range from 2 to 37 years. There were four males and two females. The characteristic clinical syndrome is one of aldosteronism with severe diastolic hypertension. All the patients have had elevated levels of plasma renin and, therefore, a secondary form of aldosteronism.

The evidence for renin production by this neoplasm includes (1) the clinical regression of the hypertension and a drop in plasma renin following surgical removal of the tumor; (2) the presence of large amounts of extractable renin in the tumor as compared to uninvolved kidney; and (3) documentation of renin secretion by proliferating tumor in tissue culture.

GROSS FEATURES. The juxtaglomerular tumors have all presented as small, well circumscribed, or encapsulated neoplasms arising in the renal cortex (pl. IX-A). None have been invasive or have metastasized. Their gross features resemble those of renal adenocarcinoma, but they are more tan to gray rather than yellow.

MICROSCOPIC FEATURES. Histologically, this tumor is composed of small, fairly uniform cells exhibiting little nuclear pleomorphism or mitotic activity. Tumor cells are arranged in large sheets and occasionally tubular structures, with many interposed vascular spaces (pl. IX-B).

Features that distinguish the juxtaglomerular tumor from renal adenocarcinoma are the presence of many cytoplasmic granules which stain deep blue to purple with the Bowie method (pl. IX-C; fig. 178), and the absence of significant amounts of cytoplasmic glycogen or lipid. A positive immunofluorescence with antihuman renin indicates that the cytoplasmic granules contain renin (fig. 179). This is borne out by the electron microscopic appearance of the membrane-bound secretion granules which are identical with those

PLATE IX*
JUXTAGLOMERULAR TUMOR
(Plate IX and Figure 178 from same case)

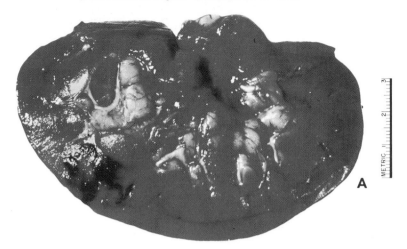

A. A kidney removed from a 26 year old man had caused renovascular hypertension due to a cortical juxtaglomerular tumor, 2 cm. in greatest diameter. The tumor is well circumscribed, light tan, and focally hemorrhagic.

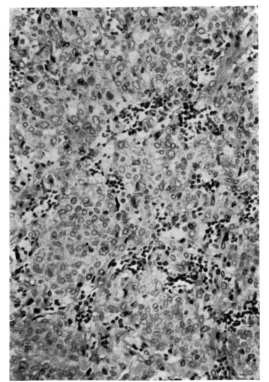

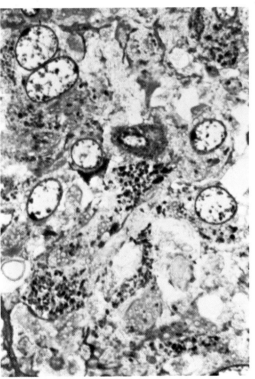

B. The central portion of the same tumor is histologically indistinguishable from a hemangiopericytoma by routine staining. X100.

C. The higher power magnification of this juxtaglomerular tumor demonstrates characteristic prominent cytoplasmic granules when stained with toluidine blue-azure II. X400.

....
*A, B, and C are figs. 1B, 3A, and 4 from Schambelan, M., Howes, E. L., Jr., Stockigt, J. R., Noakes, C. A., and Biglieri, A. G. Role of renin and aldosterone in hypertension due to a renin-secreting tumor. Am. J. Med. 55:86-92, 1973.

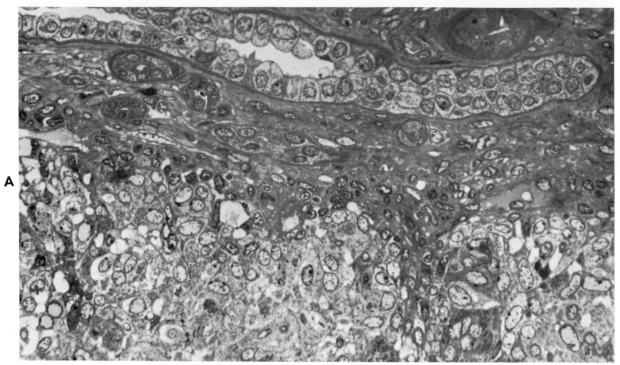

Figure 178
JUXTAGLOMERULAR TUMOR
(Figure 178 and Plate IX from same case)

A. A 1 micron thick Araldite embedded section of the tumor shown in plate IX reveals tumor cells arranged in solid sheets interspersed among renal tubules. No perivascular pattern is evident in this field. Individual tumor cells show considerable variation in nuclear size. Toluidine blue. X460.

B. This higher power magnification demonstrates abundant dark staining cytoplasmic granules. Toluidine blue. X1100.

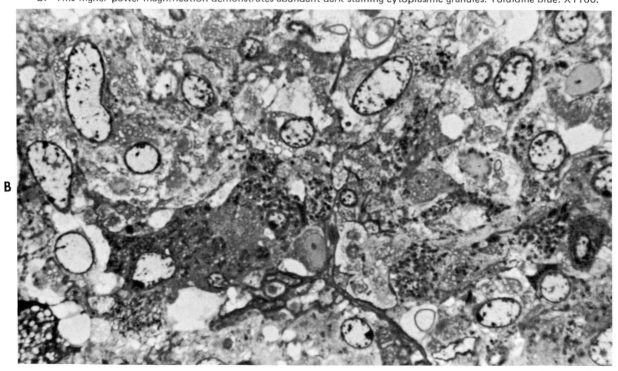

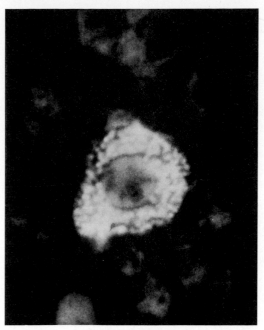

Figure 179
JUXTAGLOMERULAR TUMOR
(Figures 179 and 180 from same case)
The cell from this cortical juxtaglomerular tumor was stained with Thioflavin T to demonstrate the fluorescence of renin granules. X1250. (Fig. 7 from Robertson, P. W., Klidjian, M. B., Harding, L. K., Walters, G., Lee, M. R., and Robb-Smith, A. H. T. Hypertension due to a renin-secreting renal tumour. Am. J. Med. 43:963-976, 1967.)

of the normal juxtaglomerular (granular epithelioid) cell (Barajas; Biava and West; Faarup). Tumor and normal secretion granules have irregular polyhedral profiles with occasional rhomboid shapes and a paracrystalline lattice structure (fig. 180). Rough-surfaced endoplasmic reticulum is prominent, and occasional fibrils and pinocytotic vesicles are associated with the plasmalemma.

Juxtaglomerular (granular epithelioid) cells are thought to be derived from the smooth muscle of the afferent arteriolar media and occasionally from the extraglomerular mesangium. There is little to distinguish juxtaglomerular cells from smooth muscle cells or pericytes, aside from the presence of secretion granules in the juxtaglomerular cells (Faarup), or tumor cells of hemangiopericytoma from normal pericytes and smooth muscle cells (Hahn et al.). This cytologic and histogenetic evidence supports the concept that the juxtaglomerular tumor of the kidney is a specialized form of hemangiopericytoma, unique in its ability to secrete renin. The juxtaglomerular tumor appears to occur at a younger age and be less aggressive than nonrenin-secreting hemangiopericytomas of the kidney. Whether this represents different biologic potentials, or simply that the hormonally active tumors are detected at an earlier stage in their development, remains to be determined.

LYMPHANGIOMA

Lymphangiomas of the kidney are usually found in infants and children and are exceedingly rare (Higgins et al.; Williams). The origin of these tumors is not known. The possibility that they may represent one manifestation of some form of multisystem congenital disease is suggested by the observation that at least two patients have had a second apparently benign tumor of identical histologic type in the chest—one in the mediastinum, and one in the lung.

Renal lymphangiomas are large, unencapsulated, multicystic tumors, usually replacing a major portion of the kidney, and sometimes prolapsing into the renal pelvis. Histologically, they are composed of numerous, widely dilated, thin-walled vessels lined by a single layer of flattened endothelial cells. While these tumors become quite large, there are no cases on record of recurrence or metastases after nephrectomy. Occasionally, multilocular cystic disease of the kidney is confused with lymphangioma (see p. 81).

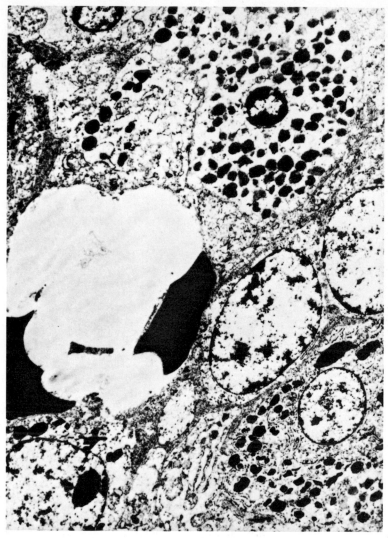

Figure 180
JUXTAGLOMERULAR TUMOR
(Figures 179 and 180 from same case)
This electron micrograph of the tumor shown in figure 179 demonstrates endothelial-lined vascular spaces surrounded by tumor cells which contain rounded to polyhedral granules of variable electron density. X6000. (Fig. 10 from Robertson, P. W., Klidjian, M. B., Harding, L. K., Walters, G., Lee, M. R., and Robb-Smith, A. H. T. Hypertension due to a renin-secreting renal tumour. Am. J. Med. 43:963-976, 1967.)

TUMORS OF FIBROUS TISSUE

FIBROMA

References in the literature to fibromas of the renal cortex give the impression that fibromas are relatively common among benign mesenchymal tumors of the kidney (Colvin). Actually, fibromas of the cortex are exceedingly rare. Xipell examined multiple sections of both kidneys from 250 consecutive autopsies and found a number of mesenchymal cortical tumors, including 13 leiomyomas, 2 lipomas, and 6 myolipomas, but no fibromas. Reese and Winstanley carried out a similar study utilizing one kidney from each of 212 patients and found 12 leiomyomas, 7 lipomas, and 13 myolipomas, but no fibromas.

There is no reason to assume that fibromas should not occur in the renal cortex, and perhaps they do on occasion, but we have never seen one. Most reports of cortical fibromas appear in the older literature and do not include results of special stains which might indicate the presence of smooth muscle.

Medullary fibroma is discussed under renomedullary interstitial cell tumor on page 231.

FIBROSARCOMA*

Prior to 1900, most malignant tumors of the kidney were diagnosed as sarcoma. Gradually, it was recognized that carcinomas made up the majority of malignant renal tumors, but little progress was made in distinguishing between different histologic types of renal sarcoma until 1919, when Berry reported the first leiomyosarcoma of the kidney. Until Berry's report, sarcomas of the kidney were diagnosed as spindle cell sarcoma or more usually, fibrosarcoma.

Because of the uncritical acceptance of the many reports of fibrosarcoma in the literature, the concept became established that fibrosarcoma was the most common form of renal sarcoma. This idea persisted well after the time when histochemical procedures were generally available, which showed otherwise. In 1937, Mintz accepted 53 examples of fibrosarcoma; in 1943, Weisel and associates discussed 29 instances of fibrosarcoma; and as late as 1948, Culp and Hartman accepted 30 reports of fibrosarcoma of the kidney. With improvements and greater use of histochemical technics, the diagnosis of renal fibrosarcoma has all but disappeared. In a thorough review of renal sarcomas among 2386 malignant renal tumors of adults from the Mayo Clinic over a period of 60 years, Farrow and associates (Part I) were unable to find any examples of fibrosarcoma among 26 sarcomas of the kidney. It would appear that the fibrosarcoma like the fibroma of the kidney is exceedingly rare, and reports of such lesions should be carefully scrutinized before acceptance.

FIBROXANTHOSARCOMA

SYNONYMS AND RELATED TERMS: Malignant xanthofibroma.

We have seen one fibroxanthosarcoma of the kidney from the files of the Los Angeles Tumor Tissue Registry. This tumor is included in the group of fibrous histiocytomas because of its dual composition of fibroblasts and histiocytes. Morphologically, the lesion is characterized by spindle cells with a collagenous stroma arranged in a storiform pattern and intermixed with plump histiocytes possessing prominent vesicular nuclei and large eosinophilic

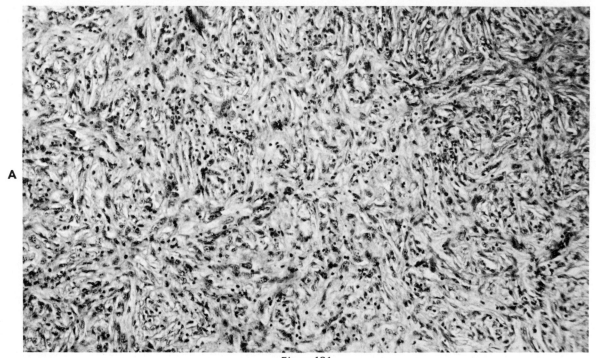

Figure 181

FIBROXANTHOSARCOMA

A. This fibroxanthosarcoma of the kidney is composed of spindle-shaped histiocytic cells arranged in a storiform pattern. Occasional large histiocytic cells are present. X185.

B. This higher power magnification demonstrates atypical multinucleated giant cells. Nucleoli are prominent and mitotic figures are abundant. X375.

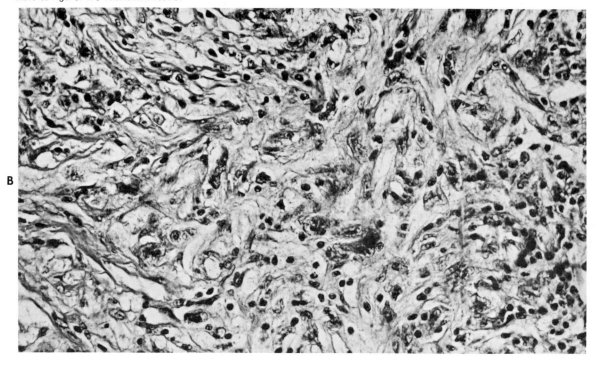

nucleoli (fig. 181). Variable amounts of lipid may be present in the cytoplasm. Scattered throughout the tumor are bizarre giant cells with an eosinophilic to ground-glass cytoplasm (Kempson and Kyriakos). The cells appear to arise from tumor histiocytes and may be multinucleated and form Touton-like giant cells. Mitotic activity is prominent and abnormal mitotic figures are frequent.

The lesions most likely to be confused with fibroxanthosarcoma are xanthogranulomatous pyelonephritis and malakoplakia (see p. 163), and retroperitoneal xanthogranuloma secondarily involving the kidney (Waller et al.). Retroperitoneal xanthogranuloma is classified along with fibroxanthosarcoma in the group of fibrous histiocytomas. They differ histologically only in the absence of a storiform pattern and giant cells in the retroperitoneal xanthogranuloma (Kempson and Kyriakos; Oberling). Biologically, both tumors are aggressive with a high frequency of recurrence and occasional metastases.

MESOBLASTIC NEPHROMA IN THE ADULT

In 1948, Culp and Hartman reported nine malignant embryonal tumors of the kidney in adults. For these tumors, they coined the term mesoblastic nephroma, advocating that it be used in place of Wilms' tumor. Later, Bolande and associates applied the term mesoblastic nephroma to a previously unrecognized congenital renal tumor of infants, characterized by a spindle-cell fibrous or smooth muscle stroma, dilated tubules, and cysts which in prior reports had been lumped with nephroblastoma (see p. 79).

Bolande and associates reported that the mesoblastic nephroma was relatively common among renal tumors in infants, particularly newborn infants, and in their series represented 10 percent of all cases originally diagnosed microscopically as nephroblastoma. To date only one well documented instance of mesoblastic nephroma in an adult has been reported (Block et al.)

RENOMEDULLARY INTERSTITIAL CELL TUMOR

SYNONYMS AND RELATED TERMS: Medullary fibroma; medullary fibrous nodule.

Renomedullary fibromas or fibrous nodules occur with equal frequency in men and women, and have been reported in from 26 to 42 percent of patients at the time of autopsy (Xipell; Zangemeister). They are usually found in patients over the age of 50 years, and almost never in individuals under the age of 30. They occur with equal frequency in men and women. The nodules are multiple in approximately 50 percent of cases, with up to eight nodules in the same kidney (Reese and Winstanley).

Grossly, the fibrous nodules are white to pale gray and usually range in size from 0.1 to 0.3 cm. in greatest diameter. They are round to oval and unencapsulated, but with well defined margins that compress the surrounding renal parenchyma (pl. VIII-B). Histologically, they are composed of variable proportions of compressed ovoid stromal cells with indistinct cellular margins and vesicular nuclei set in a loose basophilic to densely eosinophilic and often hyalinized matrix (fig. 182). Renal tubules are entrapped throughout the nodules, particularly at the periphery. Special stains reveal intracellular neutral fat, phospholipid, and acid mucopolysaccharide. The stroma contains consider-

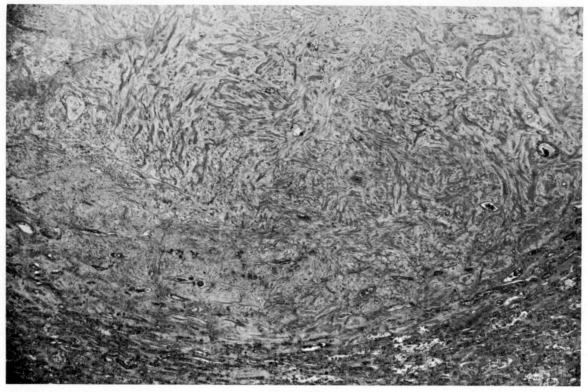

Figure 182
RENOMEDULLARY INTERSTITIAL CELL TUMOR (MEDULLARY FIBROMA)
In this renomedullary interstitial cell tumor (medullary fibroma), the nodule is not encapsulated but sharply circum-scribed, compressing the adjacent medullary stroma and collecting tubules. The interior is relatively acellular and composed predominantly of hyalinized collagenous tissue. Occasional collecting tubules are incorporated into the fibroma at the margins. X75.

able collagen, but no reticulin and no elastic tissue (pl. VIII-C). Electron microscopically, the cells of the fibrous nodules, in spite of the abundant collagen elaborated, resemble medullary interstitial cells rather than fibroblasts (Lerman et al.).

From these histologic findings, it has been concluded that these lesions are neither fibromas nor hamartomas. Whether they represent hyperplastic or neoplastic overgrowth of the interstitial cells has not been determined. However, because of the purported endocrine-like antihypertensive action of renomedullary interstitial cells, it is postulated that the stimulus or stimuli responsible for initiating an antihyper-

tensive response might also induce the hyperplastic or neoplastic transformation of these cells which produces the renomedullary interstitial cell tumor (Lerman et al.).

TUMORS OF NEUROGENIC TISSUE

Tumors of neural origin are extremely rare. All the reports we have been able to locate clearly describe the location in the renal hilum and apparent origin in the renal pelvis. These tumors are described on page 312 under mesodermal tumors of the renal pelvis and ureter.

TUMORS OF OSTEOGENIC TISSUE

A total of five osteogenic sarcomas primary in the kidney have been reported (figs. 183, 184). Two of the patients were men and three, women; their ages ranged from 52 to 82 years, with three patients over 75. Four of the patients had their tumors detected during life; all had an abdominal mass and roentgenographic evidence of calcification within their renal tumor. Three patients had gross hematuria. All five patients developed metastases and died of their tumors (Haining and Poole; Hamer and Wishard; Hudson; Johnson et al.; Soto et al.).

The origin of renal osteosarcoma is not known. Rarely, both nephroblastomas and sarcomatoid renal adenocarcinomas are accompanied by malignant bone formation; in nephroblastoma, as one line of malignant differentiation and in renal adenocarcinoma, most likely as a form of malignant metaplasia. There is no evidence to suggest that any of these osteogenic sarcomas reported in the kidney represent either nephroblastoma or renal adenocarcinoma.

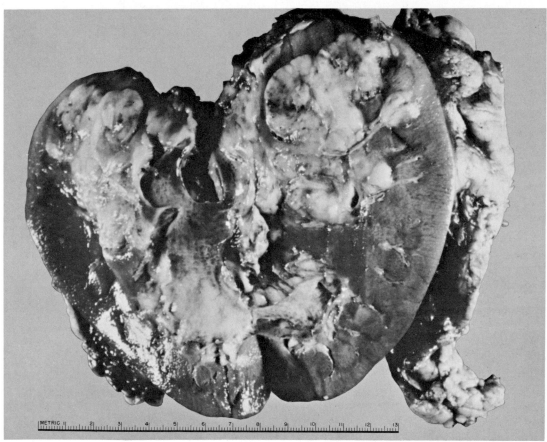

Figure 183
OSTEOGENIC SARCOMA
(Figures 183 and 184 from same case)
An osteogenic sarcoma was found in the lower pole of the right kidney in a 59 year old woman. The yellow-white variegated tumor is very well circumscribed but infiltrates the peripelvic fat. (Fig. 3 from Johnson, L. A., Ancona, V. C., Johnson, T., and Pineda, N. B. Primary osteogenic sarcoma of the kidney. J. Urol. 104:528-531, 1970.)

An origin from indifferent mesenchyme, as we postulate for renal liposarcoma and rhabdomyosarcoma, seems likely in view of the well documented potential of osteosarcoma to develop in extraosseous soft tissues.

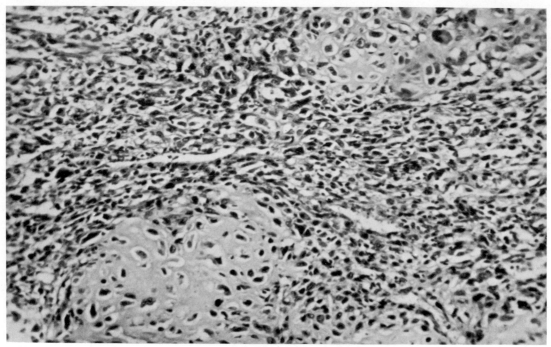

Figure 184
OSTEOGENIC SARCOMA
(Figures 183 and 184 from same case)

This is the histologic appearance of the tumor shown in figure 183. It is extremely pleomorphic with numerous small hyperchromatic spindle-shaped cells forming the bulk of the tumor, interspersed with occasional multinucleated giant cells. Clusters of calcifying osteoid tissue containing similar malignant cells are scattered throughout the tumor. X450. (Fig. 4 from Johnson, L. A., Ancona, V. C., Johnson, T., and Pineda, N. B. Primary osteogenic sarcoma of the kidney. J. Urol. 104:528-531, 1970.)

TUMORS OF HEMATOPOIETIC TISSUE

LEUKEMIA

In a review of 108 patients with leukemia, Sternby found that the kidneys were enlarged and contained leukemic infiltrates in 42 percent of those patients with lymphatic leukemia and 24 percent with myelogenous leukemia. Kirshbaum and Preuss reported a higher frequency of leukemic involvement, 63 percent, but did not report the relative frequencies of the type of leukemias producing the infiltrates.

In patients with leukemia, the kidneys are frequently enlarged, but not necessarily due to leukemic involvement. When renal leukemic infiltrates are present, the kidneys may be 2 to 3 times normal size. The leukemic infiltrates produce irregular geographic patterns or mottling of the cortex (figs. 185, 186). Normal cortical tissue appears tan, while areas of the cortex containing leukemic infiltrates are pale gray-pink or gray-white. Infiltration is usually limited to the outer cortex, with rare involvement of the inner cortex and medulla. The infiltrates, irrespective of the type of leukemia, are interstitial, diffuse or irregularly confluent, and nonnodular in contrast to infiltrates of certain lymphomas like Hodgkin's disease, which are usually discrete and nodular (fig. 187; Amromin).

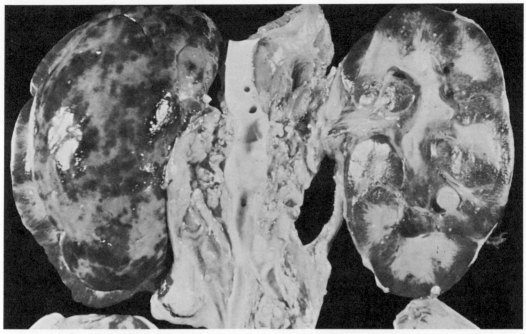

Figure 185
LYMPHOCYTIC LEUKEMIA
These grossly enlarged kidneys were removed from a patient with lymphocytic leukemia. They demonstrate mottling due to leukemic infiltrates, limited primarily to the outer cortex. (Courtesy of Dr. Seth L. Haber, Santa Clara, Calif.)

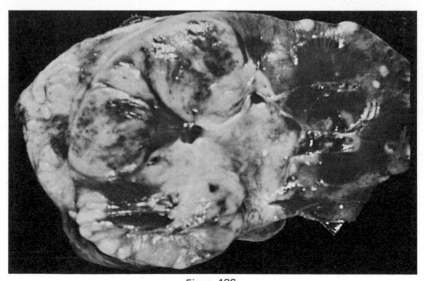

Figure 186
MALIGNANT LYMPHOMA
This typical appearance of renal infiltrates in malignant lymphoma demonstrates a pattern of palpable discrete nodules rather than diffuse infiltration. (Courtesy of Dr. Seth L. Haber, Santa Clara, Calif.)

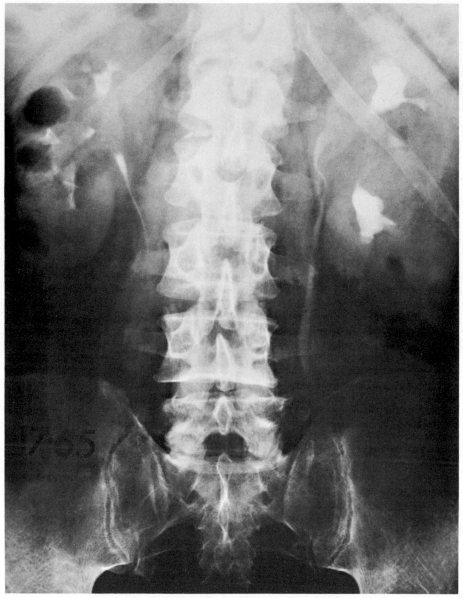

Figure 187
LYMPHOCYTIC LYMPHOMA
(Figures 187 and 188 from same case)

This excretory urogram of a 58 year old man with longstanding lymphocytic lymphoma reveals distortion of the left renal pelvis and caliceal system by an intrarenal mass. Both kidneys are enlarged.

MALIGNANT LYMPHOMA

There are very few instances in which the kidneys have been documented as the site of a primary lymphoma (Farrow et al., Part II). Some authors have flatly stated that it never occurs. However, secondary renal involvement in lymphomas, either generalized or retroperitoneal, is very common and a renal mass or symptoms referable to the urinary system may first draw attention to the disease (fig. 188;

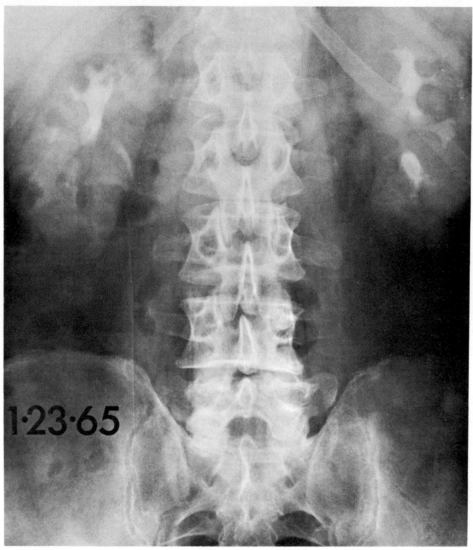

Figure 188
LYMPHOCYTIC LYMPHOMA
(Figures 187 and 188 from same case)
Another excretory urogram was taken of the same patient as shown in figure 187 following radiation therapy. The mass of the left kidney is no longer evident. (Courtesy of Dr. Joachim Burhenne, San Francisco, Calif.)

Farrow et al., Part II; Richmond et al.). Only the lung is more frequently involved than the kidneys by secondary deposits of lymphoma; among metastases to the kidney, only carcinoma of the lung and breast are the sites of the primary tumor more frequently than malignant lymphoma.

In one large autopsy series, the overall frequency of lymphomatous infiltration of the kidney in patients dying of malignant lymphoma was 33.5 percent (Richmond et al.). The renal involvement of patients with various forms of lymphoma was: Hodgkin's disease, 13 percent; lymphocytic lymphoma with marrow infiltration, 63 percent; histiocytic lymphoma, 46 percent; and mycosis fungoides, 0 percent. Of those patients with renal involvement, infiltration of the kidneys was bilateral in 74 percent of cases. No relationship was found between the frequency of involvement and age, sex, or duration of the disease.

Grossly, the lesions may be diffusely infiltrating (6 percent) or circumscribed solitary parenchymal nodules (13 percent), but are generally multiple discrete nodules (61 percent) (fig. 187). The remainder are microscopic or represent extension from adjacent organs.

MULTIPLE MYELOMA

In multiple myeloma, the lesions are not necessarily confined to the skeleton, but may also involve the reticuloendothelial structures including the lymph nodes, liver, and spleen. Diffuse or nodular lesions also have been described in the heart, lungs, thyroid, testis, ovary, gastrointestinal tract, adrenal gland, and kidneys (Churg and Gordon; Pasmantier and Azar). Rarely, primary plasma cell tumors occur in extraosseous sites and then most frequently in the mucosa or submucosa of the nasopharynx, mouth, or upper respiratory tract. Occasionally, primary multiple myeloma is reported in such sites as the lymph nodes, gastrointestinal tract, thyroid, breast, pancreas, ovary, testis, skin, and kidney (Dolin and Dewar; Farrow et al., Part II).

There are many allusions to the not infrequent occurrence of multiple myeloma infiltrating the kidney, although statistical data are scarce. In a small, but excellent review of extraosseous spread of multiple myeloma, Pasmantier and Azar demonstrated that of 57 patients with multiple myeloma, 10 had renal involvement; 7 had microscopic involvement alone, and only 3 had demonstrable gross lesions within the kidney. Involvement of the kidney was at least twice as frequent as involvement of the adrenal gland, thyroid, lung, or pancreas.

In typical multiple myeloma, diagnosis of the metastatic lesions of the kidney should present no problem (fig. 189). Primary multiple myeloma of the kidney is sufficiently rare that this possibility may not be considered if the tumor is poorly differentiated.

If the infiltrate is well differentiated, one must distinguish between myeloma and reactive plasma cell infiltration. If poorly differentiated, the tumor cells are generally large with ample cytoplasm, large nuclei, and absence of the characteristic plasma cell appearance and distinctive cartwheel aggregate of chromatin along the nuclear membrane. When this occurs, the tumor may resemble a malignant histiocytic lymphoma. This lesion can also be confused with Hodgkin's disease if large pleomorphic cells resembling Sternberg-Reed cells are present.

In patients with multiple myeloma, there may be significant renal damage

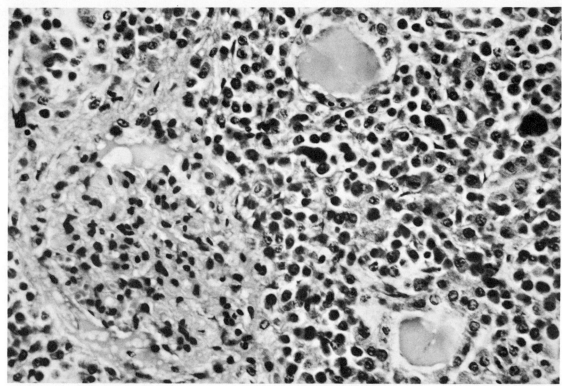

Figure 189
MULTIPLE MYELOMA
Nodular infiltration by malignant plasma cells occurred in the kidney of a patient with multiple myeloma. The majority
of the cells are well differentiated, although occasional pleomorphic plasma cells are seen. X460.

(myeloma kidney) in the absence of neo-plastic infiltration of the renal parenchyma. Over 50 percent of patients with Bence-Jones proteinuria have hard, eosinophilic protein casts in widely dilated, convoluted and collecting tubules. Tubular epithelial cell hyperplasia and syncytial epithelial giant cells are usually found around the casts. Amyloid confined to renal arteries is found in approximately 14 to 15 percent of patients with multiple myeloma (Heptinstall).

References

Abrams, H. L., Spiro, R., and Goldstein, N. Metastases in carcinoma: analysis of 1000 autopsied cases. Cancer 3:74-85, 1950.

Ackerman, L. V. Tumors of the Retroperitoneum, Mesentery and Peritoneum. Fascicles 23 and 24, Atlas of Tumor Pathology. Washington: Armed Forces Institute of Pathology, 1954.

Amromin, G. D. Pathology of Leukemia, pp. 251-257. New York: Hoeber Medical Division, Harper & Row, 1968.

Barajas, L. The development and ultrastructure of the juxtaglomerular cell granule. J. Ultrastruct. Res. 15:400-413, 1966.

Bazaz-Malik, G., and Gupta, D. N. Leiomyosarcoma of kidney: Report of a case and review of the literature. J. Urol. 95:754-758, 1966.

Beadles, R. O., Jr., and Urich, R. W. Intrarenal lipoma: Report of a case. J. Urol. 67:460-463, 1952.

Berg, J. W. Angiolipomyosarcoma of kidney (malignant hamartomatous angiolipomyoma) in a case with solitary metastasis from bronchogenic carcinoma. Cancer 8:759-763, 1955.

Berk, L. E., Erinc, A. I., and McManus, R. G. Hemangiopericytoma involving a kidney. N. Engl. J. Med. 263:1185-1187, 1960.

Berry, F. B. Report of three cases of combined tumors of the kidney in adults. J. Med. Res. 40:459-469, 1919.

Biava, C. G., and West, M. Fine structure of normal human juxtaglomerular cells. II. Specific and non-specific cytoplasmic granules. Am. J. Pathol. 49:955-979, 1966.

Black, H. R., and Heinemann, S. Hemangiopericytoma: Report of a case involving the kidney. J. Urol. 74:42-46, 1955.

Block, N. L., Grabstald, H. G., and Melamed, M. R. Congenital mesoblastic nephroma (leiomyomatous hamartoma): first adult case. J. Urol. 110:380-383, 1973.

Bolande, R. P., Brough, A. J., and Izant, R. J., Jr. Congenital mesoblastic nephroma of infancy. A report of eight cases and the relationship to Wilms' tumor. Pediatrics 40:272-278, 1967.

Bulkley, G. J., and Drinker, H. R. Malignant mesenchymoma of the kidney: case report. J. Urol. 77:583-588, 1957.

Churg, J., and Gordon, A. J. Multiple myeloma with unusual visceral involvement. Arch. Pathol. 34:546-556, 1942.

Clinton-Thomas, C. L. A giant leiomyoma of the kidney. Br. J. Surg. 43:497-501, 1956.

Colvin, S. H., Jr. Certain capsular and subcapsular mixed tumors of the kidney herein called "capsuloma." J. Urol. 48:585-600, 1942.

Critchley, M., and Earl, C. J. C. Tuberose sclerosis and allied conditions. Brain 55:311-346, 1932.

Culp, O. S., and Hartman, F. W. Mesoblastic nephroma in adults: A clinico-pathologic study of Wilms' tumors and related renal neoplasms. J. Urol. 60:552-576, 1948.

Dolin, S., and Dewar, J. P. Extramedullary plasmacytoma. Am. J. Pathol. 32:83-103, 1956.

Evans, R. W. Histological Appearances of Tumours; with a Consideration of their Histogenesis and Certain Aspects of their Clinical Features and Behaviour, 2d ed. Baltimore: Williams & Wilkins Co., 1967; Edinburgh and London: E. & S. Livingstone, Ltd., 1966.

Faarup, P. Morphological aspects of the renin-angiotensin system. Acta Pathol. Microbiol. Scand. (A) Suppl. 222:1-96, 1971.

Farrow, G. M., Harrison, E. G., Jr., Utz, D. C., and ReMine, W. H. Sarcomas and sarcomatoid and mixed malignant tumors of the kidney in adults—Part I. Cancer 22:545-550, 1968.

............, Harrison, E. G., Jr., and Utz, D. C. Sarcomas and sarcomatoid and mixed malignant tumors of the kidney in adults—Part II. Cancer 22:551-555, 1968.

............, Harrison, E. G., Jr., Utz, D. C., and Jones, D. R. Renal angiomyolipoma. A clinicopathologic study of 32 cases. Cancer 22:564-570, 1968.

Fischer, W. Die Nierentumoren bei der tuberösen Hirnsklerose. Beitr. Pathol. 50:235-282, 1911.

Friedman, P. S., and Solis-Cohen, L. Hemangioma of the kidney; its roentgen diagnosis. Am. J. Roentgenol. Radium Ther. Nucl. Med. 60:408-410, 1948.

Gordon, M. P., Jr., Kimmelstiel, P., and Cabell, C. L. Leiomyoma of the kidney. Report of a case with review of the literature. J. Urol. 42:507-519, 1939.

Gupta, O. P., and Dube, M. K. Rare primary renal sarcoma. Br. J. Urol. 43:546-571, 1971.

Hahn, M. J., Dawson, R., Esterly, J. A., and Joseph, D. J. Hemangiopericytoma. An ultrastructural study. Cancer 31:255-261, 1973.

Haining, R. B., and Poole, F. E. Osteoblastoma of the kidney, histologically identical with osteogenic sarcoma. Arch. Pathol. 21:44-54, 1936.

Hajdu, S. I., and Foote, F. W., Jr. Angiomyolipoma of the kidney: Report of 27 cases and review of the literature. J. Urol. 102:396-401, 1969.

Hamer, H. G., and Wishard, W. N., Jr. Osteogenic sarcoma involving the right kidney. J. Urol. 60:10-17, 1948.

Hartveit, F., and Hallerbraker, B. A report of three angiolipomyomata and one angiolipomyosarcoma. Acta Pathol. Microbiol. Scand. 49: 329-336, 1960.

Heptinstall, R. H. Pathology of the Kidney, 1st ed., pp. 588-589. Boston: Little, Brown and Company, 1966.

Herzog, H. Nierengeschwülste mit quergestreifter Muskulatur. Z. Krebsforsch. 48:424-446, 1939.

Higgins, T. T., Williams, D. I., and Nash, D. F. E. The Urology of Childhood. London: Mosby; Butterworth and Co., 1951.

Hudson, H. C. Osteogenic sarcoma involving the left kidney. J. Urol. 75:21-24, 1956.

Jenkins, J. D., Anderson, C. K., and Williams, R. E. Renal sarcoma. Br. J. Urol. 43:263-267, 1971.

Johnson, L. A., Ancona, V. C., Johnson, T., and Pineda, N. B. Primary osteogenic sarcoma of the kidney. J. Urol. 104:528-531, 1970.

Kempson, R. L., and Kyriakos, M. Fibroxanthosarcoma of the soft tissues. A type of malignant fibrous histiocytoma. Cancer 29:961-976, 1972.

Kirshbaum, J. D., and Preuss, F. S. Leukemia. A clinical and pathologic study of one hundred and twenty-three fatal cases in a series of 14,400 necropsies. Arch. Intern. Med. 71:777-792, 1943.

Klapproth, H. J., Poutasse, E. F., and Hazard, J. B. Renal angiomyolipomas. Report of four cases. Arch. Pathol. 67:400-411, 1959.

Lee, H. C., and Kay, S. Hemangiopericytoma: Report of a case involving the kidney with an 11-year follow up. Ann. Surg. 156:125-128, 1962.

Lerman, R. J., Pitcock, J. A., Stephenson, P., and Muirhead, E. E. Renomedullary interstitial cell tumor (formerly fibroma of renal medulla). Hum. Pathol. 3:559-568, 1972.

Loomis, R. C. Primary leiomyosarcoma of the kidney: Report of a case and review of the literature. J. Urol. 107:557-560, 1972.

Lucké, B., and Schlumberger, H. G. Tumors of the Kidney, Renal Pelvis and Ureter. Fascicle 30, Atlas of Tumor Pathology. Washington: Armed Forces Institute of Pathology, 1957.

McCrea, L. E. Hemangioma of the kidney; review of the literature. Urologic Cutan. Rev. 55:670-680, 1951.

Messinger, W. J., and Jarman, W. D. Rhabdomyosarcoma of the kidney: case report with autopsy findings. Surgery 2:26-32, 1937.

Mintz, E. R. Sarcoma of the kidney in adults. Ann. Surg. 105:521-538, 1937.

Morgan, G. S., Straumfjord, J. V., and Hall, E. J. Angio-myolipoma of the kidney. J. Urol. 65:525-527, 1951.

Oberling, C. Retroperitoneal xanthogranuloma. Am. J. Cancer 23:477-489, 1935.

Pasmantier, M. W., and Azar, H. A. Extraskeletal spread in multiple plasma cell myeloma. A review of 57 autopsied cases. Cancer 23:167-174, 1969.

Price, E. B., Jr., and Mostofi, F. K. Symptomatic angio-myolipoma of the kidney. Cancer 18:761-774, 1965.

Prince, C. L. Primary angio-endothelioma of the kidney: Report of a case and brief review. J. Urol. 47:787-792, 1942.

Reese, A. J. M., and Winstanley, D. P. The small tumour-like lesions of the kidney. Br. J. Cancer 12:507-516, 1958.

Riches, E. W., Griffiths, I. H., and Thackray, A. C. New growths of the kidney and ureter. Br. J. Urol. 23:297-356, 1951.

Richmond, J., Sherman, R. S., Diamond, H. D., and Craver, L. F. Renal lesions associated with malignant lymphomas. Am. J. Med. 32:184-207, 1962.

Robertson, P. W., Klidjian, A., Harding, L. K., Walters, G., Lee, M. R., and Robb-Smith, A. H. T. Hypertension due to a renin-secreting renal tumour. Am. J. Med. 43:963-976, 1967.

Robertson, T. D., and Hand, J. R. Primary intrarenal lipoma of surgical significance. J. Urol. 46:458-474, 1941.

Schambelan, M., Howes, E. L., Jr., Noakes, C. A., Stockigt, J. R., and Biglieri, E. G. Role of renin and aldosterone in hypertension due to a renin-secreting tumor. Am. J. Med. 55:86-92, 1973.

Seabury, J. C., Jr. Renal rhabdomyosarcoma. J.A.M.A. 201:1043-1044, 1967.

Simon, R., and Greene, R. C. Perirenal hemangioperi-cytoma. A case associated with hypoglycemia. J.A.M.A. 189:155-156, 1964.

Soto, P. J., Jr., Rader, E. S., Martin, J. M., and Gregowicz, A. Osteogenic sarcoma of the kidney: Report of a case. J. Urol. 94:532-535, 1965.

Steiner, P. E. Cancer: Race and Geography; Some Etiological, Environmental, Ethnological, and Statistical Aspects in Caucasoids, Mongoloids, Negroids, and Mexicans, pp. 9-23; 255-264. Baltimore: Williams & Wilkins Co., 1954.

Sternby, N. H. Studies in enlargement of leukaemic kidneys. Acta Haematol. 14:354-362, 1955.

Stout, A. P., and Murray, M. R. Hemangiopericytoma. A vascular tumor featuring Zimmermann's pericytes. Ann. Surg. 116:26-33, 1942.

Swan, R. H. J., and Balme, H. Angioma of the kidney; report of a case with an analysis of 26 previously reported cases. Br. J. Surg. 23:282-295, 1935.

Tannenbaum, M. Ultrastructural pathology of human renal cell tumors. Pathol. Annu. 6:249-277, 1971.

Waller, J. I., Hellwig, C. A., and Barbosa, E. Retroperitoneal xanthogranuloma associated with visceral eosinophilic granuloma. Cancer 10:388-392, 1957.

Weisel, W., Dockerty, M. B., and Priestley, J. T. Sarcoma of the kidney. J. Urol. 50:564-573, 1943.

Williams, D. I. Nephroblastoma: Clinical Picture and Diagnosis, pp. 235-254. In: Monographs on Neoplastic Disease at Various Sites, Vol. V. Tumours of the Kidney and Ureter. (Ed.) Riches, E. W. Baltimore: Williams & Wilkins Co.; London: E. & S. Livingstone, Ltd., 1964.

Williams, J. P., and Savage, P. T. Liposarcoma of the kidney. Br. J. Surg. 46:225-231, 1958.

Willis, R. A. Pathology of Tumours, 4th ed. New York: Appleton-Century-Crofts, 1968.

Xipell, J. M. The incidence of benign renal nodules (a clinicopathologic study). J. Urol. 106:503-506, 1971.

Zangemeister, W. Untersuchungen über Altersverteilung, Häufigkeit und Morphologie der Nierenfibrome unter Mitberücksichtigung der übrigen ausgereiften Tumoren. Beitr. Pathol. 97:142-183, 1936.

TUMORS OF THE RENAL PELVIS AND URETER

EPITHELIAL TUMORS

Epithelial tumors of the renal pelvis and ureter have been reported more frequently in the last decade than previously, leading to the speculation that the incidence of these tumors may be rising. It is likely that the apparent increase is due to refinement in the collection and coding of public health data as well as improvements in diagnostic technics.

Tumors of the renal pelvis and ureter are reported separately now in most registries rather than included with tumors of the kidney. This will certainly provide much more accurate data on the frequency of these tumors than previously available. Additionally, improved diagnostic technics permit earlier detection of renal pelvic and ureteral tumors before they become so advanced that their origin cannot be accurately established pathologically.

Epithelial tumors of the renal pelvis and ureter exhibit the same spectrum of histologic patterns as those of the bladder. Carcinomas of the renal pelvis and ureter appear more aggressive than their counterparts in the bladder, which is probably related more to anatomic factors than to any differences in intrinsic malignant potential. Because the epithelial tumors of the renal pelvis and ureter are so closely related anatomically, epidemiologically, and histologically, they are discussed here together.

Histogenesis

The transitional epithelium (urothelium) lining the urinary tract responds to a number of protracted noxious stimuli by various forms of reactive proliferation (Mostofi). The epithelium may become redundant as in papillary cystitis, may become cystic, and it may undergo glandular or squamous metaplasia.

A frequent response to injury or irritation is the invagination of transitional epithelium into the lamina propria, forming buds which may eventually lose their continuity with the surface, leaving discrete masses of epithelial cells sequestered in the lamina propria—Brunn's nests (fig. 190). These nests, composed of tightly packed cuboidal and fusiform epithelial cells, are usually solid, although they may contain small crevices or cavities which dilate and eventually become cystic. The largest of the cysts arising from Brunn's nests have a thin lining; often they have only a double layer of cuboidal or columnar cells (fig. 191). These cystic changes are referred to as cystitis, ureteritis, or pyelitis cystica depending upon the location in the urinary tract (Mostofi, 1954). The mechanism by which the cysts develop has not been established. The possibility of their origin through secretory activity is suggested, however, by the observation that these cystic changes are frequently accompanied by a metaplastic transformation of the epithelium lining the cystic Brunn's nests to tall columnar epithelium capable of secreting mucus into the gland lumens (fig. 192; Gordon; Salm). Again, depending upon the location in the urinary tract, the metaplastic glandular changes are referred to as cystitis, ureteritis, or pyelitis glandularis.

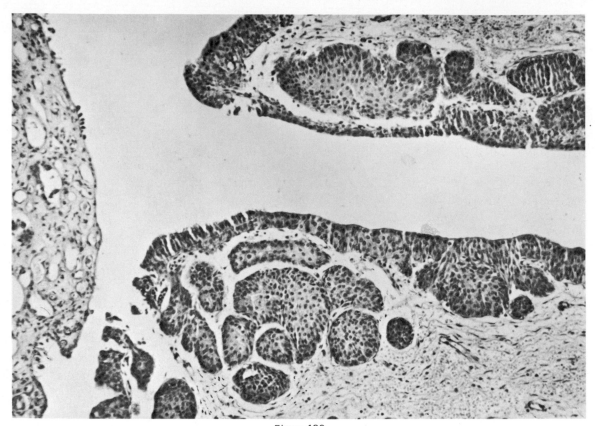

Figure 190
BRUNN'S NESTS
Brunn's nests are seen in the submucosa of the renal pelvis. X112.

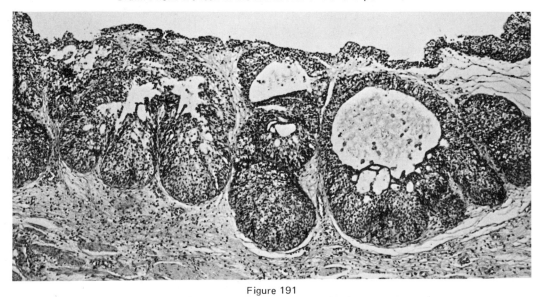

Figure 191
BRUNN'S NESTS AND IN SITU CARCINOMA
Cystic Brunn's nests show cytologic atypia and associated in situ carcinoma in the overlying renal pelvic mucosa. X40.

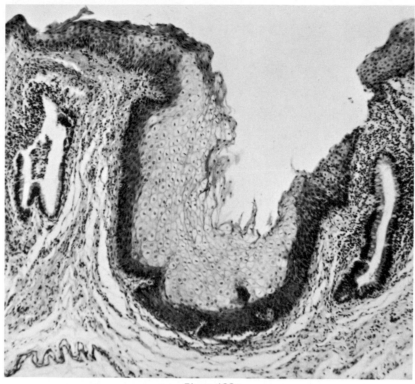

Figure 192
METAPLASIA
Squamous metaplasia of the mucosa of the renal pelvis is associated with mucinous metaplasia in submucosal Brunn's nests. X95.

This metaplastic glandular mucosa mimics that of the large intestine, and the resemblance is heightened by the occasional findings of argentaffin and Paneth cells interspersed among the metaplastic glandular cells (Gordon). The suggestion has been made that the close embryologic relation of the urinary tract and cloaca accounts for the potential of intestinal metaplasia arising in transitional epithelium of the urinary tract. In the more florid forms of glandular metaplasia, extensive replacement of the surface transitional epithelium is seen and differentiation from an adenocarcinoma may be difficult.

Squamous metaplasia occurs in the urinary tract, but more often in the bladder than the renal pelvis or the ureter. The earliest features are the formation of large, clear polygonal cells with pyknotic nuclei and numerous intercellular bridges (fig. 192). Later, accentuation of the granular layer, superficial keratinization, and even hyperkeratosis are seen (figs. 193, 194). The squamous metaplastic changes seem to occur solely on the surface epithelium, but may occur in conjunction with glandular metaplasia arising in Brunn's nests (fig. 192; Gordon).

The Brunn's nests, cysts, and glandular and squamous metaplasia generally are preceded or accompanied by irritants such as infection, inflammation, urinary calculi, and hydronephrosis. They are also found in association with cancer of the urinary tract in man (fig. 191), in experimentally induced carcinomas, and with vitamin A deficiency in laboratory animals (Evans; Ghidoni and Campbell; Gordon; Roe; Salm).

Such associations tempt one to assume that the various proliferative and neoplastic changes in the urinary tract are all due to the same stimulus or stimuli; i.e., that squamous metaplasia is a stage in the development of epidermoid carcinoma, and glandular metaplasia is a stage in the development of adenocarcinoma of the urinary tract. However, there is no direct evidence that these metaplastic changes are pre-malignant. On the contrary, most carcinomas of the urinary tract are transitional cell rather than squamous, develop without accompanying squamous metaplasia, and are rarely found arising in foci of squamous metaplasia. Because there is no satisfactory evidence that the squamous changes are premalignant, we avoid the term leukoplakia, which is histologically ambiguous and connotes to many a premalignant change. Adenocarcinoma of the urinary tract usually arises without preexisting metaplastic changes, although occasionally it may be accompanied by, or even arise in foci of glandular metaplasia (Salm).

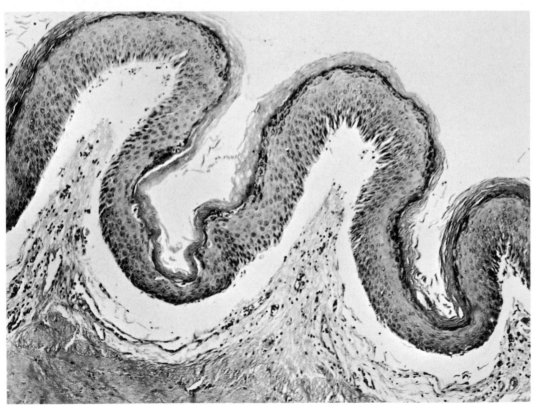

Figure 193
METAPLASIA

This shows extensive squamous metaplasia of ureteral mucosa with the formation of a granular layer and overlying hyperkeratosis. X112.

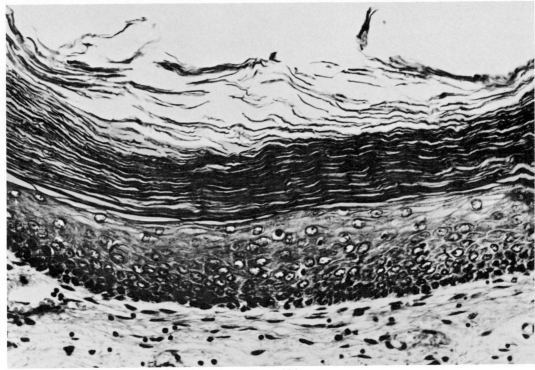

Figure 194
METAPLASIA
This illustrates desquamation of hyperkeratotic debris from metaplastic squamous epithelium in the renal pelvis. X350.

Comparative Pathology

Spontaneous Tumors in Lower Animals

While naturally occurring renal adenocarcinomas and nephroblastomas are rare, they are much more frequent than carcinomas of the renal pelvis or ureter. There are only isolated reports of renal pelvic carcinoma and to our knowledge no reported instances of ureteral carcinoma in wild, domestic, or laboratory animals. In an extensive review of the literature, Guerin and associates found one renal pelvic carcinoma in a rat and one in a mouse, but none in other laboratory animals. In the several large series of examinations of domestic animals, no renal pelvic carcinomas were reported (Monlux et al.; Sandison and Anderson).

Experimentally Induced Tumors

The frequency of renal pelvic carcinoma in laboratory animals exposed to a variety of carcinogens is relatively low compared to that of induced renal adenocarcinoma and nephroblastoma, but still significantly greater than in normal animals (Guerin et al.; Roe). To date, there are no reports of experimentally induced ureteral carcinomas.

Chemical Agents. Transitional and squamous cell carcinoma of the renal pelvis were first produced in mice and rats by direct implantation of crystals of dibenzanthracene, methylcholanthrene, and benzpyrene into the kidney. Subsequently, renal pelvic carcinomas were produced by administration of carcinogens remote from the kidney by feeding or intragastric instillation of mice with 2-acetylaminofluorene, and rats with 1-acetylaminofluorene (Guerin et al.). Recently, a promising model has been found—feeding of diets containing aflatoxin B, which elicits a fairly high frequency of renal pelvic carcinomas as well as renal adenocarcinomas (Butler and Barnes).

In addition to organic compounds, lead salts are effective in producing renal pelvic carcinomas as well as adenocarcinomas. Both lead acetate and lead phosphate administered over long periods of time are capable of inducing carcinoma of the renal pelvis in rats (Boyland et al.; Roe et al.). Other species have not yet been used successfully for the production of pelvic carcinomas with organic or inorganic carcinogens.

Physical Agents. Several investigators have induced renal pelvic carcinomas in rats with whole body X-radiation (Guerin et al.). As with chemical agents, renal adenocarcinomas are produced with much greater frequency and ureteral carcinoma apparently not at all.

Viral Agents. Recent electron microscopic studies have demonstrated the presence of a previously unknown human RNA virus in papillary transitional cell carcinomas of the renal pelvis (fig. 195), and neutralizing antibodies to the virus were found in several of the patients (Elliott et al.). Whether this virus is involved in the development of these tumors is not known; however, the relationship does appear specific for this tumor type since the same investigators have not identified this virus electron microscopically or isolated it from any other types of renal tumor.

Epidemiology

Of the tumors arising in the renal pelvis and ureter, 75 to 80 percent are malignant (Abeshouse; Grabstald et al.). These include the papillary transitional cell carcinoma, squamous cell carcinoma, undifferentiated carcinoma, adenocarcinoma, and the relatively rare sarcomas. Among the apparently benign tumors of the renal pelvis and ureter, approximately 50 percent are papillomas and the remainder include polyps, angiomas, fibromas, and myomas.

While primary malignant tumors of the renal parenchyma are uncommon, they are, however, 4 to 5 times as frequent as all malignant tumors of the renal pelvis and ureter combined. Carcinoma of the renal pelvis is approximately 2.5 times as frequent as carcinoma of the ureter (Table III).

Tumors of the ureter and renal pelvis share embryologic, morphologic, and etiologic similarities to tumors of the bladder. In these anatomic sites, papillomas and carcinomas are frequently multicentric and may arise in several areas within the renal pelvis, ureter, and bladder (Abeshouse; Grabstald et al.; Poole-Wilson; Smart). Simultaneous or sequential occurrence of papillomas or carcinomas in two or all three of these structures is not uncommon. However, multiple primary tumors involving both kidney and excretory tract do occur, but are uncommon (Sarma; Gillis et al.; Graham and Vynalek; Richardson and Woodburn; Walker and Jordan).

Carcinoma of the bladder is much more common than carcinoma of the renal pelvis or the ureter. A series of 257 malignant tumors of the urinary tract collected at the Oakland Kaiser Foundation Hospital over a period of 16 years included 238 tumors of the bladder, 14 of the renal pelvis, and 5 of the ureter; a ratio of approximately 50 to 3 to 1. One of the more intriguing theories to explain the great variation in the frequencies with which carcinomas develop in

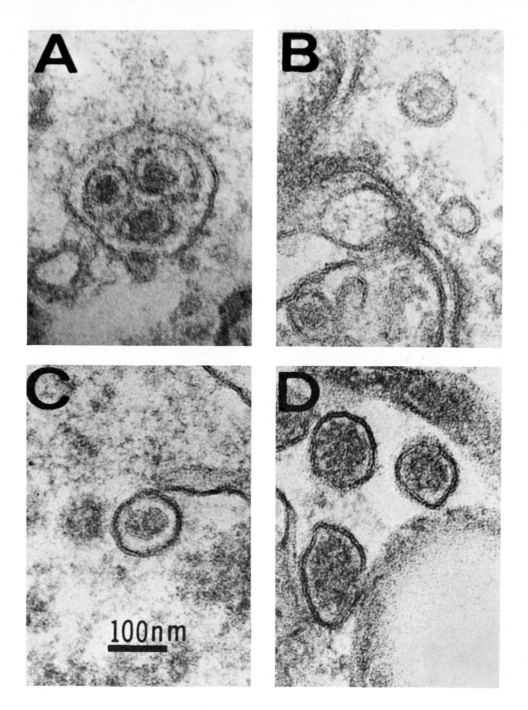

Figure 195
PAPILLARY TRANSITIONAL CELL CARCINOMA
EFMU virus particles were found in this papillary transitional cell carcinoma of the renal pelvis. (A) Extracellular particles in T_1 cells; (B) intracellular particles in T_1 cells; and (C and D) intracellular particles in T_2 cells. X154,000. (Fig. 1 from Elliott, A. Y., Fraley, E. E., Cleveland, P., Castro, A. E., and Stein, N. Isolation of RNA virus from papillary tumors of the human renal pelvis. Science 179:393-395, 1973.)

the renal pelvis, ureter, and bladder is that the likelihood of carcinomas corresponds to the surface areas of mucosa in each of these structures (Willis). This is a very attractive explanation, but that it may not be the entire answer is indicated by the fact that the distribution of tumors in the ureter is not uniform; a majority of cancers (75 percent) occur in the lower third of the ureter. There is a similar propensity for papillomas to develop in the lower third of the ureter as well.

Age

Carcinomas of the renal pelvis and ureter occur most frequently in patients in the older age groups and are rare under the age of 30. The majority of tumors are found in the sixth to eighth decades with an apparent peak in the seventh decade. When rates are standardized to a common base of 100,000 population by age intervals, a steady rise in the incidence of renal pelvic and ureteral carcinoma is seen with advancing age (Graph III).

Sex

As with renal adenocarcinoma, there is a well documented preponderance of carcinoma of the renal pelvis and ureter in men. The data from the California Tumor Registry for Alameda County indicate that renal pelvic carcinoma is three times as frequent and ureteral carcinoma twice as frequent in men as in women (figures adjusted to a base of 100,000 population by sex). These figures agree with the previously estimated frequency of these tumors by sex (Abeshouse; Grabstald et al.).

Geographic and Racial Distribution

Because carcinomas of the renal pelvis are usually included with those of the kidney, and carcinomas of the ureter completely ignored in large epidemiologic studies, no extensive data are available for the analyses of possible geographic or racial influences on the occurrence of these tumors.

A most intriguing geographic localization of carcinoma of the renal pelvis, ureter, and bladder is that occurring in Bulgaria, Rumania, and Yugoslavia in a high percentage of individuals afflicted with an endemic chronic renal disease of unknown etiology, referred to as Balkan nephropathy (Wolstenholme and Knight). The relatively high frequency of carcinoma of the urinary tract in this disease makes it an excellent source for epidemiologic studies on carcinogenesis of the renal pelvis, ureter, and bladder.

Instances of carcinoma of the renal pelvis and ureter in nonwhites residing in California have been recorded in the California Tumor Registry (Table III); however, the numbers are too small for statistical analyses of expected rates, based on census figures for Blacks, Mexicans, Indians, Chinese, and Japanese living in California.

Heredity

To our knowledge, there have been no reports of laboratory animals with high rates of spontaneously occurring tumors of the renal pelvis or ureter, and none of a familial distribution of these tumors in humans.

Unlike nephroblastoma and renal adenocarcinoma, there is no indication of any relationship between renal pelvic or ureteral carcinoma and any hereditary diseases.

Etiologic Factors

Inflammation. Glandular and squamous metaplasia of the ureteral and renal pelvic mucosa frequently accompany carcinomas arising in the same areas. In turn, both metaplastic and neoplastic changes are often associated with the presence of inflammation and/or calculi in the renal pelvis and ureter.

The interrelationships of these various pathologic alterations are not clearly established. Carcinoma of the pelvis or ureter can predispose to pyelitis or ureteritis as well as calculus formation, but the converse has not been proved. Metaplastic changes occur in areas of inflammation and in conjunction, often in continuity with cancers of the renal pelvis or ureter. It is tempting to see metaplasia as a response to inflammation or calculi, or both, which may then progress to carcinoma.

While inflammation, calculi, and metaplasia are the most frequently observed pathologic alterations associated with carcinoma of the urinary tract, such an orderly scheme of interrelationship based on a presumed sequence of events unfortunately has not been proved.

One well documented form of inflammation related to the development of carcinoma of the bladder is schistosomiasis. Involvement of the ureter as well as the bladder by *Schistosoma haematobium* is frequent. The few reports on schistosomiasis in association with carcinoma of the ureter may be due to the low incidence of ureteral carcinoma in the general population which makes even a small but significant increase inapparent (Makar).

Chemical Agents. Cancer of the urinary tract is a well established occupational hazard in certain industries, including dyestuff, rubber, cable, plastic, and gas (Cole et al.; Poole-Wilson; Sarma). The responsible carcinogenic agents have been identified as o-aminophenols (aromatic hydrocarbons with an amino radical) such as beta-naphthylamine, benzidine, 4-aminodiphenyl, and 2-acetylaminofluorene. Metabolism of these aromatic compounds is primarily through N-hydroxylation, which produces metabolites more carcinogenic than the parent compounds.

These metabolites are detoxified in the liver by conjugation with sulfuric and glucuronic acid and largely excreted in the urine. Amines such as 3-dichlorobenzidine and hydrazobenzene are rendered noncarcinogenic by the process of conjugation, although benzidine is not.

Beta-glucuronidase and sulfatase activity is elevated in the urine of patients with bladder cancer. Many of the o-aminophenols are more carcinogenic in their unconjugated state, which suggests that beta-glucuronidase activity may play an indirect role in carcinogenesis of the urinary tract. However, it is not established that beta-glucuronidase activity in the urine arises in response to the presence of chemical carcinogens prior to tumor formation. It is well documented that bladder tumors themselves elaborate large amounts of beta-glucuronidase and that levels fall to normal values following extirpation of the tumor (Sarma).

While carcinoma of the bladder occurs most frequently, carcinomas of the ureter and renal pelvis also are induced by these industrial chemical carcinogens, and much more frequently than would be expected in the normal population. The relative frequency of carcinomas of the ureter, renal pelvis, and bladder in patients exposed to several known chemical carcinogens is parallel to the ratio seen in unexposed individuals (Poole-Wilson). This strongly suggests that with chemically induced, as well as naturally occurring, tumors of the urinary tract, there is no preferential site for the development of these tumors. It does favor the hypothesis that the frequency of cancer in the various sites of the urinary tract is in part related to the surface area of transitional mucosa in the bladder, renal pelvis, and ureter.

Habits. In addition to the hazards of various industrial chemicals, there is good evidence that the intake of large amounts of phenacetin predisposes to carcinomas of the renal pelvis at rates over 40 times that expected in the normal population (Bengtsson et al.; Buch et al.). The ratio of men to women developing renal pelvic carcinomas among phenacetin abusers is the same as in nonusers, i.e., 2 to 1. Interestingly, phenacetin is a compound which is also metabolized to an o-aminophenol (2-hydroxy-4 ethoxyaniline), similar to carcinogenically active industrial amines. It is of particular interest that the site of action is selective on the renal pelvis without involvement of ureter or bladder as in other chemically induced tumors of the urinary tract. The concomitant pyelonephritis and papillary necrosis that develop in phenacetin abusers may possibly indicate that the associated inflammation in the region of the renal pelvis predisposes this mucosa to cancer formation (Bengtsson et al.; Buch et al.).

There is also the previously mentioned strong association between tobacco use, including cigarettes, pipes, and cigars, with development of tumors of the urinary tract, including carcinomas of the bladder and renal parenchyma (Sarma; Bennington and Kradjian). Evidence also points to smoking as a predisposing factor in the development of carcinoma of the renal

pelvis (Bennington and Antonius; Wynder et al.).

The possibility that coffee drinking may be associated with carcinoma of the urinary tract has been suggested by Cole.

Clinical Features

The relative frequency of the various signs and symptoms arising from tumors of the renal pelvis are almost identical to those of the ureter (Table IX; Bloom et al.; Grabstald et al.; Grace et al.; Jönsson; Newman et al.). Hematuria is the most frequent sign in tumors of both sites, appearing in 80 percent of patients, and usually taking the form of gross hematuria. Pain, abdominal mass, and pyuria appear to occur as frequently in tumors of the renal pelvis as in those of the ureter, but dysuria and urinary frequency are reported more often in patients with ureteral tumors.

Table IX

CLINICAL SIGNS AND SYMPTOMS

	Renal Pelvic Tumors (Percent)	Ureteral Tumors (Percent)
Hematuria	80 (2)	80 (1)
Pain	24 (2)	40-50 (1, 3)
Frequency or Dysuria	10 (2)	52 (1)
Abdominal Mass	10 (2)	7 (1)
Pyuria	8 (4)	8 (4)

(1) Bloom, N. A. et al., 1970.
(2) Grabstald, H. et al., 1971.
(3) Jönsson, G., 1963.
(4) Newman, D. M. et al., 1967.

These figures are derived from several small studies in which benign as well as malignant tumors have been combined, including papillomas, intraepithelial carcinomas, and invasive carcinomas. That is, they are a composite of the symptomatic conditions of all epithelial tumors of the renal pelvis and ureter. Unfortunately, a breakdown of frequencies of symptoms by tumor types and stage is not available.

Papilloma, one of the earliest recognizable neoplastic lesions of the transitional epithelium, is capable of producing symptoms, but the percentage of symptomatic renal pelvic and ureteral papillomas is not known. Gross hematuria was the presenting sign in 7 of 9 patients (77 percent) with papillomas in a series of 52 ureteral tumors (Hawtrey). A correspondingly high rate of hematuria was found in 73 percent of a large series of patients with papillomas of the bladder (Greene et al.).

A neoplasm arising in the upper urinary tract that is large enough to produce a palpable abdominal mass is assuredly evidence of a far advanced tumor. It remains to be established whether pain, frequent urination, dysuria, and pyuria are sufficiently uncommon in papillomas to distinguish them from carcinomas clinically.

Nonspecific Findings

There are few reports of nonurologic systemic symptoms associated with tumors of the renal pelvis or ureter as compared with renal adenocarcinoma. We are aware of reports of one instance of unexplained hypercalcemia (Bourne et al.), one of secondary amyloidosis associated with transitional cell carcinoma of the renal pelvis (Clinicopathological Conference), and one of a male who had high levels of human chorionic gonadotropins associated with a primary pleomorphic carcinoma of the renal pelvis (Golde et al.). The physiologic basis for these systemic effects is not known.

Laboratory Findings

Urinary Cytologic Findings

The value of cytologic studies of the urine as an aid to the diagnosis of malignant tumors of the bladder is well established, with an average reported accuracy of nearly 72 percent and a false-positive rate ranging from 1.3 to 11.9 percent (Sarnacki et al.). Since cells of transitional cell carcinoma and squamous cell carcinoma are relatively resistant to degenerative changes, exfoliated cells from carcinomas of the upper urinary tract retain their characteristic cytologic features and are detected with an accuracy which approaches that of tumors of the bladder. In general, the cytologic features of the exfoliated cells reflect the extent of anaplasia of the tumor (fig. 196). Recently, Sarnacki and associates published their results from a cytologic study of 2400 urine specimens. Within the study, there were 22 patients with transitional cell carcinoma of the renal pelvis and 10 patients with transitional cell carcinoma of the ureter. Fifty-nine percent of the carcinomas in the renal pelvis and 70 percent of those in the ureter were detected cytologically. Factors contributing to false-negative cytologic diagnoses in carcinomas of the renal pelvis and ureter include: inadequate specimens, nonfunctioning kidneys, and obstructed ureters (Wagle et al.).

In cancers of the renal pelvis and ureter, urinary cytologic examination appears to be a valuable adjunct to the diagnosis of

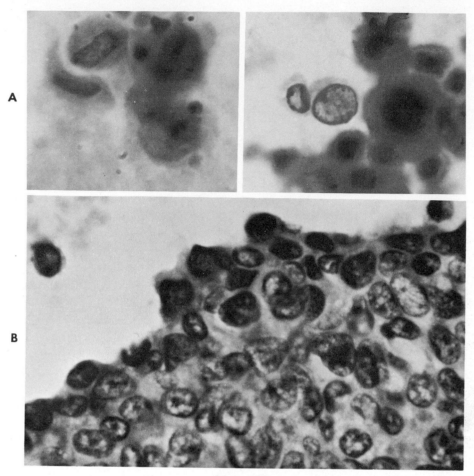

Figure 196
PAPILLARY TRANSITIONAL CELL CARCINOMA

A. These photomicrographs show exfoliated malignant cells from a papillary transitional cell carcinoma of the renal pelvis which were obtained from the patient's urine.

B. This histologic section demonstrates the similarity of individual cells in a carcinoma to those detected cytologically in the urine. X775. (Courtesy of Dr. P. N. Cowen, Leeds, England.)

symptomatic patients and should be regarded as an excellent screening technic in the asymptomatic, high risk patient.

Chemical Tests

A recent finding that serum levels of carcinoembryonic antigen, although not specific for this tumor, are elevated in patients with transitional cell carcinoma of the bladder raises the possibility that this test may be of some use in the diagnosis of transitional cell carcinomas of the renal pelvis and ureter (Hall et al.). Although there are numerous reports of elevated levels of lysosomal enzymes in the urine, as well as a variety of tryptophan metabolites in patients with urinary tract carcinomas, the results have not proved sufficiently specific to warrant their consideration as diagnostic procedures.

Radiographic Findings

Tumors of the ureter frequently obstruct the ureter, producing hydronephrosis or a nonfunctioning kidney. Therefore, excretory urography is frequently not sufficient to establish a diagnosis. Retrograde urography is much more likely to demonstrate the presence of a lesion and define its margin (fig. 197). The radiologic appearance of the filling defect produced by the tumor may be represented by a uniform narrowing of the ureteral lumen secondary to mural infiltration or it may be goblet-shaped due to the presence of a pedunculated tumor projecting into the lumen. Because filling defects caused by ureteral calculi, inflammatory strictures, and extrinsic tumors are often indistinguishable from neoplasms, the accuracy of radiologic diagnosis for tumors of the ureter does not exceed 50 percent.

On the other hand, tumors of the renal pelvis are usually diagnosed with the excretory urogram (figs. 198–200). In a series of 70 patients with renal pelvic tumors reported by Grabstald and associates, a total of 77 urograms were performed with one reported as negative, 17 as nondiagnostic, and the remainder as showing hydronephrosis and/or a filling defect, a mass, or a nonfunctioning kidney.

Scintigraphy

Scintigraphy may be useful in the demonstration of lesions obstructing the renal pelvis and ureter when radiographic procedures are nondiagnostic. Glomerular filtration rate agents, such as 99m technetium DTP, can generally produce diagnostic images in spite of severe obstruction and loss of renal function.

Pathologic Features

There are many classifications for tumors arising from the transitional epithelium of the urinary tract, the most complicated of which recognizes 22 histologic variants (Scott). To be useful, a classification must be simple, based on readily recognizable features, and convey meaningful information between the pathologist and the surgeon as well as other therapists. We believe the classification we use fulfills these requirements. It is readily augmented by the inclusion of information on histologic grade and stage of the tumor (Table X).

Table X

CLASSIFICATION OF RENAL PELVIC AND URETERAL EPITHELIAL TUMORS

Epithelial Tumors
  Benign
    Papilloma
  Malignant
    Transitional cell carcinoma
    Transitional cell carcinoma with differentiation
      Squamous differentiation
      Glandular differentiation
      Mixed squamous and glandular differentiation
    Squamous cell carcinoma
    Adenocarcinoma
    Undifferentiated carcinoma

Multicentricity

One important theme that runs through the discussion of all epithelial tumors of the urinary tract is that of multicentricity. This applies to papillomas (fig. 201) as well as carcinomas (figs. 202–204) involving the renal pelvis, ureter, and bladder.

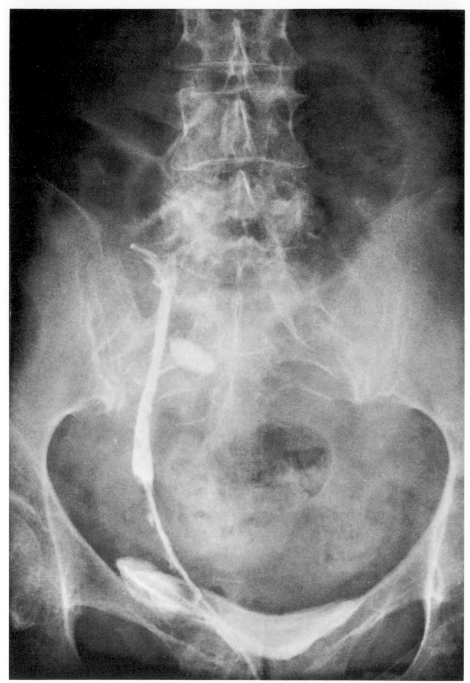

Figure 197
SQUAMOUS CELL CARCINOMA
(Figures 197 and 215 from same case)
This retrograde urogram illustrates abrupt narrowing in the midportion and proximal dilatation of the ureter produced by squamous cell carcinoma found in a 66 year old woman. The gross appearance of this tumor is seen in figure 215. (Courtesy of Dr. Bradford Young, San Francisco, Calif.)

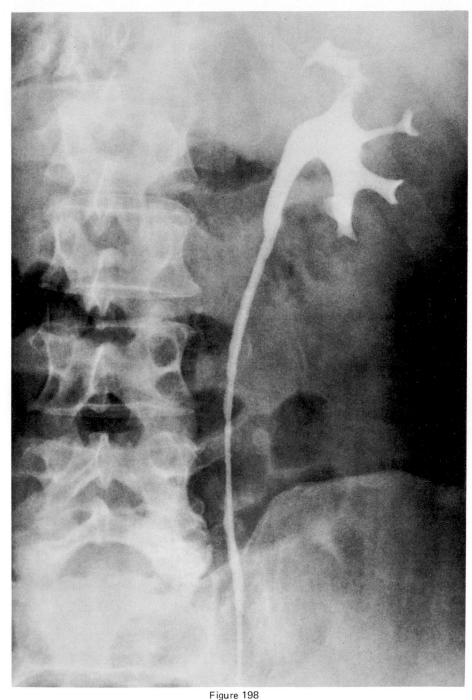

Figure 198
PAPILLARY TRANSITIONAL CELL CARCINOMA
(Figure 198 and Plate X-B from same case)
This retrograde urogram reveals distortion and a filling defect in the superior pole calix of a 57 year old man. The tumor was a papillary transitional cell carcinoma. The gross appearance is shown in plate X-B.

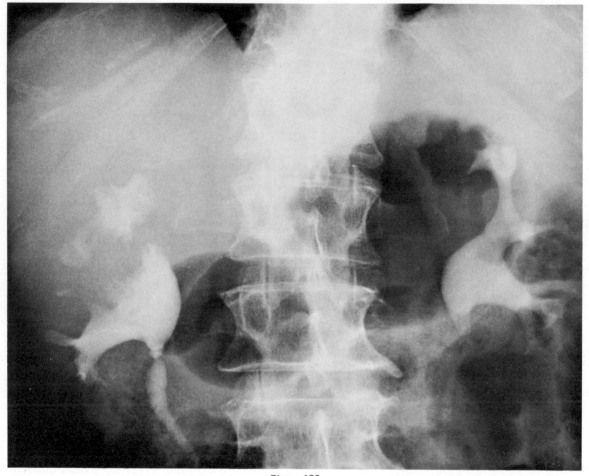

Figure 199
PAPILLARY TRANSITIONAL CELL CARCINOMA
An excretory urogram demonstrates a filling defect in the right pelvocaliceal area of a 57 year old man with a 2-year history of intermittent hematuria and chronic pyelonephritis. Because of the long duration of symptoms, xanthogranulomatous pyelonephritis was strongly suspected; however, the lesion proved to be a papillary transitional cell carcinoma.

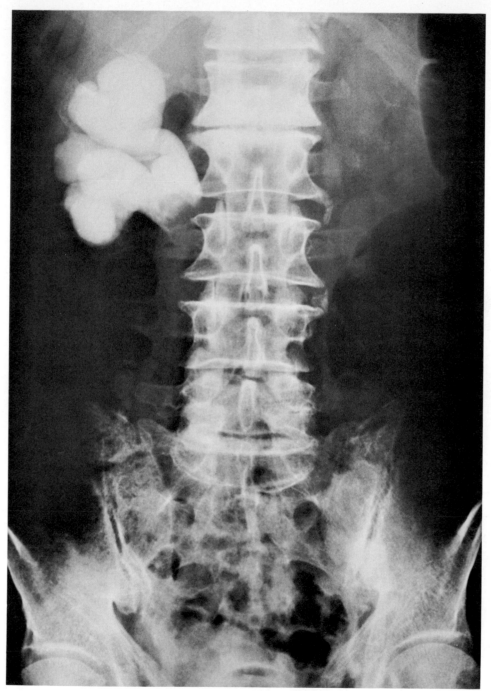

Figure 200
TRANSITIONAL CELL CARCINOMA

An excretory urogram of a 58 year old man shows the outline of a mass projecting into the renal pelvis. This transitional cell carcinoma of the ureteropelvic junction produced obstruction with dilatation of the renal pelvis. (Courtesy of Dr. Joachim Burhenne, San Francisco, Calif.)

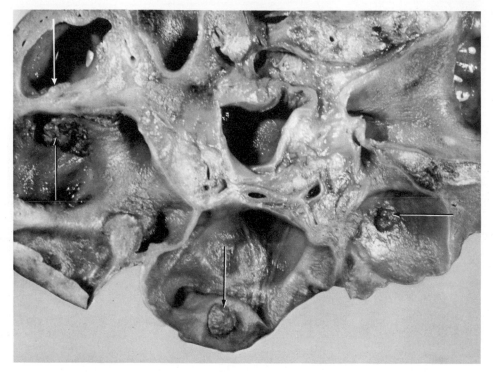

Figure 201
MULTIPLE PAPILLOMAS
Multiple papillomas (arrows) may be observed in the calices of a hydronephrotic kidney. (Fig. 149 from Lucke, B., and Schlumberger, H. G. Tumors of the Kidney, Renal Pelvis and Ureter. Fascicle 30, Atlas of Tumor Pathology, First Series. Washington: Armed Forces Institute of Pathology, 1957.)

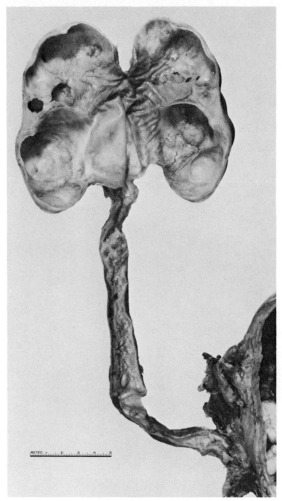

Figure 202

Figure 202
MULTIPLE CARCINOMAS
Multiple carcinomas of the urinary tract are shown involving the renal pelvis, ureter, and bladder. (Fig. IB from Wallace, D. M. Total cystectomy. An editorial overview. Cancer 32:1078-1083, 1973.)

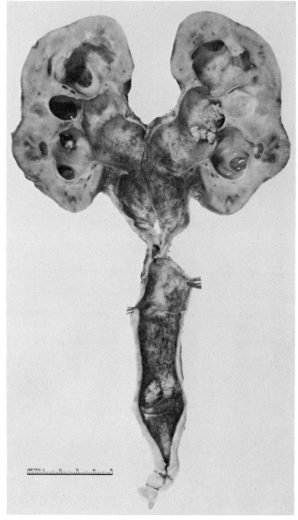

Figure 203
MULTIPLE CARCINOMAS
This right hydronephrosis and hydroureter are from a 44 year old man with multiple papillary transitional cell carcinomas of the calices and lower ureter, including the distal resected margin. The kidney showed chronic pyelonephritis. (Courtesy of Dr. Roger Pugh, London, England.)

Figure 203

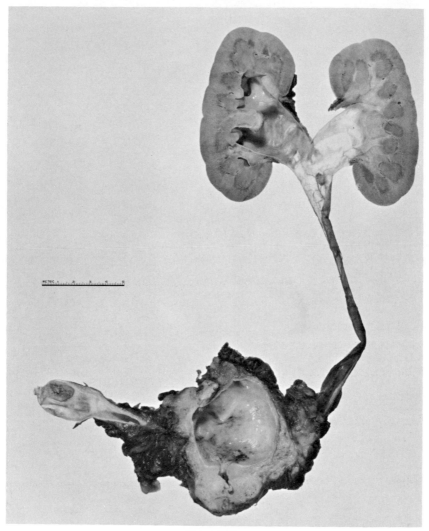

Figure 204
MULTIPLE CARCINOMAS
This nephrouretero cystectomy specimen illustrates cancer of the bladder and bilateral carcinomas of the ureter. The patient subsequently developed a carcinoma of the urethra four years later. (Fig. IC from Wallace, D. M. Total cystectomy. An editorial overview. Cancer 32:1078-1083, 1973.)

Grabstald and associates reviewed 70 patients with renal pelvic tumors. Thirteen of the tumors were papillomas, of which six (46 percent) were multiple papillomas. Three patients had bilateral renal pelvic papillomas, and five had papillomas in the ureters and/or bladder as well as in the renal pelvis.

More importantly, three of the six patients with multiple papillomas also had one or more carcinomas in the urinary tract. Two patients had in situ carcinomas of the bladder, one of which subsequently became invasive, and a third had a papillary carcinoma of the bladder as well as a focally invasive carcinoma of the ureter.

Whatever the biologic potential of the papilloma, whether located in the renal pelvis, ureter, or bladder, it appears to have an ominous portent. Nearly 25 percent of the patients who presented with a renal pelvic papilloma subsequently developed a carcinoma. Of those patients with multiple papillomas, 50 percent developed a carcinoma.

Among patients with carcinoma of the renal pelvis or the ureter, the frequency of multicentric carcinomas approached 50 percent (Grabstald et al.; Wagle et al.). Hvidt and Feldt-Rasmussen found that of those carcinomas apparently primary in the renal pelvis, 30 percent were multicentric, with simultaneous carcinomas present in the ureter in 26 percent of the patients and in the bladder in 4 percent. Of carcinomas apparently primary in the ureters, 40 percent were multicentric with simultaneous carcinomas in the renal pelvis in 32 percent; in the bladder, 2 percent; and at other sites in the ureter in 6 percent.

While the multicentric origin of renal pelvic, ureteral, and bladder carcinomas is well established, it is generally not appreciated that patients with carcinoma of the renal pelvis or ureter may have bilateral carcinomas, i.e., a second carcinoma of either the contralateral renal pelvis or ureter (fig. 204). The fact that there are relatively few reports of bilateral carcinomas has been advanced as evidence for the highly unlikely possibility that multiple tumors result from implantation metastases rather than that they represent multicentric independent primary carcinomas. On the contrary, a substantial number of bilateral carcinomas do occur which helps to substantiate the concept that multiple simultaneous tumors found in the urinary tract represent multicentric independent tumors. Grabstald and associates found that 3.5 percent of patients, and Wagle and associates found that 4 percent of patients with renal pelvic carcinoma had bilateral renal pelvic carcinomas; Sharma and associates reported 4 of 17 patients (23 percent), and Schade and associates, 2 of 13 patients (15 percent) with carcinoma in situ of the ureter had bilateral ureteral carcinomas; and Poole-Wilson found that 4 of 22 patients (18 percent) with upper urinary tract cancer had bilateral carcinomas.

Factors which weigh against the discovery of a contralateral carcinoma of the upper urinary tract are: (1) the relatively short overall survival of patients with carcinoma of the renal pelvis and ureter; (2) a reluctance to operate on patients developing a lesion or obstruction of the contralateral renal pelvis or ureter, presupposing the patient to have metastatic spread; and (3) inadequate examination of the contralateral renal pelvis and ureter at autopsy.

PAPILLOMA

SYNONYMS AND RELATED TERMS: Papillary carcinoma, grade I.

Transitional cell papillomas of the renal pelvis and ureter are histologically identical to those seen in the bladder. They are approximately three times as common in men as women and have rarely been reported in patients under the age of 50 (Grabstald et al.; Hawtrey). No data are available on a predilection for any particular areas of the renal pelvis or ureter.

Since tumors of the renal pelvis and ureter are relatively uncommon and papillomas account for no more than 16 to 18 percent of the total, pathologists infrequently encounter such papillomas (Bloom et al.; Grabstald et al.; Hawtrey; Meyer; Wagle et al.). In spite of the fact that papillomas of the renal pelvis and ureter are rare, they are important and of interest because of their uncertain biologic potential, their association with carcinomas elsewhere in the urinary tract, and their histologic similarity to well differentiated papillary transitional cell carcinomas.

The malignant potential of papillomas is much discussed. Many authors feel that papillomas represent a nonmalignant neoplastic proliferation of transitional epithelial cells, of interest primarily because of their association with independent carcinomas in the renal pelvis, ureter, or bladder. Others have taken a dimmer view of the "papilloma," regarding it as an already malignant tumor, and use the term "papilloma" synonymously with low grade papillary transitional cell carcinoma (Hawtrey).

This issue may remain undecided for some time, since papillomas are part of the constellation of multicentric neoplastic changes which are so characteristic of transitional epithelium of the urinary tract. As a result, it is usually difficult or impossible for the pathologist to determine whether the appearance of a carcinoma subsequent to a papilloma represents a recurrence or a new primary tumor (Greene et al.). The only hope of resolving this question requires the use of strict criteria for the diagnosis of papillomas.

Pathologic Features

We use the following criteria for classifying a papilloma. The papilloma is composed of long, delicate, villous cylindrical processes which represent prolongations of the transitional epithelium, each carrying with it a fibrovascular core of lamina propria. Cut longitudinally, the sides of each villous process are parallel from base to tip. The covering transitional epithelium ranges from 5 to 10 cells thick and is indistinguishable from normal transitional epithelium in its maturation pattern, size, and shape of cells and their nuclei, and the number of mitoses (fig. 205). Loss of a normal polarity, disruption of the normal maturation pattern, pleomorphism, or increase in the frequency of mitoses are regarded as indicative of papillary carcinoma.

The typical papilloma, as described above, arises from a narrow base and is usually only a few millimeters in diameter, although it may extend laterally, or multiple foci may coalesce to form a tumor up to several centimeters in diameter. It usually draws attention to itself by hemorrhage from a damaged villous tip, but is also capable of producing obstruction, hydronephrosis, and infection if located in the ureter or ureteropelvic junction (figs. 201, 206).

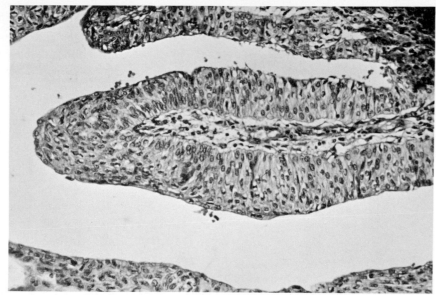

Figure 205
PAPILLOMA

This papilloma resembles a prolongation of normal transitional epithelium with a fibrovascular core. The sides are parallel for the full length of the papilloma. The epithelium is approximately eight cells thick and shows normal maturation with no atypia. X160.

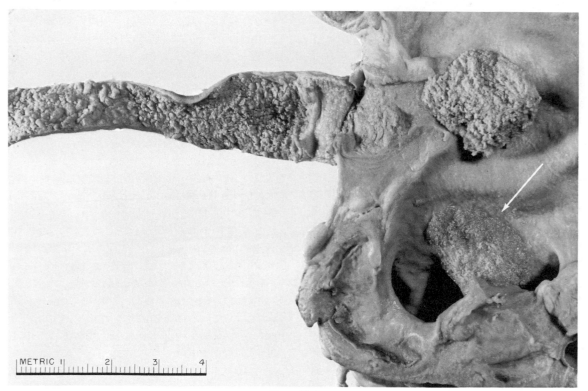

Figure 206
TRANSITIONAL CELL CARCINOMA

This transitional cell carcinoma of the ureteropelvic junction produced obstruction and hydronephrosis. Multiple papillomas are present in the ureter distal to the obstruction. (Fig. 153 from Lucke, B., and Schlumberger, H. G. Tumors of the Kidney, Renal Pelvis and Ureter. Fascicle 30, Atlas of Tumor Pathology, First Series. Washington: Armed Forces Institute of Pathology, 1957.)

In the final analysis, it may be that "papillomas" are indeed carcinomas merely clad in a benign disguise. However, before accepting this conclusion, it seems well worth the effort to make every use of the histologic features which generally serve to distinguish benign from malignant neoplasms to classify papillary tumors of the transitional epithelium for correlation with their biologic behavior.

CARCINOMA

SYNONYMS AND RELATED TERMS: **Transitional cell carcinoma**; papillary carcinoma; papillary carcinoma with invasion; urothelial carcinoma; squamous cell carcinoma; adenocarcinoma.

Pathologic Features

Cell Type

The histologic types of renal pelvic and ureteral carcinoma reflect the capacity of transitional epithelium to differentiate into malignant squamous and glandular epithelium as well as to undergo benign squamous and glandular metaplasia (see p. 243). Reports of the relative frequency of the various histologic types of carcinoma found in the renal pelvis and ureter are usually in the range of 91 to 92 percent transitional cell, 8 percent squamous cell, and less than 1 percent adenocarcinoma and undifferentiated carcinoma (Bloom et al.; Grabstald et al.). However, these estimates of the frequency of squamous cell carcinoma and adenocarcinoma are undoubtedly high since transitional cell carcinomas with foci of squamous change are frequently mistaken for squamous cell carcinoma, and those with glandular change for adenocarcinoma.

Squamous change occurs in over 20 percent of transitional cell carcinomas of the upper urinary tract, a figure which corresponds with the 18 to 20 percent found in invasive transitional cell carcinomas of the bladder (Pugh, 1959). Estimates of the frequency of squamous cell carcinoma from routine pathologic examination of cancers of the bladder run as high as 6 to 7 percent. However, in studies in which transitional cell carcinomas with foci of squamous change were not diagnosed as squamous cell carcinoma, only 1 to 1.6 percent were found to be squamous cell carcinomas (Pugh, 1973). It is likely that focal metaplastic squamous changes are being confused with pure squamous cell carcinoma in tumors of the upper urinary tract as well as those of the bladder, and that the frequency of squamous cell carcinoma is comparably low in both the renal pelvis and the ureter.

Transitional cell carcinomas with foci of squamous change (fig. 207) should be designated as transitional cell carcinoma with squamous metaplasia, reserving the term squamous cell carcinoma for those carcinomas showing an epidermoid pattern throughout. The distinction is important if valid comparisons of the intrinsic biologic behavior of transitional and squamous cell carcinomas are to be made.

Metaplastic squamous change usually occurs in transitional cell carcinomas of the bladder which have become invasive (Pugh, 1959). We have observed the same features in transitional cell carcinomas of the renal pelvis and ureter. Unfortunately, keratinization has been regarded as a hallmark of a malignant tumor; that is, the tumor invades because it is keratinizing rather than that keratinization occurs subsequent to invasion (Grabstald et al.).

There is some indication that, in the bladder, squamous cell carcinomas offer a better prognosis than transitional cell carcinomas of comparable stage. Among tumors

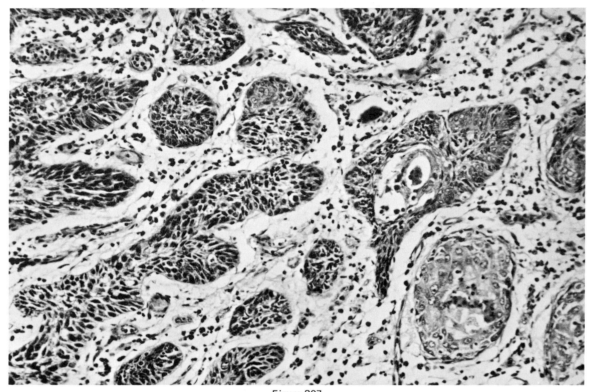

Figure 207
TRANSITIONAL CELL CARCINOMA
A transitional cell carcinoma of the ureter shows focal areas of keratinization in individual cells as well as keratin pearl formation in areas of stromal invasion. X185.

of the bladder, well differentiated squamous cell carcinomas grow more slowly and metastasize later to the regional lymph nodes than transitional cell carcinomas with squamous metaplasia (Pugh, 1959). However, the results of one study suggest that while less frequently multifocal in the ureter, bladder, and urethra, and less frequently metastatic to lymph nodes, squamous cell carcinomas of the renal pelvis more frequently invade peripelvic structures than transitional cell carcinomas arising in that area (Rafla).

Invasive transitional cell carcinomas may also be accompanied by tubular or glandular metaplasia complete with mucus production (fig. 208; pl. X-D). Glandular meta-

plasia which may occur alone, or in combination with squamous metaplasia, was reported by Meyer in 24 percent of transitional cell carcinomas of the ureter, and is also seen in the renal pelvis (fig. 209). The presence of glandular metaplasia can lead the unwary into making a diagnosis of adenocarcinoma. These tumors with focal glandular change should be diagnosed as transitional cell carcinomas with glandular metaplasia. The term adenocarcinoma should be used exclusively for those tumors which are predominantly glandular.

In addition to these three cell types, i.e., transitional, squamous, and glandular, there is a fourth type occasionally encountered

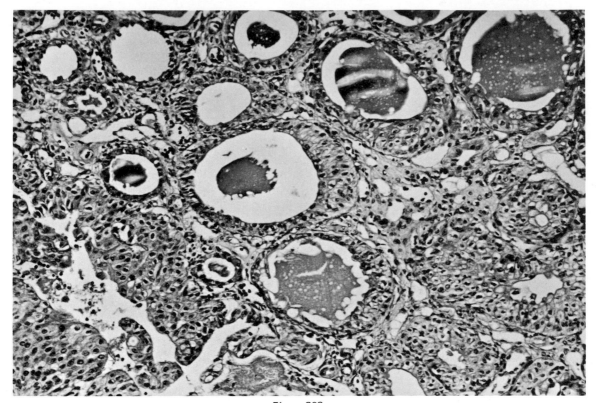

Figure 208
TRANSITIONAL CELL CARCINOMA
This transitional cell carcinoma of the renal pelvis exhibits multiple foci of tubular change. The cells lining the tubular structures are undergoing metaplastic differentiation into columnar mucosecretory cells. X185.

in carcinomas of the renal pelvis, ureter, and bladder. For this fourth cell type which shows no evidence of transitional, squamous, or glandular differentiation, Mostofi (1968) has proposed the term "undifferentiated cell." It should be emphasized that the term undifferentiated implies only a lack of maturation toward a recognizable cell type and carries no connotation of anaplasia, although undifferentiated tumors are frequently markedly anaplastic.

The authors follow the World Health Organization classification for epithelial carcinomas of the upper urinary tract which is based on these four cell types. Using this classification, the possible histologic diagnoses are: transitional cell carcinoma; transitional cell carcinoma with squamous or glandular change, or both; squamous cell carcinoma; adenocarcinoma; and undifferentiated carcinoma. The degree of anaplasia, pattern of growth, and extent of invasion are recorded independently of the histologic type as an adjunct to the diagnosis.

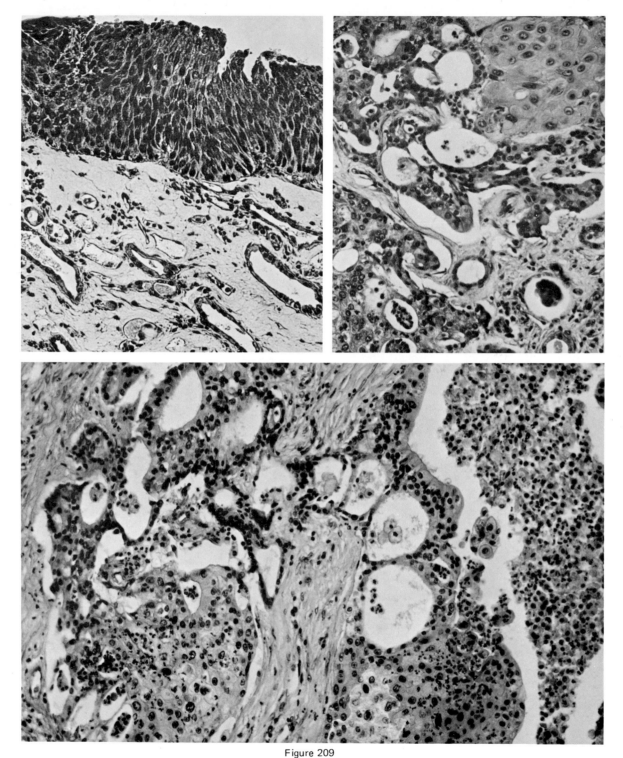

Figure 209
TRANSITIONAL CELL CARCINOMA
WITH GLANDULAR AND SQUAMOUS COMPONENTS
A composite carcinoma of the renal pelvis was found in a 75 year old man. In addition to transitional cell carcinoma, there are glandular and squamous components scattered throughout the tumor. X185. (Figs. I, 2A, and 2B from Kohout, N. D., and Goldman, R. L. An unusual composite carcinoma of the renal pelvis. J. Urol. 109:567-568, 1973.)

Growth Pattern

Carcinomas arising in the renal pelvis and ureter fall into one of four distinct growth patterns. They are (1) planar (non-papillary) and intraepithelial (figs. 210, 211); (2) papillary and intraepithelial (fig. 212); (3) papillary and infiltrating (fig. 213); and (4) planar and infiltrating (fig. 214).

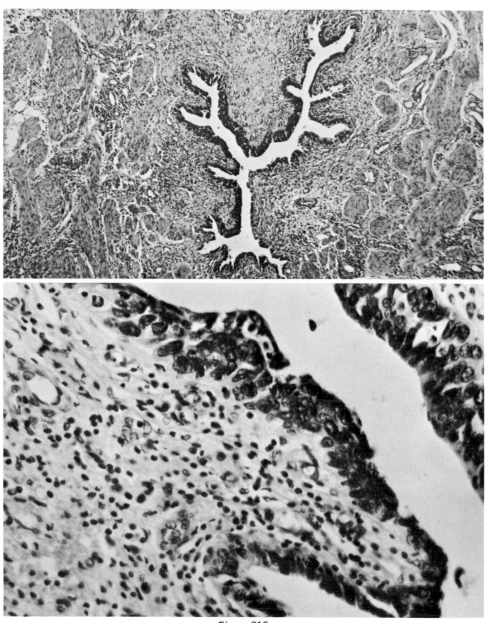

Figure 210
IN SITU CARCINOMA
This in situ carcinoma of the ureter shows no evidence of papillary proliferation. The number of cell layers is not increased, but there is marked nuclear pleomorphism, hyperchromasia, and cellular disorganization. Upper, X45; lower, X310.

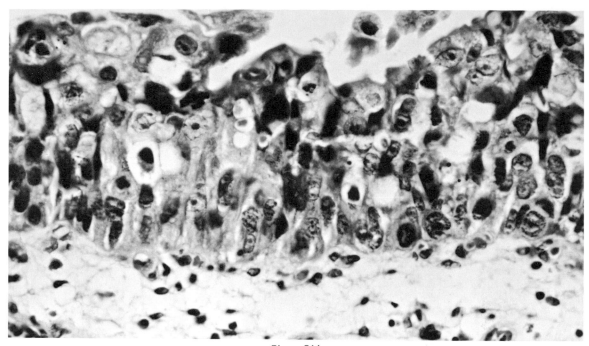

Figure 211
IN SITU TRANSITIONAL CELL CARCINOMA
This nonpapillary in situ transitional cell carcinoma of the renal pelvis shows marked disorganization of the maturation pattern as well as an increased number of mitoses and many bizarre hyperchromatic, pleomorphic cells. X550.

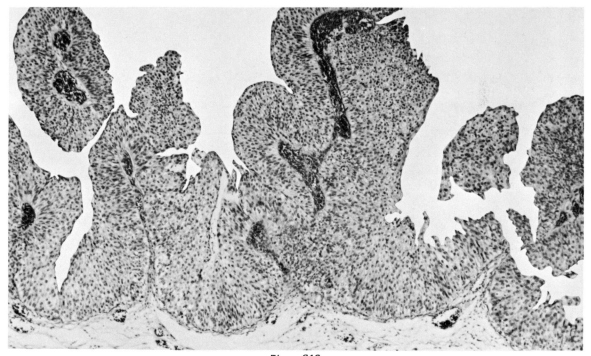

Figure 212
PAPILLARY TRANSITIONAL CELL CARCINOMA
The papillary transitional cell carcinoma of the renal pelvis illustrated here does not exhibit any evidence of invasion in the underlying stroma. X95.

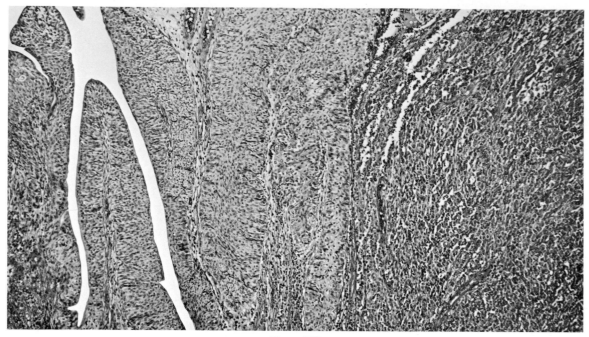

Figure 213

PAPILLARY TRANSITIONAL CELL CARCINOMA

At the surface, this papillary transitional cell carcinoma is Grade I to II. In the underlying invasive portion on the right, the carcinoma is anaplastic and not recognized as transitional cell in origin. X72.

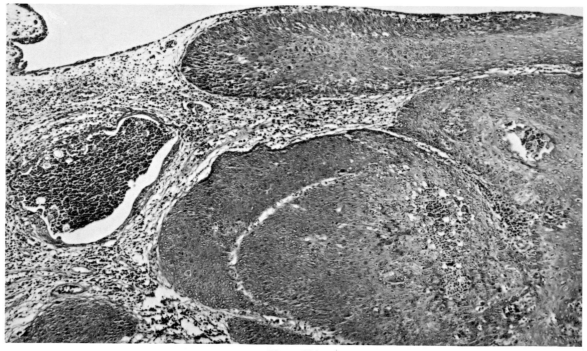

Figure 214

SQUAMOUS CELL CARCINOMA

This nonpapillary squamous cell carcinoma of the ureter shows extensive intramural invasion. X112.

It is our impression that the growth pattern is largely a function of the cell type of the carcinoma and its degree of anaplasia. The mechanisms involved are not understood, but, in general, low grade transitional carcinomas are more likely to be intraepithelial, either papillary or planar, than high grade transitional cell carcinomas, and transitional cell carcinomas of all grades are more likely to be papillary than squamous, undifferentiated, or adenocarcinomas.

The description of the growth pattern must be included as part of the histologic diagnosis to provide the surgeon or radiotherapist with the maximum amount of information on the likely behavior of the tumor and the patient's prognosis. This is discussed further in the section on tumor staging on page 309.

Gross Features

Nonpapillary, noninfiltrating carcinomas of the renal pelvis and ureter are asymptomatic and, therefore, rarely seen by the pathologist. From the observations of intraepithelial nonpapillary foci of carcinoma at the margins of more typical papillary transitional cell carcinomas, we know that nonpapillary intraepithelial cancers may show no gross change or only minimal changes, including slight thickening, roughening, and hyperemia or hemorrhage of affected mucosa (fig. 215).

Papillary transitional cell carcinomas, which represent the vast majority of transitional cell carcinomas (85 percent), are usually soft, bulky, tan-pink, translucent, and glistening (pl. X-B); they may have an arborescent, occasionally lobular surface which is formed by a myriad of delicate filiform projections of the neoplastic epithelium (figs. 216, 217). They are usually sessile (pl. X-B; fig. 218), but are occasionally pedunculated (fig. 219). They occur with equal frequency on the right and left in the renal pelvis and ureters. While these carcinomas may arise anyplace in the renal pelvis, they are more likely to be discovered while relatively small when they cause obstruction by their location in the calix or near the ureteropelvic junction (pl. X-C). Tumors which, because of their location, do not produce obstruction may grow quite large and even fill the entire renal pelvis before they are discovered (figs. 220, 221). Large carcinomas, particularly those which are invasive, are often focally hemorrhagic and associated with underlying fibrosis, supervening infection, and hydronephrosis which modifies the tumor and the surrounding mucosa. Transitional cell carcinomas occur most commonly in the lower third of the ureter (74 percent) (figs. 202, 203, 215, 222; Abeshouse). Because intraluminal proliferation quickly fills the lumen of the ureter, these tumors are frequently associated with hydroureter and hydronephrosis (figs. 202, 203, 222; pl. XI-A). The predilection of these tumors for the distal ureter and their multicentricity explain the relatively frequent recurrence in the ureteral stump after partial ureterectomy for a carcinoma arising higher in the ureter or renal pelvis, and are the basis for complete nephroureterectomy and removal of a cuff of bladder for transitional cell carcinoma of the renal pelvis or ureter (Abeshouse; Bloom et al.; Kimball and Ferris; Newman et al.).

Squamous cell carcinomas and **undifferentiated carcinomas** tend to be solid and extensive, flat, slightly raised or rounded rather than papillary, and are often ulcerated (fig. 215). Invasion of the underlying structures accompanying fibrosis and

PLATE X

ANAPLASTIC TRANSITIONAL CELL CARCINOMA
(Plate X-A and Figure 232 from same case)

A. This is a poorly vascular tumor of the kidney from a 76 year old woman. The cut surface is gray, and there is no evidence of necrosis or hemorrhage. The margins are irregular; the pelvis is obliterated and the renal capsule involved.

PAPILLARY TRANSITIONAL CELL CARCINOMA
(Plate X-B and Figure 198 from same case)

B. This papillary transitional cell carcinoma of the renal calix is sessile, tan-pink, and soft; it is composed of small, blunted villous projections. The tumor is demonstrated radiographically in figure 198.

TRANSITIONAL CELL CARCINOMA

C. This pedunculated transitional cell carcinoma of the ureteropelvic junction produced intermittent obstruction.

TRANSITIONAL CELL CARCINOMA

D. This is a grade I transitional cell carcinoma of the renal pelvis, with extensive glandular metaplasia. Intracellular and intraluminal mucus is demonstrated by the mucicarmine stain. X115. (Courtesy of the Armed Forces Institute of Pathology, Washington, D. C.)

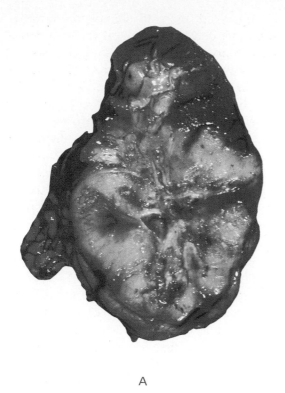

A

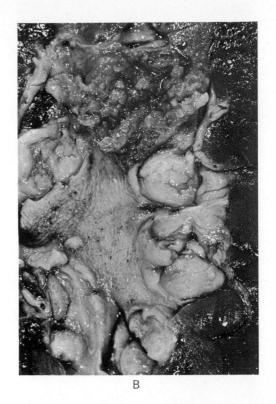

B

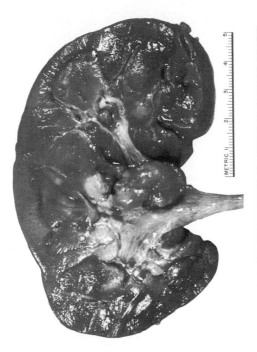

C

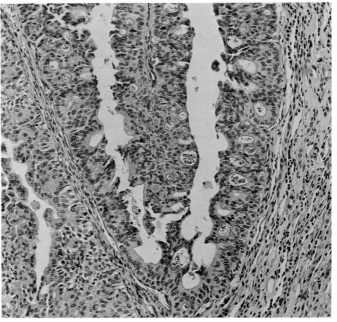

D

PLATE X

275

inflammation contribute to the tendency of these tumors to be firm and fixed. There are no reports of any predilection for the right or left or a particular location in the renal pelvis or ureter.

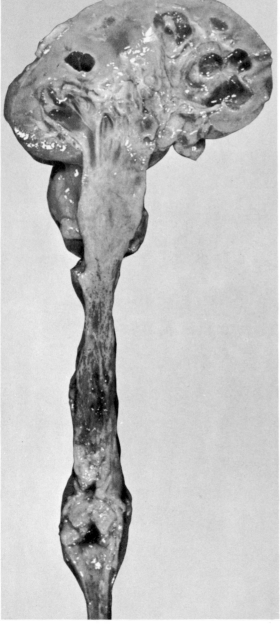

Figure 215

Since less than 35 adenocarcinomas of the renal pelvis and none of the ureter have been reported, there are few gross descriptions of upper urinary tract adenocarcinomas (Quattlebaum and Shirley; Ragins and Rolnick; Aufderheide and Streitz). In general, they appear to conform to the gross appearance of colonic adenocarcinomas. The usual description is that of a heaped up nodular mass of glistening mucoid tumor, apparently arising from the mucosa, which may obstruct the renal pelvis or ureter, producing hydronephrosis and pyelonephritis (fig. 247). We have personally seen two instances of adenocarcinoma of the ureter (figs. 244—246).

Features of particular interest are the relatively higher frequency of calculi, squamous metaplasia, and longstanding pyelonephritis associated with squamous cell carcinomas and adenocarcinomas compared to transitional cell carcinomas of the upper urinary tract. The suggestion that the presence of calculus and accompanying inflammation plays a role in the genesis of these two types of carcinoma has not been substantiated.

Figure 215
SQUAMOUS CELL CARCINOMA
(Figures 197 and 215 from same case)
This squamous cell carcinoma of the ureter is demonstrated radiographically in figure 197. The tumor was firm, with slightly rolled edges and an ulcerated center. Proximally, the ureter is roughened, hyperemic, and focally hemorrhagic for a distance of several centimeters over an area which proved to be carcinoma in situ. (Courtesy of Dr. Bradford Young, San Francisco, Calif.)

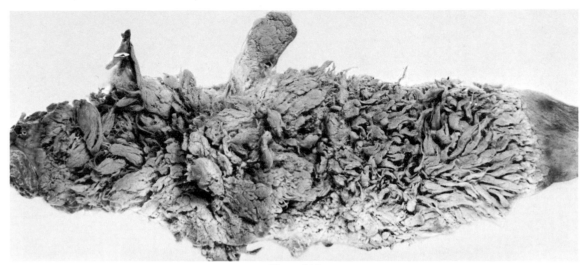

Figure 216
PAPILLARY TRANSITIONAL CELL CARCINOMA
(Figures 216 and 217 from same case)
This papillary transitional cell carcinoma of the ureter, removed from a 60 year old man, is composed predominantly of elongated filiform projections. Similar tumors were present in the bladder. (Fig. 170 from Lucke, B. and Schlumberger, H. G. Tumors of the Kidney, Renal Pelvis and Ureter. Fascicle 30, Atlas of Tumor Pathology, First Series. Washington: Armed Forces Institute of Pathology, 1957.)

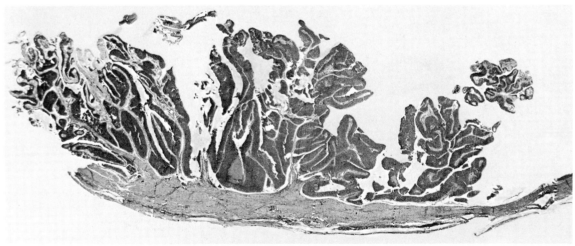

Figure 217
PAPILLARY TRANSITIONAL CELL CARCINOMA
(Figures 216 and 217 from same case)
This is a longitudinal section of the papillary transitional cell carcinoma shown in figure 216. In spite of the extensive involvement of the ureter, there is no evidence of stromal invasion. (Fig. 171 from Lucke, B. and Schlumberger, H. G. Tumors of the Kidney, Renal Pelvis and Ureter. Fascicle 30, Atlas of Tumor Pathology, First Series. Washington: Armed Forces Institute of Pathology, 1957.)

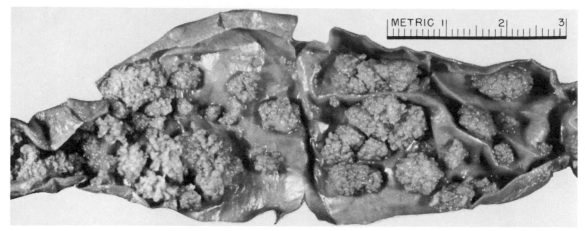

Figure 218
TRANSITIONAL CELL CARCINOMA

This transitional cell carcinoma of the ureter is characterized by multiple discrete mulberry-like masses of tumor. Similar tumors were subsequently removed from the bladder five months later. (Fig. 172 from Lucke, B. and Schlumberger, H. G. Tumors of the Kidney, Renal Pelvis and Ureter. Fascicle 30, Atlas of Tumor Pathology, First Series. Washington: Armed Forces Institute of Pathology, 1957.)

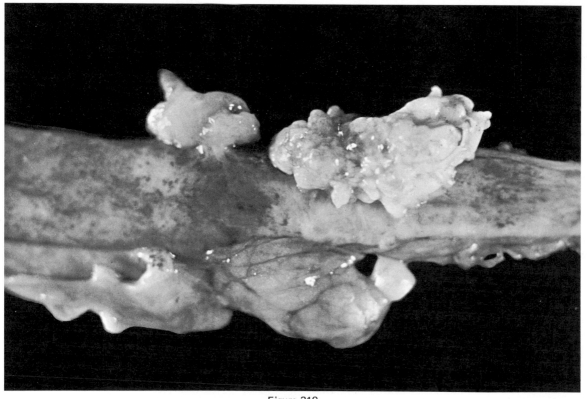

Figure 219
TRANSITIONAL CELL CARCINOMA

Illustrated is a transitional cell carcinoma of the ureter, forming two pedunculated intraluminal masses, each supported by short slender stalks.

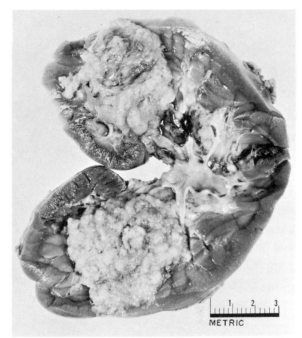

Figure 220
PAPILLARY TRANSITIONAL CELL CARCINOMA
This demonstrates a papillary transitional cell
rcinoma filling the calices and a major portion of the
nal pelvis. (Courtesy of the Armed Forces Institute of
athology, Washington, D. C.)

Figure 220

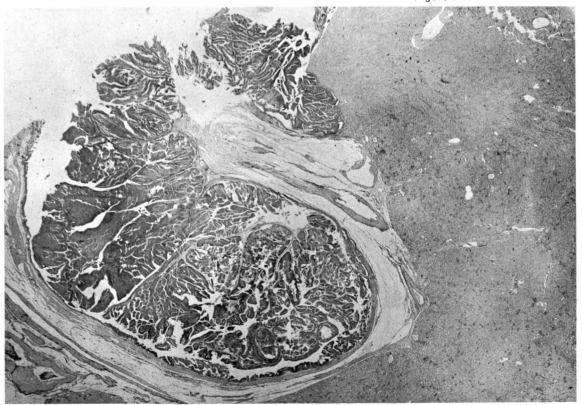

Figure 221
PAPILLARY TRANSITIONAL CELL CARCINOMA
This papillary transitional cell carcinoma occupied much of the renal pelvis, but in spite of the extensive involvement, there was no evidence of invasion. X4. (Courtesy of Dr. P. N. Cowen, Leeds, England.)

279

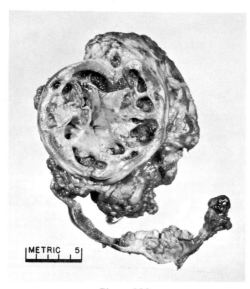

Figure 222
PAPILLARY CARCINOMA
This nephroureterectomy specimen demonstrates a papillary carcinoma located in the lower third of the ureter, which obstructed the lumen and produced hydro-ureter and hydronephrosis. (Courtesy of the Armed Forces Institute of Pathology, Washington, D. C.)

Histologic Features

The noninfiltrating **transitional cell carcinomas** may be either papillary (figs. 212, 223) or nonpapillary (figs. 210, 211). It is tempting to think of the nonpapillary carcinomas as precursors of the papillary carcinoma, but this has not been documented. On the contrary, the intraepithelial transitional cell carcinoma frequently shows no increase in the number of cell layers and is conspicuous only by its marked cellular atypia, hyperchromatism, and substantial number of mitoses—features which are not found in early or low grade papillary carcinomas. We have observed nonpapillary intraepithelial changes at the margins of invasive squamous cell carcinomas which raise the possibility that the nonpapillary intra-epithelial carcinoma may be an early stage in the evolution of the squamous cell carcinoma.

Intraepithelial nonpapillary changes in the transitional mucosa of a different type are often seen adjacent to papillary transitional cell carcinomas. However, these changes are primarily those of an increased number of cell layers and mild atypism, as seen in the frankly papillary portions of transitional cell carcinomas.

Papillary carcinomas tend to be larger than papillomas, with thicker villi and broader bases. They are further distinguished from papillomas by their less orderly pattern of growth, including irregular stratification, and some loss of polarity and maturation (figs. 223, 224). The parallel orientation of the overlying epithelium to the accompanying fibrovascular core along the long axis of each villous process is not well maintained, and the papillary pattern may be obscured by coalescence of adjacent villi and diminution of the fibrovascular core by compression (fig. 225). Occasionally, the papillary proliferation is inverted rather than projecting into the lumen of the renal pelvis or ureter (fig. 226).

More anaplastic forms of transitional cell carcinoma show an increase in cytologic atypia (figs. 227, 228) and, occasionally, spindle cell change (fig. 229), which causes such tumors to be confused with sarcomas or sarcomatoid renal adenocarcinomas. Sarcomatoid changes have been observed in transitional cell carcinomas (fig. 230), but whether they represent an expression of further differentiation in the tumor cells or an induction by the tumor of sarcomatous change in the stroma has not been determined (Evans).

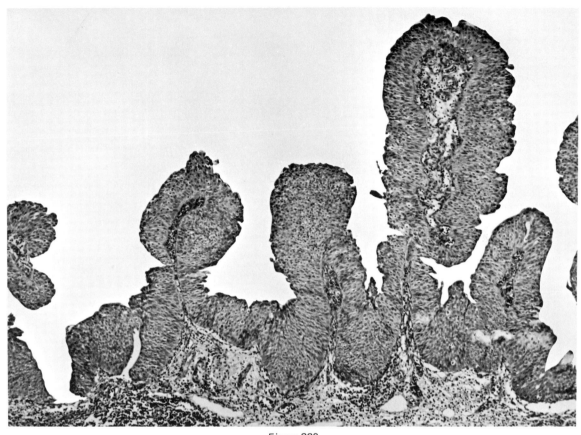

Figure 223
PAPILLARY TRANSITIONAL CELL CARCINOMA
The papillary projections of this carcinoma of the renal pelvis have irregular contours with correspondingly irregular fibrovascular cores. The epithelium varies in thickness from 15 to 20 cells. The maturation pattern is disorganized. X72.

Figure 224

TRANSITIONAL CELL CARCINOMA, GRADE I

There is minimal histologic deviation from normal transitional epithelium in this transitional cell carcinoma, grade I. Tumors of this grade are characterized by an increased number of cell layers, slight irregularity of cell stratification, and loss of normal polarity and maturation. Mitotic figures are more numerous than in normal transitional epithelium. X460.

Figure 225

PAPILLARY TRANSITIONAL CELL CARCINOMA

This papillary transitional cell carcinoma of the renal pelvis shows no evidence of invasion. Extensive crowding of papillary processes has caused a loss of the usual delicate villous pattern, and compression of the fibrovascular stroma. X8.

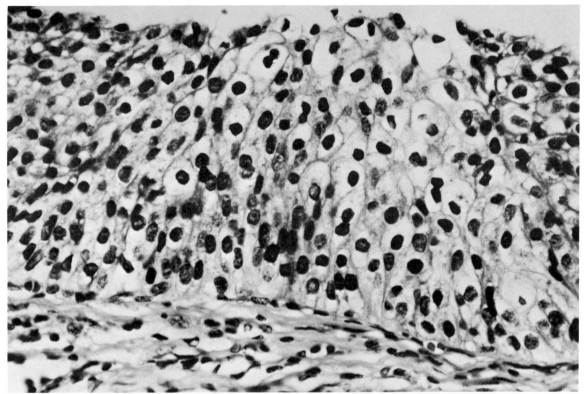

Figure 224

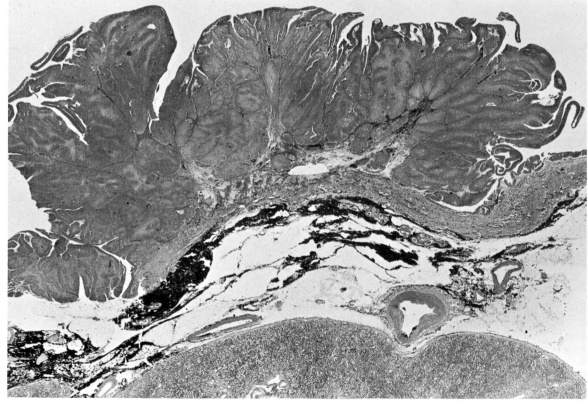

Figure 225

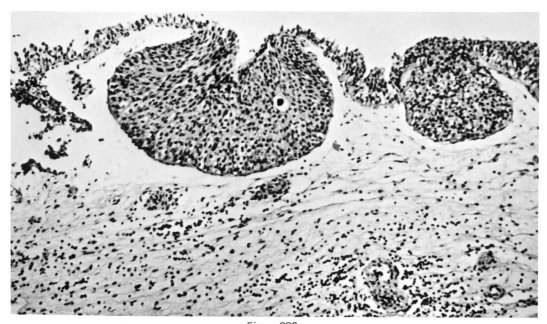

Figure 226
TRANSITIONAL CELL CARCINOMA, GRADE I
This transitional cell carcinoma, grade I of the renal pelvis forms a papillary projection inverted into the lamina propria. X120.

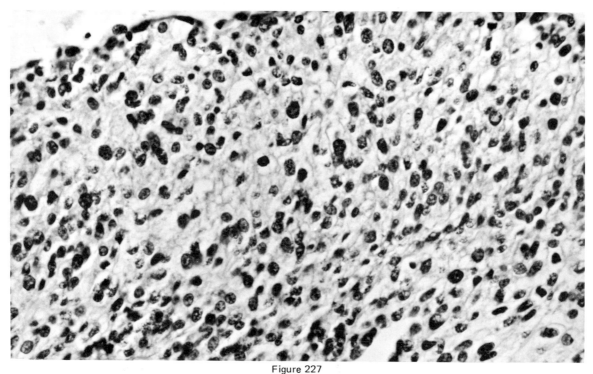

Figure 227
TRANSITIONAL CELL CARCINOMA, GRADE II
In this tumor, the anaplasia, i.e., cellular pleomorphism and disorganization, is intermediate between that of grade I and grade III transitional cell carcinomas. X460.

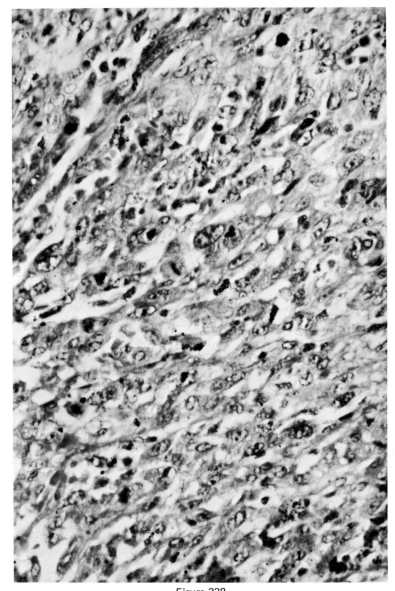

Figure 228
TRANSITIONAL CELL CARCINOMA, GRADE III
The tumor is markedly anaplastic, but still recognizable as a transitional cell carcinoma. Organization is haphazard and individual cells show marked variation in size, shape, and staining characteristics. X460.

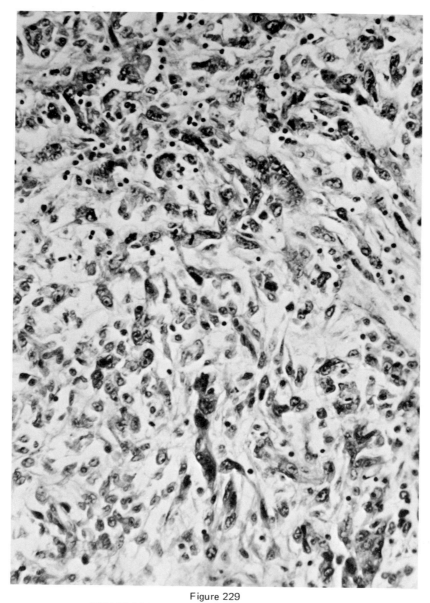

Figure 229
TRANSITIONAL CELL CARCINOMA, GRADE III
The majority of cells in this carcinoma are spindle shaped. The tumor is anaplastic, but still recognizable as transitional cell in origin. X268.

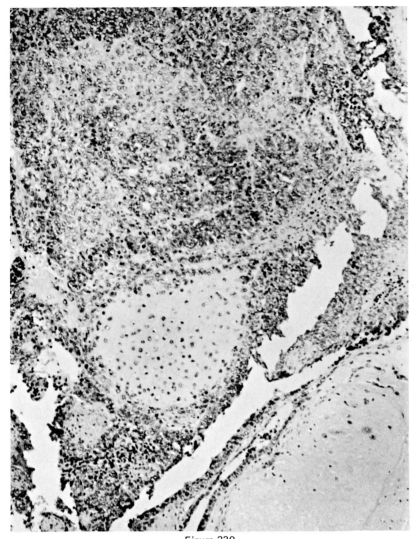

Figure 230
TRANSITIONAL CELL CARCINOMA, GRADE III
This transitional cell carcinoma of the renal pelvis shows chondromatous sarcomatoid change in multiple areas of the tumor. X120.

It must be kept in mind that simultaneous renal parenchymal adenocarcinomas and renal pelvic transitional cell carcinomas do occur in the same kidney, although rarely (Gillis et al.; Graham and Vynalek; Richardson and Woodburn; Walker and Jordan; Wagle et al.). When both the renal pelvis and renal parenchyma are involved, it may be impossible to tell whether there are one or two primary tumors (fig. 231). Both renal adenocarcinoma and renal pelvic transitional cell carcinoma can be sarcomatoid and sufficiently anaplastic to obscure their true origin (pl. X-A; fig. 232). Furthermore, transitional cell carcinomas may undergo clear cell change which mimics histologically, but not histo-chemically, clear cell renal adenocarcinoma (fig. 233).

The electron microscopic features of the normal transitional epithelium of the renal pelvis and ureter (p. 13) are also seen in the well differentiated transitional cell carcinoma; i.e., attachment of basal cells to the basement membrane is by hemidesmosomes, connection of lateral cell surfaces by discrete attachments (maculae adherentes), and of luminal cells by circumferential watertight junctions (zonulae occludens), intracellular tonofilaments, and lateral intracellular spaces (lateral cisternae) formed by infoldings of the lateral cell membranes (figs. 234, 235).

While the ultrastructural features of

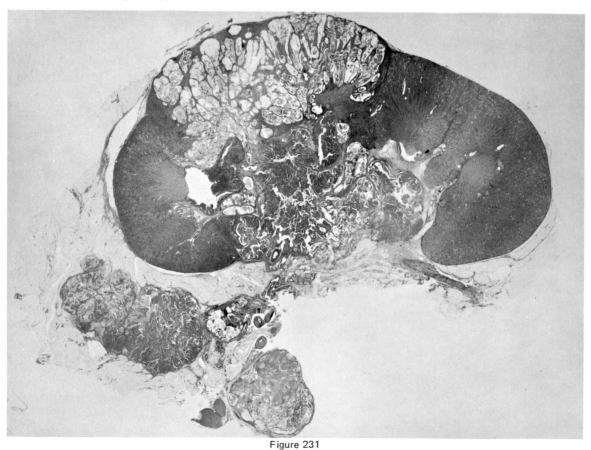

Figure 231

TRANSITIONAL CELL CARCINOMA WITH METASTASES

This whole mount of a kidney and regional lymph nodes demonstrates extensive involvement of the renal pelvis, renal parenchyma, and metastases to the adjacent lymph nodes from a transitional cell carcinoma arising in the renal pelvis. (Courtesy of Dr. Carlos Perez-Mesa, Columbia, Mo.)

carcinomas arising in the epithelium of the urinary tract have not been extensively studied, it appears, in general, that ultrastructural features of normal transitional epithelium persist in the well differentiated grades of transitional cell carcinoma. No changes are seen to indicate that the epithelium is malignant. In less well differentiated transitional cell carcinomas, nuclear pleomorphism and mitotic figures are seen, while the characteristic lateral cisternae are reduced in number or lost completely, presumably a function of anaplasia. In the undifferentiated carcinomas arising in the renal pelvis or ureter which we have examined electron microscopically, we have been unable to find any distinguishing features to indicate the cell of origin of the carcinoma.

Invasion is not always easy to recognize, especially in well differentiated papillary transitional cell carcinomas. Frequently in these tumors, there is a submucosal infiltrate of lymphocytes and plasma cells, often complete with well formed germinal centers (fig. 236). This inflammation is not indicative of invasion, but may obscure the interface between the epithelium and lamina propria, making it difficult to determine whether or not invasion is present. Many well oriented, thin, and adequately stained sections are essential for the proper evaluation of invasion in apparently noninvasive carcinomas. When invasion is piecemeal in the form of small cords, nests, or even individual cells (fig. 237), a form referred to by Mostofi (1968) as tentacular, the prognosis is more ominous but the presence of invasion is easily recognized. When the tumor invades en bloc as a broad expansile mass (fig. 238), it may be more difficult to determine that invasion has taken place, but fortunately this form of invasion carries a better prognosis. Attention should also be directed to the lamina propria, muscularis, and adventitia in the vicinity of the tumor. Even in the absence of detectable local invasion, there may be spread via the small lymphatics in these layers (fig. 239). Foci of squamous and glandular change, or both, may be seen in a transitional cell carcinoma which has become invasive; it should be recorded as transitional cell carcinoma with metaplastic change (figs. 207, 208) rather than diagnosed as squamous cell carcinoma or adenocarcinoma.

Squamous cell carcinomas are composed of sheets of rounded to polygonal cells infiltrating the stroma as irregular, crooked, branching, and anastomosing projections. Cells in the basal layer near the stroma are usually small with hyperchromatic nuclei occupying a large portion of the cell. Cells further away from the basal layer usually show features reminiscent of maturation in normal squamous epithelium, i.e., increase in cell size, reduction in the nuclear cytoplasmic ratio, increased eosinophilia of the cytoplasm, intercellular bridges, and keratinization (figs. 240, 241).

Undifferentiated carcinomas are characterized by solid sheets of small oval cells with hyperchromatic nuclei which bear a strong resemblance to the small cell undifferentiated carcinoma of the lung (fig. 242). They show all degrees of anaplasia which suggests that this is probably a tumor of a distinct cell line and not merely an anaplastic transitional cell carcinoma. Occasionally, one sees a highly anaplastic carcinoma in which the cell type is not identifiable (fig. 243). In such circumstances, it is preferable and more honest to indicate that the tumor is a highly anaplastic carcinoma of indeterminate cell type rather than to classify it arbitrarily as a transitional cell or undifferentiated carcinoma.

Figure 232
ANAPLASTIC TRANSITIONAL CELL CARCINOMA
(Figure 232 and Plate X-A from same case)
This is the histologic appearance of the same tumor shown in plate X-A; individual cells are clear and range from polygonal to spindle-shaped. Histochemically, no fat was identified. Electron microscopically, the tumor was unlike renal adenocarcinoma and compatible with transitional cell carcinoma. The sparing of glomeruli (B) and invasion of collecting tubules (C) are much more typical of a tumor of renal pelvis than parenchymal origin. X180.

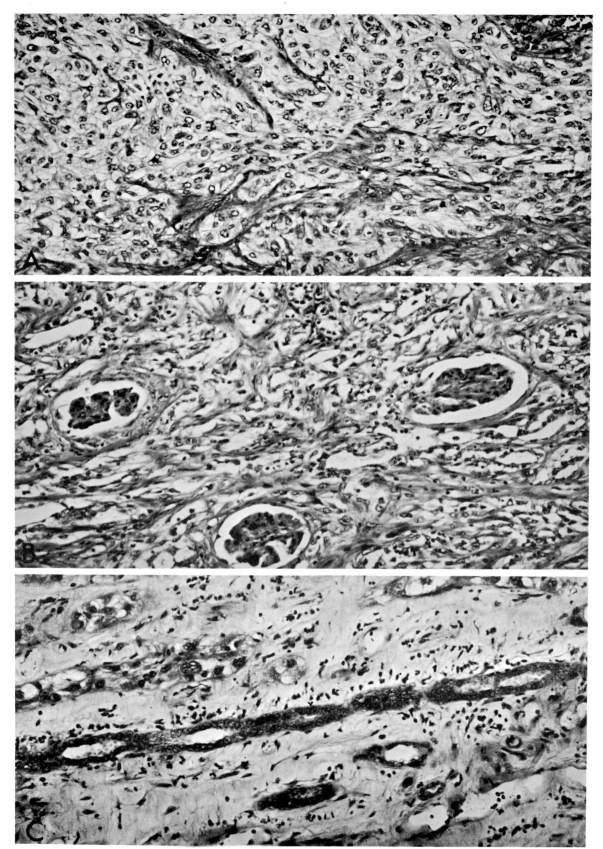

Figure 232

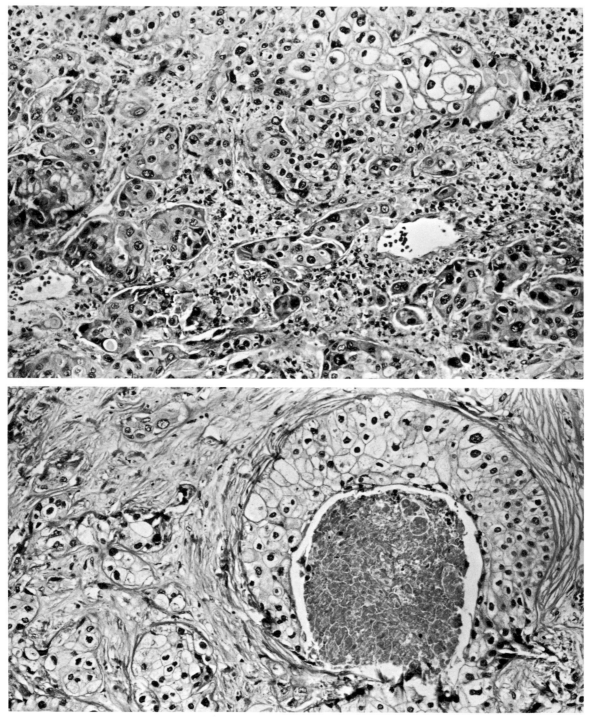

Figure 233

Figure 233
TRANSITIONAL CELL CARCINOMA

In this transitional cell carcinoma of the renal pelvis, an area of grade II-III carcinoma is easily recognizable as transitional cell in origin (upper). The clear cell change seen in areas throughout this tumor closely mimics the appearance of renal adenocarcinoma (lower). X290.

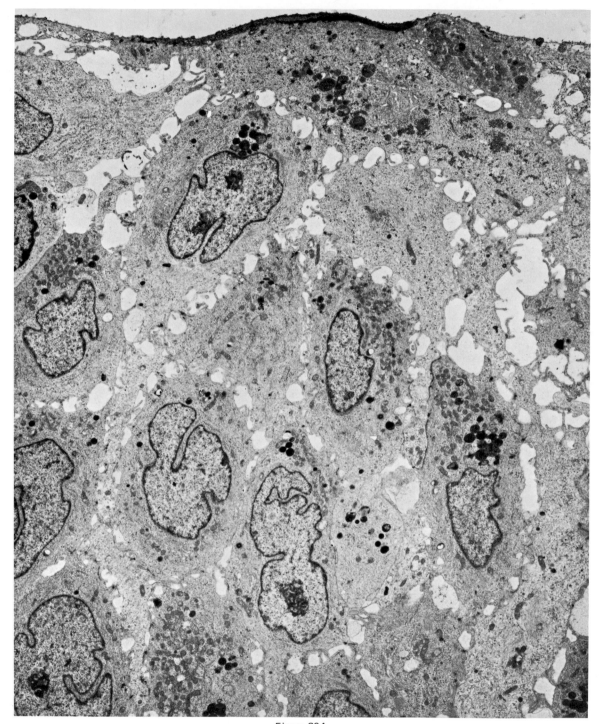

Figure 234
TRANSITIONAL CELL CARCINOMA
(Figures 234 and 235 from same case)
There is preservation of intracellular cisternae seen as dilated spaces about the tumor cells in this electron micrograph of a transitional cell carcinoma. Nuclear irregularity is a manifestation of the nuclear pleomorphism seen by light microscopy. X4680.

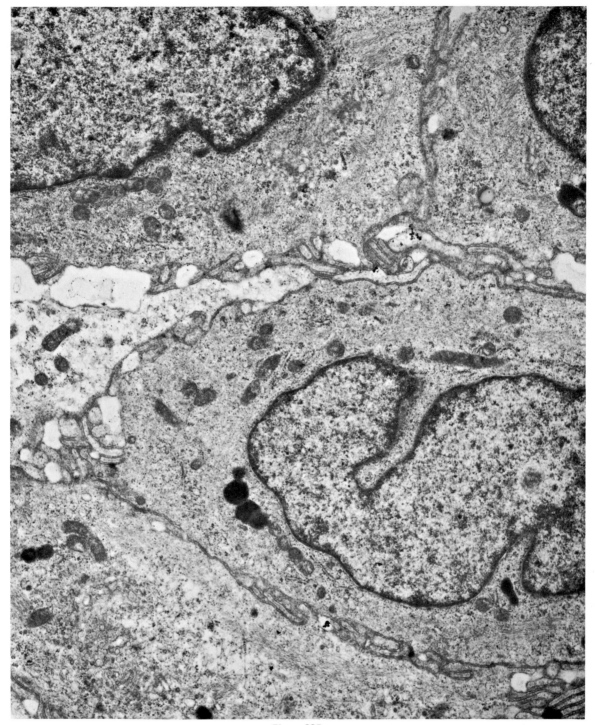

Figure 235
TRANSITIONAL CELL CARCINOMA
(Figures 234 and 235 from same case)
Higher magnification of figure 234 demonstrates the elaborate folded and interdigitating cell membrane characteristic of the transitional cells which bound the lateral cisternae. X14,630.

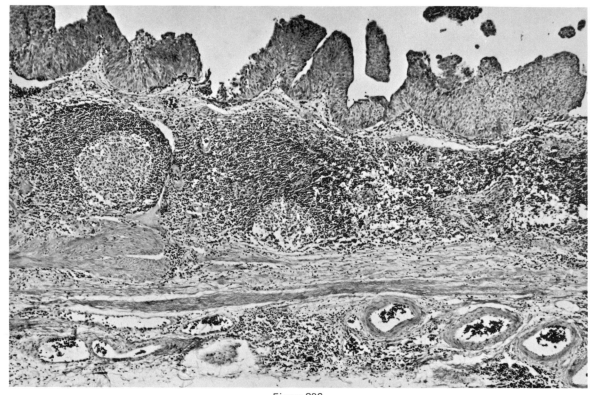

Figure 236
NONINVASIVE TRANSITIONAL CELL CARCINOMA
This noninvasive transitional cell carcinoma of the renal pelvis exhibits lymphoid infiltrates and lymphoid follicles in the underlying stroma. X75.

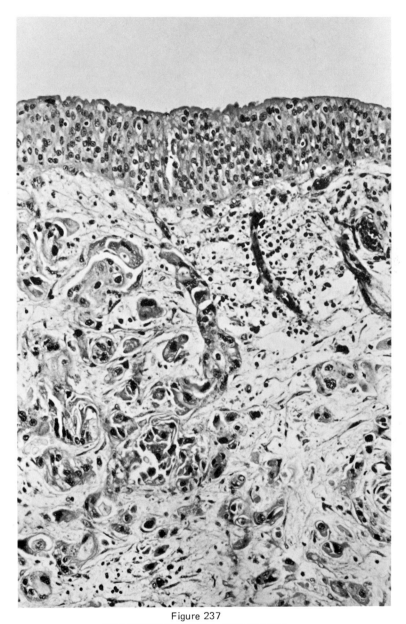

Figure 237
TRANSITIONAL CELL CARCINOMA
An example of piecemeal or tentacular invasion of the lamina propria is seen in this transitional cell carcinoma. X185.

Figure 238
TRANSITIONAL CELL CARCINOMA, GRADE I
An example of en bloc or pushing type of invasion is seen in this transitional cell carcinoma, grade I. The subjacent stroma is compressed by the advancing mass of tumor. X185.

Figure 239
INVASIVE CARCINOMA
Invasive carcinoma of the ureter is illustrated showing permeation of mural lymphatic vessels in the region of the tumor. X185.

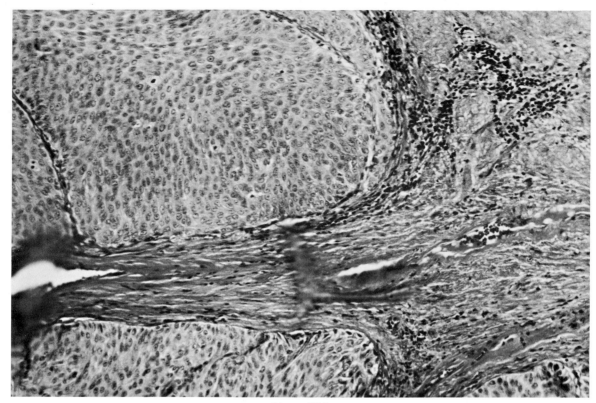

Figure 238

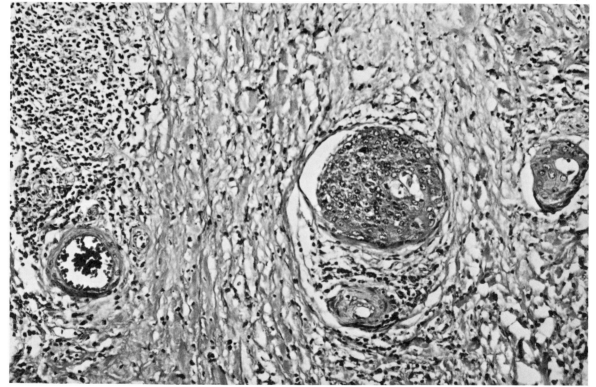

Figure 239

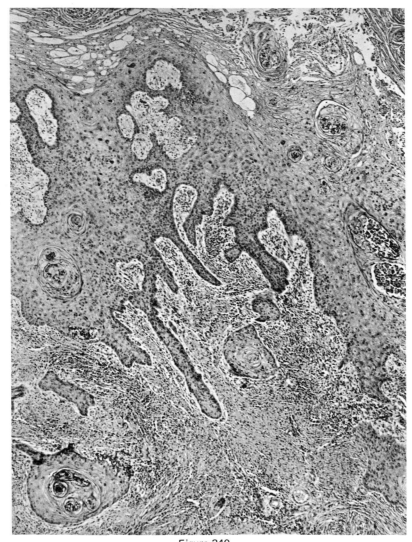

Figure 240
SQUAMOUS CELL CARCINOMA
(Figures 240 and 241 from same case)
Squamous cell carcinoma of the renal pelvis shows little anaplasia, but extensive stromal invasion. X75.

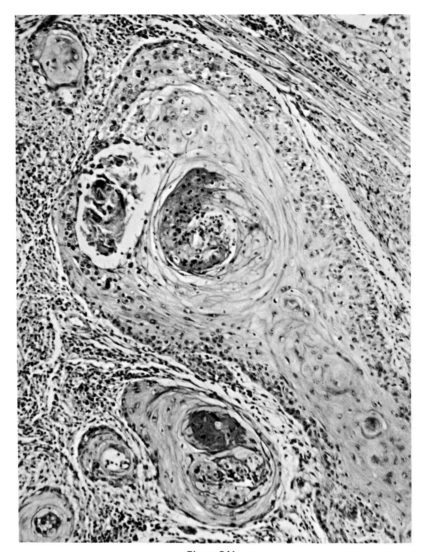

Figure 241
SQUAMOUS CELL CARCINOMA
(Figures 240 and 241 from same case)
Higher magnification of figure 240 shows a lack of anaplasia in the invasive foci. X185.

Figure 242
UNDIFFERENTIATED CARCINOMA OF RENAL PELVIS
This carcinoma of the renal pelvis is composed of small, haphazardly arranged, oval to spindle cells containing small regular, round to oval nuclei. Cell membranes are indistinct and cytoplasm is scanty. This tumor most closely resembles a small cell (oat cell) carcinoma of the lung. X290.

Figure 243
ANAPLASTIC CARCINOMA
Because of the marked pleomorphism, it is not possible to determine the cell of origin of this highly anaplastic carcinoma of the renal pelvis. X460.

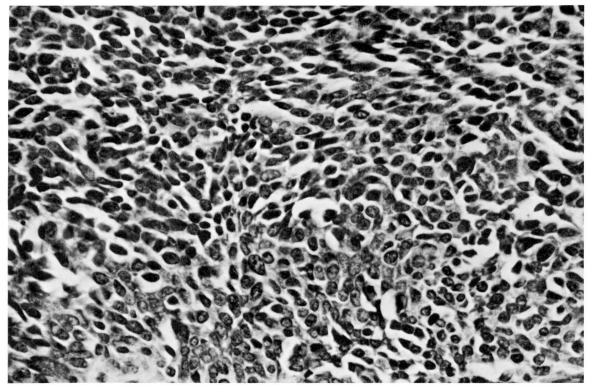

Figure 242

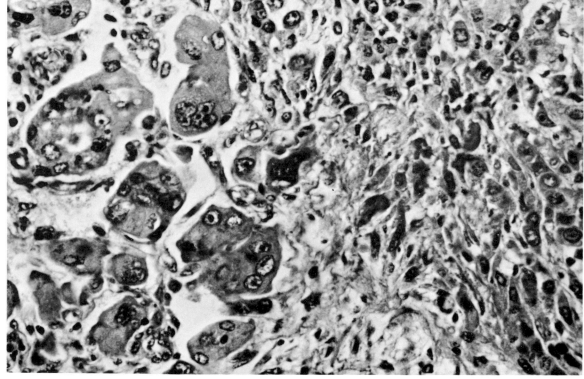

Figure 243

Adenocarcinoma may show so little anaplasia as to be difficult to distinguish from pyelitis or ureteritis glandularis (fig. 192) and may be difficult to differentiate from transitional cell carcinoma with mucinous metaplasia (fig. 208; pl. X-D). Characteristically, they are composed of tall, cylindrical mucosecretory cells with hyperchromatic, generally basally oriented nuclei (figs. 244–246). The spectrum of these tumors bears a strong resemblance to mucinous tumors of the ovary and, indeed, a stage analogous to mucinous cystadenoma may exist, although our experience has been insufficient with such glandular tumors of the renal pelvis and ureter to be certain of this point. On the other hand, we have seen invasion in glandular tumors of the renal pelvis showing little deviation from that seen in metaplastic glandular change (fig. 247); therefore, we feel the presence of nuclear pseudostratification, hyperchromasia, and irregularity, and any piling up of cells should be regarded as extremely suspicious for carcinoma.

Tumor Grade

The term anaplasia should be distinguished from the type of differentiation. We have used differentiation to indicate that the tumor recapitulates a recognizable cell type, while anaplasia denotes the

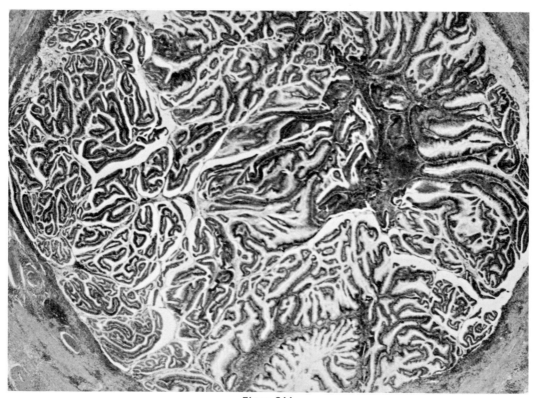

Figure 244
MUCOSECRETORY ADENOCARCINOMA
(Figures 244 and 245 from same case)
This illustrates a cross section of a ureter filled by a well differentiated mucosecretory adenocarcinoma. X50.

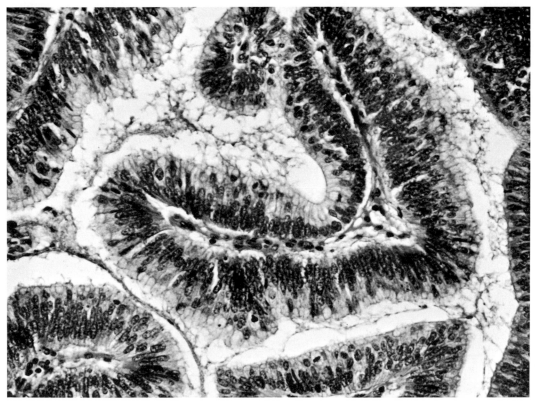

Figure 245
MUCOSECRETORY ADENOCARCINOMA
(Figures 244 and 245 from same case)
Higher magnification of figure 244 reveals that the tumor is composed of tall, cylindrical, columnar cells with pseudo-stratified nuclei which are large and vesicular and hyperchromatic. X460.

extent to which the tumor cells have deviated from the typical cytologic features of that cell type. The degree of anaplasia is usually expressed by a numerical tumor grade. While Broders originally used four grades, and others have used up to seven, for assessing anaplasia, we feel that three grades are sufficient for routine purposes.

Analytically, the pathologist takes into account such features as the extent to which there is loss of cell polarity and maturation, the degree of hyperchromasia, cell crowding, nuclear and cellular pleomorphism, and an increase in the number of cell layers, as well as the mitotic rate in grading the tumor. After reviewing a number of sections, the pathologist can readily and fairly reproducibly determine whether the worst area of the tumor is only slightly anaplastic (grade I) (fig. 224), markedly anaplastic (grade III) (fig. 228), or somewhere in between (grade II) (fig. 227). Results of such grading convey useful information to the clinician in terms of what can be expected in the tumor's behavior and the patient's prognosis. The correlation between tumor grading and patient survival is discussed under prognosis on page 309.

Figure 246

TWO PRIMARY CARCINOMAS

A. Simultaneous carcinomas are shown arising in a double ureter (upper). Squamous cell carcinoma is present in one ureter and adenocarcinoma in the other. X8.

B. Higher magnification of the squamous cell carcinoma is seen in the lower left. X100. Higher magnification of the squamous cell carcinoma and the adenocarcinoma shows little anaplasia, but reveals invasion of the underlying stroma (lower right). X100.

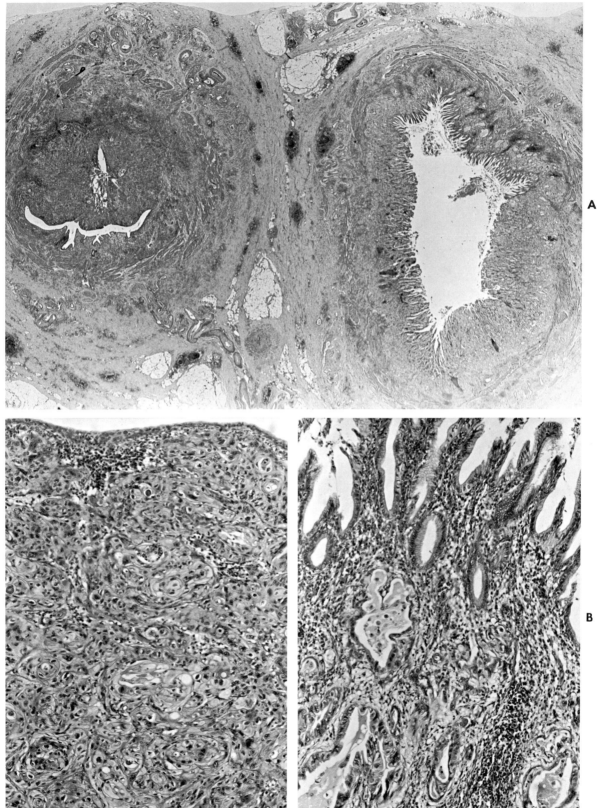

A

B

Figure 246

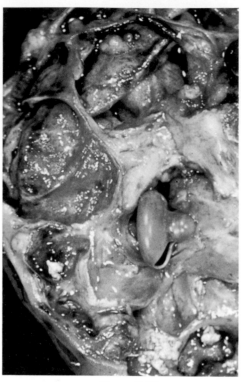

Figure 247
ADENOCARCINOMA

This adenocarcinoma of the renal pelvis was found in a 57 year old man in whom bilateral staghorn calculi were discovered in the renal pelvis. The opened kidney reveals greatly dilated calices lined by a mucoid granular tumor. A dePezzer's catheter lies within the lumen of the renal pelvis. The patient developed a right hemiparesis and died six months postoperatively. At autopsy, there was direct extension to the adrenal gland and widespread metastases. (Fig. 167 from Lucke, B., and Schlumberger, H. G. Tumors of the Kidney, Renal Pelvis and Ureter. Fascicle 30, Atlas of Tumor Pathology, First Series. Washington: Armed Forces Institute of Pathology, 1957.)

Figure 247

Tumor Stage

The extent of invasion is also important in predicting the behavior of the tumor and assessing the patient's prognosis. While there is a close correlation between the degree of anaplasia (tumor grade) and the extent of invasion (tumor stage), exceptions do occur. When the tumor is markedly anaplastic but only superficially invasive, or when the tumor is deeply invasive but only slightly anaplastic, the tumor stage rather than the histologic grade is, in our opinion, a better guide to prognosis.

No official system for pathologic staging of upper urinary tract cancers has been adopted, although studies based on proposed staging systems for tumors of the renal pelvis and ureter have clearly demonstrated their usefulness in evaluating prognosis (Grabstald et al.; Wagle et al.; Bloom et al.). Until an official staging system has been adopted, we propose the following for staging cancers of both the renal pelvis and ureter:

Stage I   Papillary or planar (nonpapillary) carcinoma with no evidence of invasion.

Stage II   Papillary or planar carcinoma, superficially invasive but with invasion limited to the lamina propria.

Stage III   Papillary or planar carcinoma, extending to the level of the muscularis (may extend beyond the muscularis in the intrarenal portions of the renal pelvis if confined to the kidney).

Stage IV   Papillary or planar carcinoma extending to the adventitial surface, involving adjacent structures and/or metastatic.

Since the walls of the ureter and renal pelvis are quite thin, extension through the wall occurs earlier than in carcinomas of the bladder (pl. XI-B). Therefore, further refinement of the system into additional stages seems unlikely to produce any real differences in survival figures between successive stages. The correlation between tumor stage and patient survival is discussed further in the section on prognosis.

Distribution of Metastases

Hematogenous spread of metastases is less common in patients with carcinoma of the renal pelvis and ureter compared to its relative frequency in patients with adenocarcinoma of the renal parenchyma. The lamina propria, muscularis, and adventitia of the renal pelvis and ureter are richly supplied with lymphatic vessels which become invaded early by infiltrating tumor. Extension through the wall of the ureter into the retroperitoneum is quite common once the tumor has become invasive. We are not aware of any reports from any large series on the distribution of metastases of renal pelvic carcinomas. However, Abeshouse reported the distribution of metastases among 45 patients who died of carcinoma of the ureter as follows: retroperitoneal lymph nodes, 31 percent; generalized metastases, 31 percent; bones, 27 percent; lungs, 20 percent; inguinal lymph nodes, 11 percent; brain, 2 percent; and spleen, 2 percent. Unfortunately, there have been too few cases analyzed to give statistically significant information on the effect of cell type on the distribution of metastases and the relative frequency of metastases at comparable stages.

Prognosis

Important factors in assessing prognosis include the cell type, tumor grade, tumor stage, type of invasion, and mode of therapy. The significance of cell type has already been mentioned. Squamous cell carcinomas appear to have a shorter natural history than transitional cell carcinomas of the renal pelvis with recurrences usually within the first year (Rafla). In general, all carcinomas of the renal pelvis and ureter are thought to be radioresistant; however, data from Rafla suggest a role for radiotherapy postoperatively in patients with transitional cell carcinoma of the renal pelvis.

Tumor Grade

Bloom and associates demonstrated an excellent correlation between tumor grade and the extent of invasion in their study of patients with ureteral carcinoma. They were able to show that the 5-year survival was 83.5 percent for patients with grade I carcinomas, 51.7 percent for grade II, 18.2 percent for grade III, and 12.5 percent for grade IV carcinomas. These figures correspond closely with those reported by Mostofi (1968) for the 5-year survival rates of patients with carcinomas of the bladder, i.e., 80 percent for grade I and 20 percent for grade III tumors.

Tumor Stage

Staging that is based on an actual measurement has the advantage of being more accurate than tumor grading that is somewhat subjective. However, to obtain the greatest accuracy in pathologic staging, it is essential for the pathologist to take many properly oriented full-thickness sections to ensure that the maximum depth of invasion has been determined.

The relationship between stage and survival can be seen in the results obtained by Bloom and associates, who found that the 5-year survival in patients with carcinoma of the ureter, staged pathologically were as follows: Stage I, 61.8 percent; Stage II, 25 percent; Stage III, 33 percent; and Stage IV, 0 percent. We are not aware of any survival figures based on pathologic staging for patients with renal pelvic carcinoma.

Invasion

There is some evidence that the form of invasion is also significant in evaluating survival. Infiltration of the carcinoma as small nests or individual cells appears to carry a poorer prognosis than when the tumor invades as a broad, well circumscribed mass which pushes and compresses the adjacent stroma as it advances.

Tumor/Host Response

A prominent inflammatory reaction in the lamina propria at the base of transitional cell carcinomas is seen frequently in the renal pelvis and ureter, as well as in the bladder. The inflammatory reaction, which is composed predominantly of lymphocytes and which may form lymphoid follicles, occurs in preinvasive as well as invasive carcinomas (fig. 236). The prognostic significance of these inflammatory infiltrates in the renal pelvis and ureter has not been established. However, in studies of bladder carcinomas, Sarma found that collections of lymphocytes were associated with a better prognosis than the tumors that lacked such an infiltrate. On the other hand, Pomerance has suggested that the presence of plasma cells is a more reliable indicator of a favorable prognosis.

Eventually, with the aid of computer-assisted multivariant analysis, it should be possible to generate a prognostic index with greater reliability than any one of the individual factors which are known to affect prognosis.

Treatment

Because tumors of the renal pelvis and ureter are often multicentric, and ureteral carcinomas have a marked propensity for the distal third of the ureter, recurrences are likely in patients treated surgically with less than a total nephroureterectomy, including a segment of bladder cuff (fig. 248). The value of combined nephroureterectomy and excision of a segment of bladder cuff in the treatment of carcinoma of the ureter or renal pelvis is highlighted by the report of Kimball and Ferris, who studied 74 patients with papillary carcinoma of the renal pelvis associated with similar tumors of the ureter and bladder developing after incomplete operation. They found that when subsequent carcinomas appeared in the ureter or bladder, which occurred in 50 cases (68 percent), the ureteral orifices were involved in 48 percent; the ureteral orifice and adjacent bladder, in 36 percent; the bladder alone, in 14 percent; and the ureter alone, in 2 percent. It is important to note that no recurrences were observed in a group of 24 patients with papillary carcinoma of the renal pelvis and ureter treated by combined nephroureterectomy and partial cystectomy.

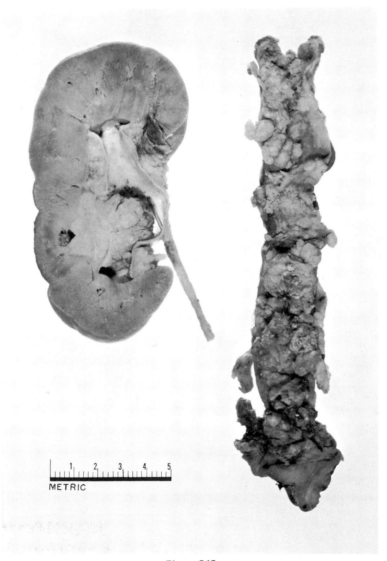

Figure 248
RECURRENT ANAPLASTIC CARCINOMA
The kidney and upper portion of ureter (left) were removed from a middle-aged man for an anaplastic carcinoma of the renal pelvis. Four years later, the patient developed recurrence of hematuria. The residual 17 cm. of ureter (right) was removed. The entire mucosal surface was replaced by tumor, histologically similar to the original carcinoma. (Courtesy of Dr. Roger Pugh, London, England.)

MESODERMAL TUMORS OF THE RENAL PELVIS AND URETER

Benign nonepithelial tumors arising in the wall of the ureter and renal pelvis are quite rare. They include the fibroepithelial polyp, leiomyoma, neurilemoma, and angioma. With the exception of the fibroepithelial polyp, only occasional examples of each are found in the literature.

Malignant nonepithelial tumors of the renal pelvis and ureter are also rare; the most frequently reported is the leiomyosarcoma. Too few reports are available to draw any conclusions about the epidemiology and clinical behavior of these tumors. Hematuria, dysuria, and flank pain are the symptoms most often reported.

TUMORS OF SMOOTH MUSCLE

LEIOMYOMA *

Among 144 benign ureteral tumors reported by Scott, three were classified as leiomyomas, although just one is a convincing example. Since his review, only one well documented leiomyoma (fig. 249) and one bizarre tumor of smooth muscle, a leiomyoblastoma (fig. 250) have been reported (de Jager). We have been able to find only one description of a leiomyoma of the renal pelvis, although we have personally examined a second case from the files of the Los Angeles Tumor Tissue Registry (fig. 251; pl. XI-C), which radiologically mimicked a renal adenocarcinoma (figs. 252, 253; Litzky et al.).

LEIOMYOSARCOMA *

In addition to two cases of leiomyosarcoma reported by Abeshouse, there have been four additional reports of ureteral leiomyosarcomas and six reports of leiomyosarcoma of the renal pelvis (Kao et al.; Kendall and Lakey; Shah and Kothari; Tolia et al.).

TUMORS OF NEUROGENIC TISSUE

Tumors of nerve sheath origin arising from the renal pelvis are extremely rare. There are two reports which represent benign neurilemomas arising in the renal pelvis (fig. 254; Fein and Hamm; Phillips and Baumrucker). We are not aware of any well documented reports of malignant neurogenic tumors of the renal pelvis in which invasion or metastases were documented.

TUMORS OF VASCULAR TISSUE

Angiomas involving the upper urinary tract are distinctly uncommon and frequently asymptomatic, and are, therefore, rarely reported. Those that are discovered are usually found in the renal parenchyma at the tips of renal papillae (McCrea; Bartone and Grieco). They usually produce nodular elevations of the caliceal mucosa, but may occasionally protrude into the lumen of the renal pelvis as a polypoid mass. The most frequent symptoms are gross hematuria and colic, secondary to the passage of clots; however, angiomas of the kidney are a rare cause of hematuria.

Only isolated instances of angiomas arising in the mucosa of the renal pelvis or ureter have been reported. To our knowledge, there are no well documented instances of angiosarcoma of the renal pelvis or ureter.

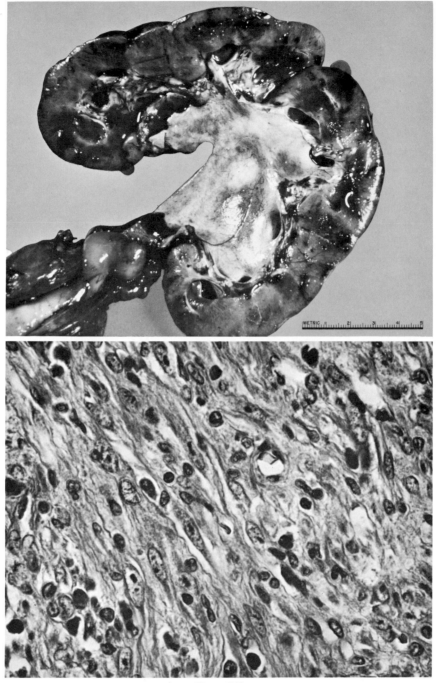

Figure 249
LEIOMYOMA

This nephroureterectomy specimen demonstrates a pedunculated mass in the upper ureter which proved to be a leiomyoma. The tumor projected into the lumen producing obstruction and hydronephrosis (upper). Histologically, the tumor is composed of elongated cells with prominent oval nuclei. The myomatous origin of the tumor was demonstrated histochemically and by immunofluorescence (lower). X460. (Fig. 2 from Kao, V., Graff, P. W., and Rappaport, H. Leiomyoma of the ureter: A histologically problematic rare tumor confirmed by immuno-histochemical studies. Cancer 24:535-542, 1969; (lower) courtesy of Dr. P. W. Graff, Chicago, Ill.)

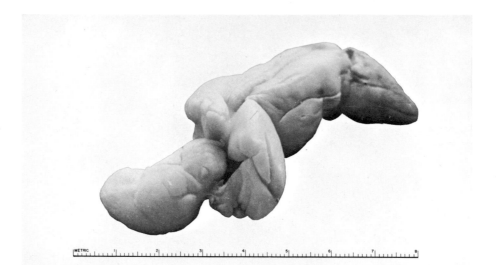

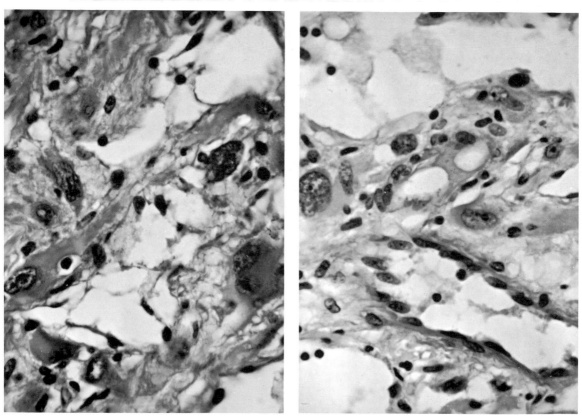

Figure 250
LEIOMYOBLASTOMA

   This leiomyoblastoma, which was found in a 55 year old woman, was attached to the right ureteral wall by a slender stalk (upper). The tumor is characterized by a bizarre appearance of the tumor cells. There is marked variation in the size and shape of individual cells and pronounced pleomorphism and hyperchromasia of nuclei, but only rare mitotic figures are seen (lower). X960. (Figs. 1 and 2 from de Jager, H. Bizarre smooth-muscle tumor of the ureter. J. Pathol. 87:424-425, 1964.)

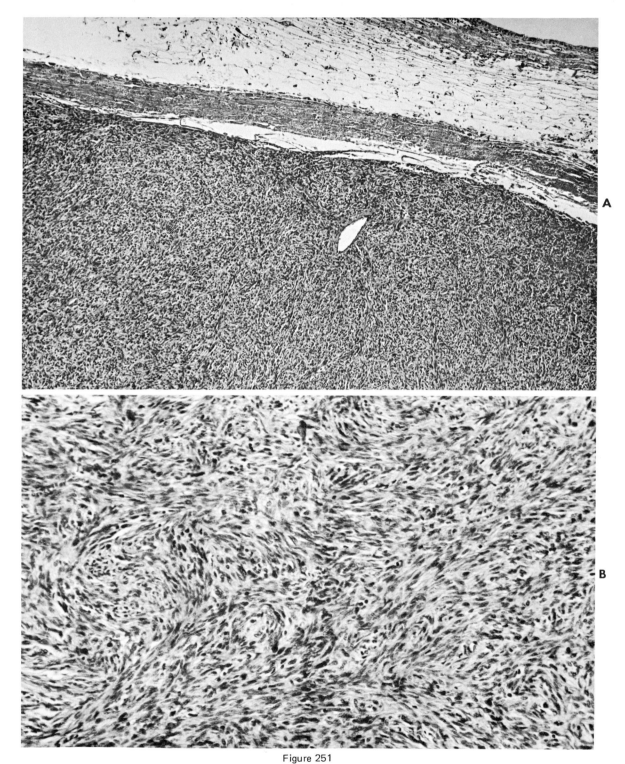

Figure 251
LEIOMYOMA
(Figures 251—253 and Plate XI-C from same case)
The tumor is arising from the renal pelvis and is composed of interlacing fascicles of tightly compacted smooth muscles.
A, X70; B, X185. (Courtesy of Dr. R. Kempson, Stanford, Calif.)

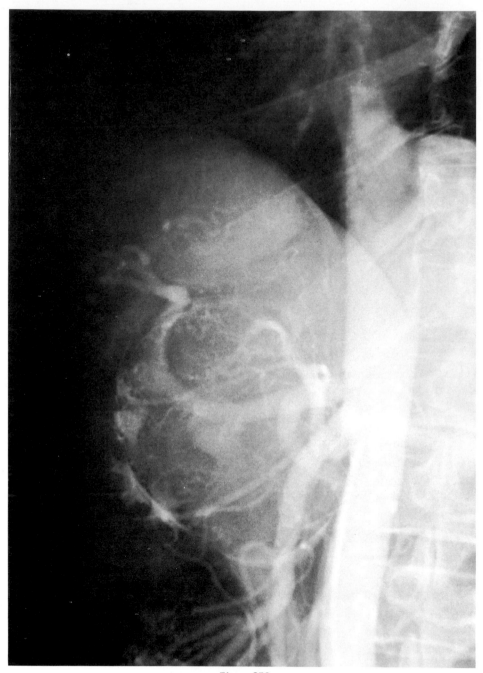

Figure 252
LEIOMYOMA
(Figures 251—253 and Plate XI-C from same case)

This is an arterial phase of a midstream abdominal aortogram (AP view) taken of the patient with the leiomyoma shown in figure 251. Multiple tortuous, enlarged, and irregular vessels occupy the area of the renal sinus and extend peripherally nearly to the renal cortical margins. There is extension of this neovascularity into the extrarenal tissues medial to the upper pole. The main renal artery supplying the lower pole is stretched around the inferior margins of the mass. (Courtesy of Dr. R. Kempson, Stanford, Calif.)

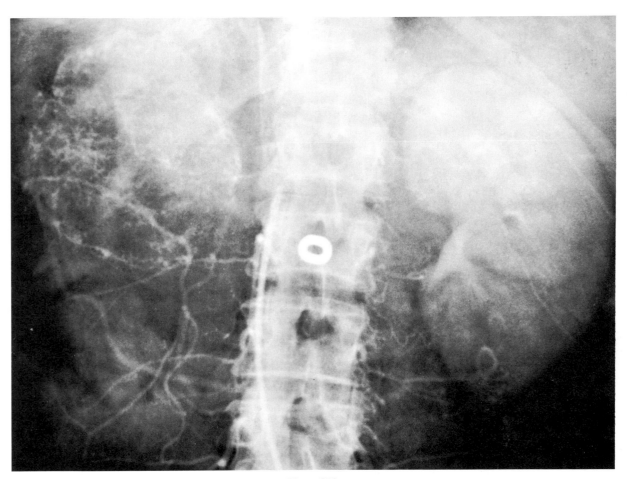

Figure 253
LEIOMYOMA
(Figures 251—253 and Plate XI-C from same case)
This is an oblique aortogram of the same patient shown in figure 252. Note the stretched, displaced, and distorted contrast-filled calices outlining the margins of the central mass inferiorly. Displacement of the renal arteries and early filling of neoplastic appearing vessels can be seen. Radiologic appearance of the tumor mimics that of a renal adeno-carcinoma. (Courtesy of Dr. R. Kempson, Stanford, Calif.)

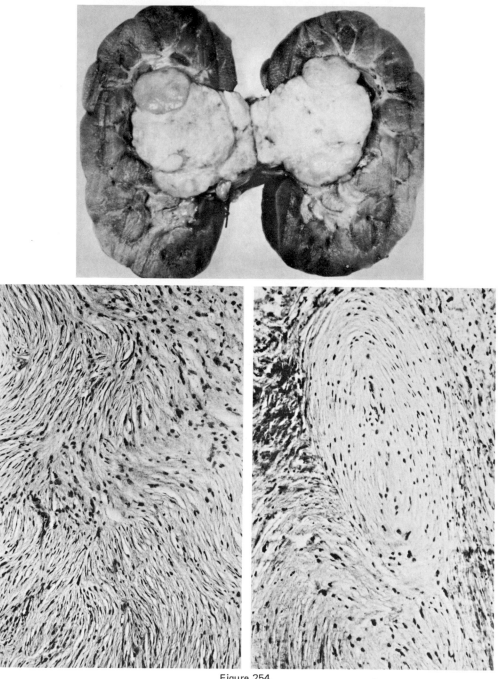

Figure 254
NEURILEMOMA

This illustrates a neurilemoma arising in, and filling the renal pelvis. The pedunculated tumor is attached to the wall of the pelvis by a narrow stalk (upper). Histologically, the tumor is composed of elongated wavy cells which show focal nuclear palisading. There is nuclear pleomorphism of the tumor, but these changes are frequently seen in neurilemomas and are not necessarily indicative of malignancy (lower). X180. (Figs. 2, 4, and 5 from Fein, R. L., and Hamm, F. C. Malignant schwannoma of the renal pelvis: A review of the literature and a case report. J. Urol. 94:356-361, 1965.)

SECONDARY TUMORS INVOLVING THE RENAL PELVIS AND URETER

Secondary involvement of the renal pelvis by local extension of a renal adenocarcinoma from the adjacent renal parenchyma, or from a sarcoma invading from the retroperitoneum, occurs in a substantial number of cases. However, judging from the few reports in the literature, metastasis to the renal pelvis from distant sites is extremely rare.

Invasion of the ureter by direct extension from carcinoma of the cervix is relatively common in patients with invasive cervical carcinoma and is a frequent cause of death. Spread to the ureter from tumors arising in the retroperitoneum is also

common, and includes carcinoma of the pancreas, sarcomas, lymphomas, and neuroblastomas.

There are many more reports of metastases to the ureter than to the renal pelvis, but it is not clear whether this is because metastases occur more frequently to the ureter or are more dramatic when found in this location (Lucké and Schlumberger; Presman and Ehrlich).

Metastases to the ureter are most frequently from carcinomas (fig. 255), although an appreciable number are from lymphomas (fig. 256). We have found just one report of a lymphoma that was primary in the ureter (Braun et al.). The relative frequency of primary tumors among reported metastases to the ureter is shown in Table XI.

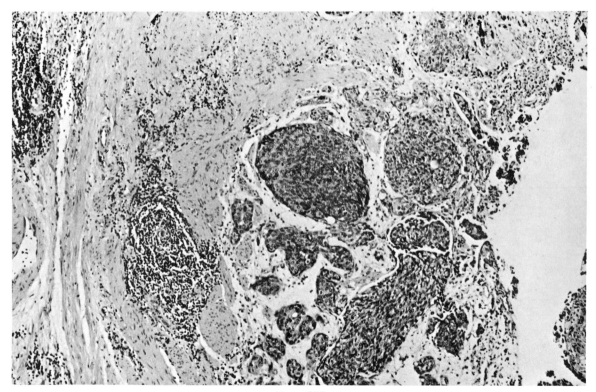

Figure 255
METASTATIC CARCINOMA
This metastatic carcinoma in the ureter originated from a primary squamous cell carcinoma of the anus. X70.

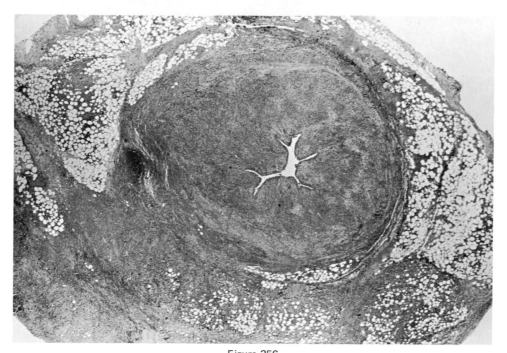

Figure 256
MALIGNANT HISTIOCYTIC LYMPHOMA
This malignant histiocytic lymphoma involving the ureter was found in a 71 year old woman with widespread histiocytic lymphoma. X12.

Table XI

PRIMARY SITE IN 99 INSTANCES OF METASTASES TO THE URETER*

Stomach	19
Prostate	17
Kidney	15
Breast	9
Lymphoma	9
Lung	7
Colon	7
Uterus	3
Cervix	3
Bladder	2
Ovary	2
Urethra	2
Vagina	1
Ureter	1
Testis	1
Skin	1
Total	99

*See references: Lucké, B., and Schlumberger, H. G., 1957; Presman, D., and Ehrlich, L., 1948.

TUMOR-LIKE LESIONS OF THE RENAL PELVIS AND URETER

FIBROEPITHELIAL POLYP

SYNONYMS AND RELATED TERMS: Fibrous polyp; fibroma; ureteral polyp.

Among the mesodermal tumors of the upper urinary tract, the fibroepithelial polyp is most numerous. This tumor is usually found in the ureter and designated as a ureteral polyp, although six cases have been reported in the renal pelvis (Colgan et al.; Crum; DeKlotz and Young; Evans and Stevens; Cassimally). The fibroepithelial polyp occurs most often in young adults and more frequently in men than women. Multiple polyps are occasionally found in the same ureter, but bilateral lesions have not been reported.

Clinical findings are chiefly those of

intermittent flank pain and, less frequently, dysuria and hematuria. Radiographically, fibroepithelial polyps produce a long, narrow, radiolucent filling defect with little evidence of accompanying renal damage. The majority of these lesions are found in the upper third of the ureter; this helps to distinguish them from transitional cell carcinomas, which are usually found in the lower third.

Grossly, most fibroepithelial polyps are long slender projections up to 5 cm. in length (fig. 257). They are occasionally polypoid with multiple projections sprouting from a single stalk (fig. 258). Typically, they are solid and firm with a gray, smooth, intact mucosal surface. Histologically, they are characterized by a loose vascular, edematous fibrous stroma which

may be inflamed (fig. 259). The overlying transitional epithelium is generally unremarkable, although benign hyperplasia has been reported. Such factors as obstruction, allergy, trauma, and exogenous carcinogens, and hormonal imbalance have been proposed as causative agents. However, the etiologic factors of these tumors are still unknown. Conservative treatment in the form of local resection by electrocoagulation—partial or complete resection of the ureteral wall containing the lesion—is recommended except when hydronephrosis or multiple polyps necessitate nephroureterectomy (Colgan et al.; DeKlotz and Young).

There do not appear to be any well documented reports of fibrosarcoma arising in the renal pelvis.

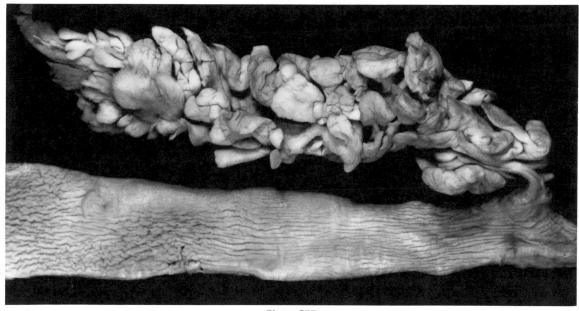

Figure 257
FIBROEPITHELIAL POLYP
(Figures 257 and 259 from same case)
This fibroepithelial polyp of the ureter was removed from a 38 year old woman. The solitary, elongated, and lobulated polyp is attached to the ureteral wall by a slender stalk. (Courtesy of Dr. Beecher-Smith, Columbus, Ohio; also fig. 182 from Lucké, B., and Schlumberger, H. G. Tumors of the Kidney, Renal Pelvis and Ureter. Fascicle 30, Atlas of Tumor Pathology, First Series. Washington: Armed Forces Institute of Pathology, 1957.)

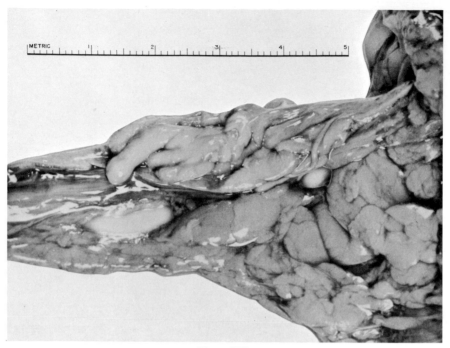

Figure 258
FIBROEPITHELIAL POLYP
This nephroureterectomy specimen was opened to show a branching fibroepithelial polyp of the upper ureter which was found in a 25 year old man. (Fig. 2 from Crum, P. M. Benign ureteral polyps. J. Urol. 102:678-682, 1969.)

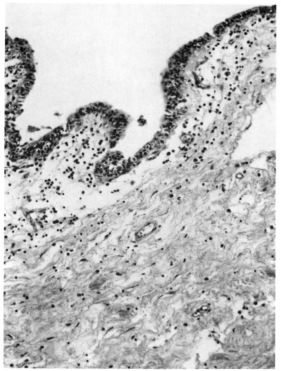

Figure 259

Figure 259
FIBROEPITHELIAL POLYP
(Figures 257 and 259 from same case)
Histologic features of this fibroepithelial polyp include a loose, edematous, richly vascular stroma which forms the bulk of the polyp and an intact but thin overlying mucosa. X90. (Courtesy of Dr. Beecher-Smith, Columbus, Ohio; also fig. 183 from Lucke, B., and Schlumberger, H. G. Tumors of the Kidney, Renal Pelvis and Ureter. Fascicle 30, Atlas of Tumor Pathology, First Series. Washington: Armed Forces Institute of Pathology, 1957.)

MALAKOPLAKIA

Malakoplakia is most frequently seen in the bladder, renal pelvis, and ureter; it occurs less frequently in the retroperitoneum, prostate, testis, epididymis and renal parenchyma. In the kidney, malakoplakia can be confused with carcinoma clinically, radiologically, and morphologically. These features, including the etiologic factors and pathogenesis and the origin of Michaelis-Gutmann bodies, are discussed under renal adenocarcinoma on page 166.

In many cases, malakoplakia of the renal pelvis and ureter is silent and discovered only at autopsy. Those cases that are clinically apparent are usually characterized by dysuria, urinary frequency, pyuria, and hematuria (Schneiderman and Simon). When the granulomatous plaques which characterize this entity are located in the ureter or ureteropelvic junction, they are likely to produce flank pain and fever, with hydronephrosis and pyelonephritis. Radiographically, there are no distinctive features of malakoplakia of the renal pelvis and ureter; because of their configuration, they are difficult to distinguish from carcinomas arising in these sites.

The morphologic appearance of malakoplakia involving the renal pelvis and ureter is that of multiple raised, discrete, yellow-gray or tan-pink plaques scattered about the mucosa (pl. XI-D). Individual plaques range from less than 1 mm. up to 3 cm. in greatest diameter, but multiple plaques may coalesce to produce large confluent areas of involvement (Schneiderman and Simon).

Histologically, these lesions are characterized by submucosal infiltrates of large rounded histiocytes with pink foamy cytoplasm, small dark rounded nuclei, and intracellular basophilic laminated (Michaelis-Gutmann) bodies. There is usually little or no apparent fibrovascular stroma, and cells show little cohesion and no evidence of any organization. Although lesions are fairly characteristic, the entity is rare and could easily be overlooked in favor of such diagnoses as metastatic clear cell carcinoma, most likely from the kidney, some form of histiocytic neoplasm such as fibroxanthosarcoma or malignant xanthogranuloma, or an early phase of retroperitoneal fibrosis.

RETROPERITONEAL FIBROSIS

Retroperitoneal fibrosis is included here because, while an uncommon disease, it is capable of producing ureteral obstruction, and biopsy material could conceivably be confused with retroperitoneal sarcoma or lymphoma. This entity is a chronic fibrosing, inflammatory process which is predominantly periaortic in distribution. It is frequently associated with inflammatory and fibrotic lesions in other sites as well as systemic disease. The retroperitoneal changes are most likely one manifestation of a larger disease complex for which the name systemic idiopathic fibrosis has been proposed.

In a series of 40 patients with retroperitoneal fibrosis collected by Mitchinson, there were 30 men and 10 women. The age range was 17 to 83 years, with a mean of 53 years. No data are available covering the social or geographic distribution of the disease, and there is no evidence to suggest any hereditary influence.

The usual mode of presentation is abdominal or flank pain, anemia, high sedimentation rate, and uremia secondary to

PLATE XI

PAPILLARY TRANSITIONAL CELL CARCINOMA

A.   This cross section of a ureter demonstrates complete filling of the lumen by multiple papillary projections of a transitional cell carcinoma. X8. (Courtesy of the Armed Forces Institute of Pathology, Washington, D. C.)

B.   This is a cross section of a ureter at the site of involvement by a papillary transitional cell carcinoma. There is widespread circumferential invasion to the depth of the muscularis. X11. (Courtesy of the Armed Forces Institute of Pathology, Washington, D. C.)

LEIOMYOMA
(Plate XI-C and Figures 253–255 from same case)

C.   This leiomyoma was a pale tan, smooth, firm pedunculated mass arising from the wall of the renal pelvis and largely filling the renal sinus. (Courtesy of Dr. R. Kempson, Stanford, Calif.)

MALAKOPLAKIA

D.   This nephroureterectomy specimen was taken from a 53 year old woman with a history of recurrent urinary tract infections. On the surface of the opened ureter, there are multiple, raised, smooth yellow nodules which proved histologically to be caused by malakoplakia involving the submucosa. (Courtesy of Dr. D. C. Schneiderman, Montreal, Canada.)

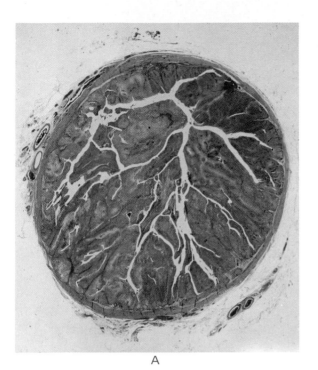

A

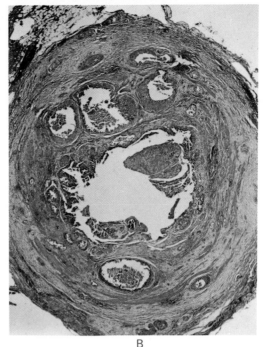

B

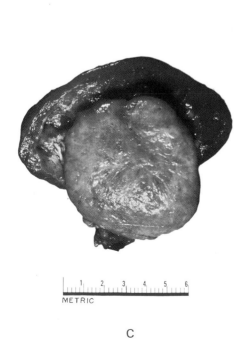

C

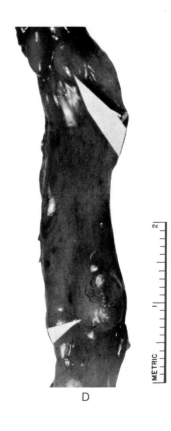

D

PLATE XI

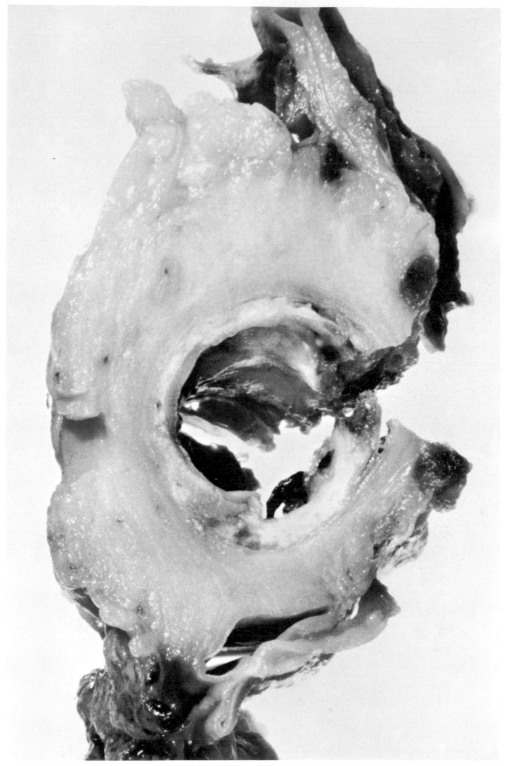

Figure 260
RETROPERITONEAL FIBROSIS
A cross section of the lower abdominal aorta demonstrates retroperitoneal fibrosis encircling the aorta. (Fig. I (right) from Mitchinson, M. J. The pathology of idiopathic retroperitoneal fibrosis. J. Clin. Pathol. 23:681-689, 1970.)

ureteral obstruction (Jones et al.). Excretory urograms typically reveal dilatation of the renal calices, pelvis, and ureter proximal to the obstruction of the affected side. The obstruction is usually bilateral, with narrowing at the lumbar level.

Conditions which are related to retroperitoneal fibrosis include: **idiopathic mediastinal fibrosis; aortitis of unknown cause; Riedel's thyroiditis; pseudotumors of the orbit**; and **sclerosis cholangitis.** Raynaud's phenomenon and alterations in plasma proteins are found in association with these various manifestations of systemic idiopathic fibrosis (Mitchinson).

Various etiologic agents have been proposed as being responsible for retroperitoneal fibrosis including trauma, infection, lymphatic and venous obstruction, vitamin E deficiency, inflammation of adipose tissue, toxoplasmosis, leakage of blood from the aorta, systemic connective tissue disorders, and drug therapy such as Methysergide. Treatment is basically surgical, although corticosteroid therapy has been effective in a few cases.

Pathologic Features

In retroperitoneal fibrosis, the basic pathologic process is fibrosis which centers around, and may encircle the aorta (fig. 260). Extension below the pelvic brim or above the renal arteries is unusual (fig. 261). In later stages, the fibrosis extends superiorly and laterally (fig. 262) drawing the ureters toward the aorta (fig. 263) and, occasionally, surrounding the ureter.

Histologically, one can distinguish early and late stages of the inflammatory process. The early stage is characterized by proliferation of active, occasionally pleomorphic fibroblasts interspersed with collagenous bundles and infiltrated by variable numbers of lymphocytes, plasma cells, eosinophils, and small numbers of mast cells. Russell bodies are frequently quite numerous (fig. 264). Adipose tissue and skeletal muscles outside the areas of fibrosis are frequently infiltrated by lymphocytes, but show no evidence of vasculitis or necrosis.

In older lesions, presumably less active, the collagenous tissue is relatively acellular, avascular, and frequently calcified with little accompanying inflammation (fig. 265).

It is important to keep this entity in mind, since a biopsy of the ureter and surrounding tissue may be misdiagnosed as a malignant neoplasm, particularly lymphoma (Kendall and Lakey).

AMYLOID TUMOR

Amyloid deposits which appear to represent primary localized amyloidosis have been reported for many sites in the urinary tract including: renal parenchyma, renal pelvis, ureter, bladder, prostate, urethra, and seminal vesicles (Gardner et al.; Johnson and Ankenman; Tripathi and Desautels).

This condition is quite rare and its etiologic factors and pathogenesis are unknown. To date, neither dysproteinemia nor significant systemic plasmacytosis have been found in association with these tumors. The ureter seems to be most frequently involved, although fewer than 50 cases have been reported.

Amyloid deposits are of interest to pathologists, radiologists, and clinicians because they can mimic a carcinoma clinically. This is especially so in the ureter where, when unilateral (fig. 266), the clinical diagnosis is usually a primary or metastatic carcinoma.

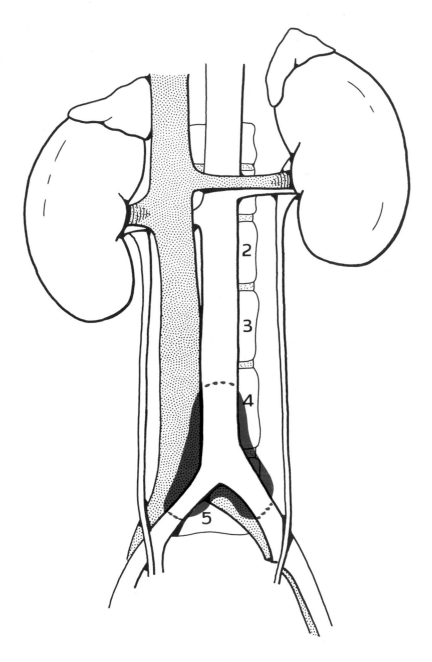

Figure 261
RETROPERITONEAL FIBROSIS
This is a graphic representation of the distribution of retroperitoneal fibrosis in its early stages. (Fig. 2 from Mitchinson, M. J. The pathology of idiopathic retroperitoneal fibrosis. J. Clin. Pathol. 23:681-689, 1970.)

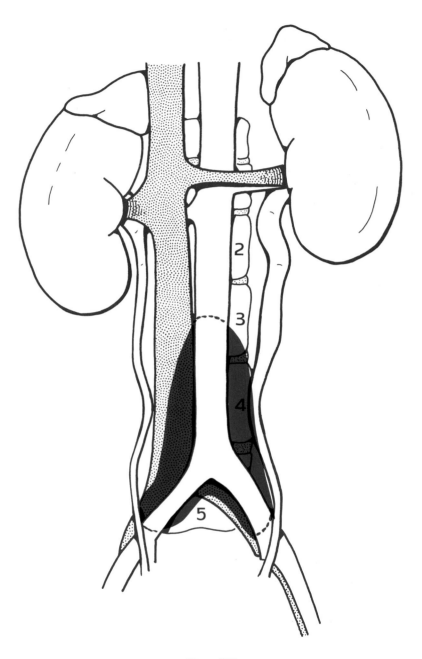

Figure 262
RETROPERITONEAL FIBROSIS
This graphic representation of the distribution of retroperitoneal fibrosis in its later stages shows the extension of fibrosis superiorly and laterally, but rarely below the pelvic brim or above the renal arteries. (Fig. 3 from Mitchinson, M. J. The pathology of idiopathic retroperitoneal fibrosis. J. Clin. Pathol. 23:681-689, 1970.)

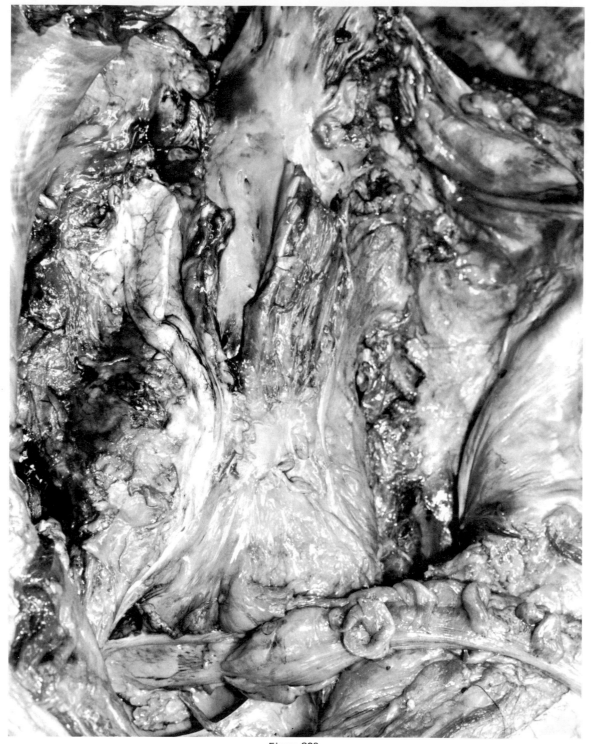

Figure 263
RETROPERITONEAL FIBROSIS
An autopsy demonstration of a typical case of retroperitoneal fibrosis reveals medial deviation of the ureters toward the aortic bifurcation. (Fig. 4 from Mitchinson, M. J. The pathology of idiopathic retroperitoneal fibrosis. J. Clin. Pathol. 23:681-689, 1970.)

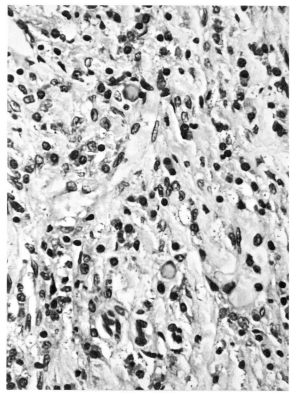

Figure 264

Figure 264
RETROPERITONEAL FIBROSIS
Histologic features of the active phase of retroperitoneal fibrosis include proliferation of immature, fibrous,
connective tissue, and accompanying chronic inflammation. X400.

Figure 265
RETROPERITONEAL FIBROSIS
This is the histologic appearance of the old or inactive
phase of retroperitoneal fibrosis. In this stage, the
processes are predominantly characterized by acellular
eosinophilic, slightly hyalinized, collagenous tissue, with
relatively little accompanying inflammation. X400.

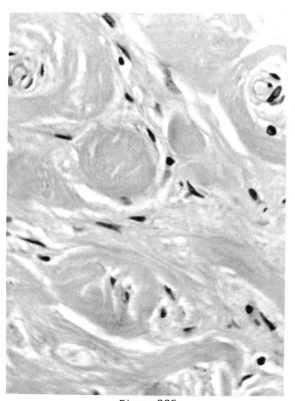

Figure 265

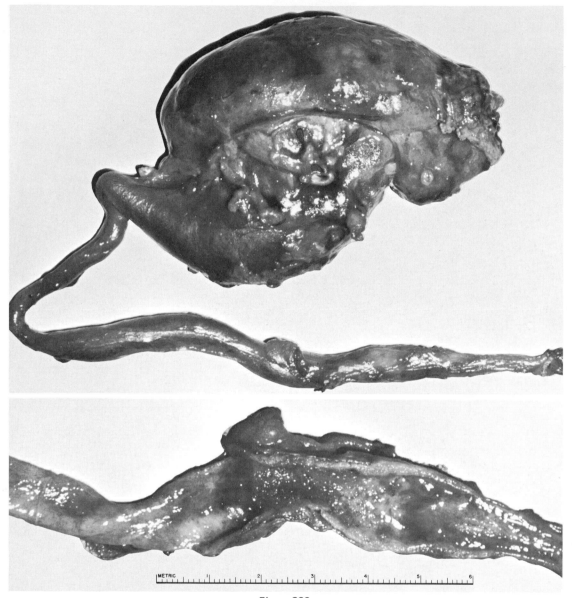

Figure 266
AMYLOID TUMOR
(Figures 266 and 267 from same case)
This nephroureterectomy specimen was taken from a 73 year old woman. There is dilatation of the renal pelvis proximal to a ureteral mass which was produced by a local accumulation of amyloid (upper). A close-up of the ureteral lesion shows a thickening of the ureteral wall and a granular mucosa (lower). (Figs. 2 and 3 from Pear, B. L. Penrose Cancer Seminar, Vol. IV, No. 5, 1971.)

Microscopically, the characteristic findings in the involved areas are diffuse interstitial and perivascular infiltrates of amorphous, eosinophilic, proteinaceous material (fig. 267). There may be an accompanying infiltrate of lymphocytes and plasma cells and a granulomatous reaction with multinucleated giant cells.

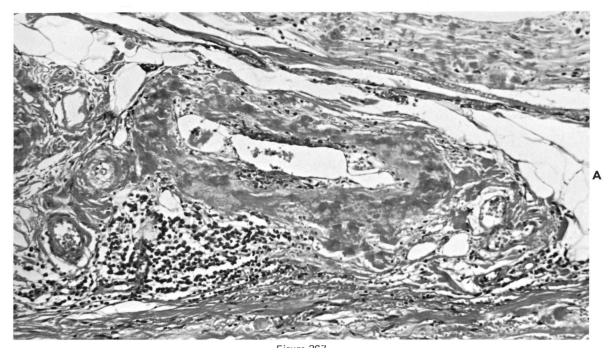

Figure 267
AMYLOID TUMOR
(Figures 266 and 267 from same case)

A. This is the histologic appearance of the amyloid tumor of the ureter in figure 266 showing a large confluent mass of amyloid in the ureteral wall, with accompanying lymphocytic and granulomatous inflammation. X140.

B. This is a higher magnification of the perivascular aggregates of amyloid in the ureteral wall and their associated lymphocytic infiltrates. X360. (Courtesy of Dr. B. L. Pear, Denver, Colo.)

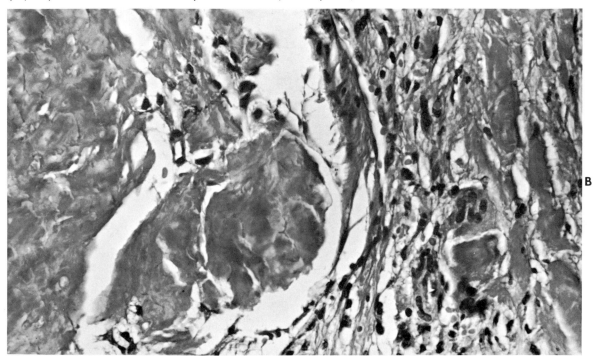

The proteinaceous material gives the usual reactions for amyloid, including staining with crystal violet and congo red, red-green dichroism under plane polarized light, and light green fluorescence under ultraviolet light after staining with Thioflavin T.

References

Abeshouse, B. S. Primary benign and malignant tumors of the ureter. A review of the literature and report of one benign and 12 malignant tumors. Am. J. Surg. 91:237-271, 1956.

Aufderheide, A. C., and Streitz, J. M. Mucinous adenocarcinoma of the renal pelvis. Report of two cases. Cancer 33:167-173, 1974.

Bartone, N. F., and Grieco, R. V. Renal hemangioma. J.A.M.A. 205:118-121, 1968.

Bengtsson, U., Angervall, L., Ekman, H., and Lehmann, L. Transitional cell tumors of the renal pelvis in analgesic abusers. Scand. J. Urol. Nephrol. 2:145-150, 1968.

Bennington, J. L., and Antonius, J. Unpublished results.

............, and Kradjian, R. M. Renal Carcinoma. Philadelphia: W. B. Saunders Co., 1967.

Bloom, N. A., Vidone, R. A., and Lytton, B. Primary carcinoma of the ureter: A report of 102 new cases. J. Urol. 103:590-598, 1970.

Bourne, H. E., Tremblay, R. E., and Ansell, J. S. Stupor, hypercalcemia and carcinoma of the renal pelvis. N. Engl. J. Med. 271:1005-1006, 1964.

Boyland, E., Dukes, C. E., Grover, P. L., and Mitchley, B. C. V. The induction of renal tumours by feeding lead acetate to rats. Br. J. Cancer 16:283-288, 1962.

Braun, E., Manley, C., Liao, K., and Boyarsky, S. Intrinsic Hodgkin's disease of the ureter. J. Urol. 107:952-954, 1972.

Buch, H., Häuser, H., Pfleger, K., and Rüdiger, W. Bestimmung von Phenacetin und N-Acetyl-p-aminophenol über Stoffwechselprodukte im Harn. Z. Klin. Chem. Klin. Biochem. 4:288-290, 1966.

Butler, W. H., and Barnes, J. M. Carcinogenic action of groundnut meal containing aflatoxin in rats. Food Cosmet. Toxicol. 6:135-141, 1968.

Cassimally, K. A. Fibroma filling the renal pelvis: Report of a case. Can. J. Surg. 14:350-352, 1971.

Clinicopathological Conference. Persistent fever in an elderly man. Br. Med. J. 1:1131-1138, 1962.

Cole, P. Coffee-drinking and cancer of the lower urinary tract. Lancet 1:1335-1337, 1971.

............, Hoover, R., and Friedell, G. H. Occupation and cancer of the lower urinary tract. Cancer 29:1250-1260, 1972.

Colgan, J. R., III, Skaist, L., and Morrow, J. W. Benign ureteral tumors in childhood: A case report and a plea for conservative management. J. Urol. 109:308-310, 1973.

Crum, P. M. Benign ureteral polyps. J. Urol. 102:678-682, 1969.

de Jager, H. Bizarre smooth-muscle tumor of the ureter. J. Pathol. 87:424-425, 1964.

DeKlotz, R. J., and Young, B. W. Conservative surgery in the management of benign ureteral polyps. A case report. Br. J. Urol. 36:375-379, 1964.

Elliott, A. Y., Frawley, E. E., Cleveland, P., Castro, A. E., and Stein, N. Isolation of RNA virus from papillary tumors of the human renal pelvis. Science 179:393-395, 1973.

Evans, A. T., and Stevens, R. K. Fibroepithelial polyps of ureter and renal pelvis: A case report. J. Urol. 86:313-315, 1961.

Evans, R. W. Histological Appearances of Tumours; with a Consideration of their Histogenesis and Certain Aspects of their Clinical Features and Behaviour, 2d ed., p. 1170. Baltimore: Williams & Wilkins Co., 1966.

Fein, R. L., and Hamm, F. C. Malignant schwannoma of the renal pelvis: A review of the literature and a case report. J. Urol. 94:356-361, 1965.

Gardner, K. D., Jr., Castellino, R. A., Kempson, R., Young, B. W., and Stamey, T. A. Primary amyloidosis of the renal pelvis. N. Engl. J. Med. 284:1196-1198, 1971.

Ghidoni, J. J., and Campbell, M. M. Fine structure of metaplastic cornified squamous epithelium in the urinary bladder of rats. J. Pathol. 97:665-670, 1969.

Gillis, D. J., Finnerty, P., and Maxted, W. C. Simultaneous occurrence of hypernephroma and transitional cell carcinoma with development of transitional cell carcinoma in the opposite kidney: case report. J. Urol. 106:646-647, 1971.

Golde, D. W., Schambelan, M., Weintraub, B. D., and Rosen, S. W. Gonadatropin-secreting renal carcinoma. Cancer 33:1048-1053, 1974.

Gordon, A. Intestinal metaplasia of the urinary tract epithelium. J. Pathol. 85:441-444, 1963.

Grabstald, H., Whitmore, W. F., and Melamed, M. R. Renal pelvic tumors. J.A.M.A. 218:845-854, 1971.

Grace, D. A., Taylor, W. N., Taylor, J. N., and Winter, C. C. Carcinoma of the renal pelvis: A 15-year review. J. Urol. 98:566-569, 1968.

Graham, J. B., and Vynalek, W. J. Renal cell and transitional cell carcinomas in the same kidney. J. Urol. 76:137-141, 1956.

Greene, L. F., Hanash, K. A., and Farrow, G. M. Benign papilloma or papillary carcinoma of the bladder? J. Urol. 110:205-207, 1973.

Guérin, M., Chouroulinkov, I., and Rivière, M. R. Experimental Kidney Tumors, pp. 199-268. In: The Kidney: Morphology, Biochemistry, Physiology, Vol. II. (Eds.) Rouiller, C., and Muller, A. F. New York and London: Academic Press, 1969.

Hall, R. R., Laurence, D. J., Neville, A. M., and Wallace, D. M. Carcinoembryonic antigen and urothelial carcinoma. Br. J. Urol. 45:88-92, 1973.

Hawtrey, C. E. Fifty-two cases of primary ureteral carcinoma: A clinical-pathologic study. J. Urol. 105:188-193, 1971.

Hvidt, V., and Feldt-Rasmussen, K. Primary tumours in the renal pelvis and ureter with particular attention to the diagnostic problems. Acta Chir. Scand. (Suppl.) 433:91-101, 1973.

Johnson, H. W., and Ankenman, G. J. Bilateral ureteral primary amyloidosis. J. Urol. 92:275-277, 1964.

Jones, J. H., Ross, E. J., Matz, L. R., Edwards, D., and Davies, D. R. Retroperitoneal fibrosis. Am. J. Med. 48:203-208, 1970.

Jönsson, G. Primary tumours of the ureter: Report of 17 cases. Acta Chir. Scand. 126:368-378, 1963.

Kao, V. C. Y., Graff, P. W., and Rappaport, H. Leiomyoma of the ureter: A histologically problematic rare tumor confirmed by immunohistochemical studies. Cancer 24:535-542, 1969.

Kendall, A. R., and Lakey, W. H. Sclerosing Hodgkin's disease vs. idiopathic retroperitoneal fibrosis. J. Urol. 86:217-221, 1961.

Kimball, F. N., and Ferris, H. W. Papillomatous tumor of the renal pelvis associated with similar tumors of the ureter and bladder. Review of literature and report of two cases. J. Urol. 31:257-301, 1934.

Litzky, G. M., Seidel, R. F., and O'Brien, J. E. Leiomyoma of the renal pelvis. J. Urol. 105:171-173, 1971.

Lucké, B., and Schlumberger, H. G. Tumors of the Kidney, Renal Pelvis and Ureter. Fascicle 30, Atlas of Tumor Pathology. Washington: Armed Forces Institute of Pathology, 1957.

Makar, N. Bilharzial ureter; some observations on surgical pathology and surgical treatment. Br. J. Surg. 36:148-155, 1948.

McCrea, L. E. Hemangioma of the kidney; review of the literature. Urologic Cutan. Rev. 55:670-680, 1951.

Meyer, P. C. The histological grading of primary epithelial neoplasms of the ureter. J. Urol. 102:30-36, 1969.

Mitchinson, M. J. The pathology of idiopathic retroperitoneal fibrosis. J. Clin. Pathol. 23:681-689, 1970.

Monlux, A. W., Anderson, W. A., and Davis, C. L. A survey of tumors occurring in cattle, sheep, and swine. Am. J. Vet. Res. 17:646-677, 1956.

Mostofi, F. K. Pathological aspects and spread of carcinoma of the bladder. J.A.M.A. 206:1764-1769, 1968.

............, Potentialities of bladder epithelium. J. Urol. 71:705-714, 1954.

Newman, D. M., Allen, L. E., Wishard, W. N., Jr., Nourse, M. H., and Mertz, J. H. O. Transitional cell carcinoma of the upper urinary tract. J. Urol. 98:322-327, 1967.

Phillips, C. A. S., and Baumrucker, G. Neurilemmoma (arising in the hilus of left kidney). J. Urol. 73:671-673, 1955.

Pomerance, A. A prognostic index for carcinoma of the bladder based on histopathological findings in cystectomy material. Br. J. Urol. 44:459-460, 1972.

Poole-Wilson, D. S. Occupational tumours of the renal pelvis and ureter arising in the dye-making industry. Proc. R. Soc. Med. 62:93-94, 1969.

Presman, D., and Ehrlich, L. Metastatic tumors of the ureter. J. Urol. 59:312-325, 1948.

Pugh, R. C. B. The Pathology of Bladder Tumours, pp. 116-156. In: Monographs on Neoplastic Disease at Various Sites, Vol. II. Tumours of the Bladder. (Ed.) Wallace, D. M. Edinburgh: E. & S. Livingstone, Ltd., 1959.

............, The pathology of cancer of the bladder. An editorial overview. Cancer 32:1267-1274, 1973.

Quattlebaum, R. B., and Shirley, S. W. Adenocarcinoma of the renal pelvis. J. Urol. 99:384-386, 1968.

Rafla, S. Tumors of the upper urothelium. Am. J. Roentgen. Radium Ther. Nucl. M. 123:540-551, 1975.

Ragins, A. B., and Rolnick, H. C. Mucus producing adenocarcinoma of the renal pelvis. J. Urol. 63:66-73, 1950.

Richardson, E. J., and Woodburn, R. L. Dissimilar primary tumors in the right upper urinary tract: Case report. J. Urol. 90:253-255, 1963.

Roe, F. J. C. An illustrated classification of the proliferative and neoplastic changes in mouse bladder epithelium in response to prolonged irritation. Br. J. Urol. 36:238-253, 1964.

............, Boyland, E., Dukes, C. E., and Mitchley, B. C. V. Failure of testosterone or xanthopterin to influence the induction of renal neoplasms by lead in rats. Br. J. Cancer 19:860-866, 1965.

Salm, R. Combined intestinal and squamous metaplasia of the renal pelvis. J. Clin. Pathol. 22:187-191, 1969.

Sandison, A. T., and Anderson, L. J. Tumors of the kidney in cattle, sheep and pigs. Cancer 21:727-742, 1968.

Sarma, K. P. Proliferative and lymphoid reactions in bladder cancer. Invest. Urol. 10:199-207, 1972.

............, Tumors of the Urinary Bladder. Epidemiology of Bladder Cancer, pp. 163-204. New York: Appleton-Century-Crofts; London: Butterworth, 1969.

Sarnacki, C. T., McCormack, L. J., Kiser, W. S., Hazard, J. B., McLaughlin, T. C., and Belovich, D. M. Urinary cytology and the clinical diagnosis of urinary tract malignancy: A clinicopathologic study of 1,400 patients. J. Urol. 106:761-764, 1971.

Schade, R. O. K., Serck-Hanssen, A., and Swinney, J. Morphological changes in the ureter in cases of bladder carcinoma. Cancer 27:1267-1272, 1971.

Schneiderman, C., and Simon, M. A. Malacoplakia of the urinary tract. J. Urol. 100:694-698, 1963.

Scott, W. W. Tumors of the Ureter, pp. 999-1026. In: Urology, 2d ed. (Ed.) Campbell, M. F. Philadelphia and London: W. B. Saunders Company, 1963.

Shah, J. P., and Kothari, A. B. Leiomyosarcoma of the ureter. J. Urol. 105:505-506, 1971.

Sharma, T. C., Melamed, M. R., and Whitmore, W. F., Jr. Carcinoma in-situ of the ureter in patients with bladder carcinoma treated by cystectomy. Cancer 26:583-587, 1970.

Smart, J. G. Renal and ureteric tumours in association with bladder tumours. Br. J. Urol. 36:380-390, 1964.

Tolia, B. M., Hajdu, S. I., and Whitmore, W. F., Jr. Leiomyosarcoma of the renal pelvis. J. Urol. 109:974-976, 1973.

Tripathi, V. N. P., and Desautels, R. E. Primary amyloidosis of the urogenital system: A study of 16 cases and brief review. J. Urol. 102:96-101, 1969.

Wagle, D. G., Moore, R. H., and Murphy, G. P. Primary carcinoma of the renal pelvis. Cancer 33:1642-1648, 1974.

Walker, D., and Jordan, W. P., Jr. Renal carcinoma and transitional cell carcinoma in the same kidney. South. Med. J. 61:829-832, 1968.

Willis, R. A. Pathology of Tumours, 4th ed., pp. 456-485. New York: Appleton-Century-Crofts, 1968.

Wolstenholme, G. E. W., and Knight, J. The Balkan Nephropathy (CIBA Foundation Study Group No. 30). Boston: Little Brown and Company, 1967.

Wynder, E. L., Kiyohiko, M., and Whitmore, W. P. Epidemiology of cancer of the kidney. (In preparation)

INDEX

PROFESSIONAL NOTES AND FINDINGS

PROFESSIONAL NOTES AND FINDINGS